LEGAL AND ETHICAL ASPECTS OF HEALTHCARE

LEGAL AND ETHICAL ASPECTS OF HEALTHCARE

S.A.M. McLEAN

LLB, MLitt, PhD, LLD, (Abertay, Edin) FRSE, FRCP (Ed), FRSA
Director, Institute of Law and Ethics in Medicine
School of Law
University of Glasgow

J.K. MASON

CBE, MD, LLD, FRCPath, FRCP(Ed), FRSE
Professor (Emeritus) of Forensic Medicine
The Edinburgh Law School
University of Edinburgh

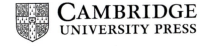

CAMBRIDGE UNIVERSITY PRESS

CAMBRIDGE UNIVERSITY PRESS
Cambridge, New York, Melbourne, Madrid, Cape Town, Singapore, São Paulo, Delhi

Cambridge University Press
The Edinburgh Building, Cambridge CB2 8RU, UK

Published in the United States of America by Cambridge University Press, New York

www.cambridge.org
Information on this title: www.cambridge.org/9780521734509

First published 2003
Digitally reprinted by Cambridge University Press 2009

A catalogue record for this publication is available from the British Library

ISBN 978-0-521-73450-9 paperback

CONTENTS

ACKNOWLEDGEMENTS

It is never possible to complete this sort of project without a great deal of assistance – present and past. We, therefore, wish to express our thanks – in no particular order – to Betty, Beth, Bill, Sandy and all of our families, colleagues and friends for their help in many ways over many years.

Dedication

This book celebrates a close and enduring friendship

PREFACE

There have, of course, always been 'doctors' or healers. In the past, they were very different from those who minister to our health today. Priests, mystics and local 'wise women' historically held control over our health, even following the time of Hippocrates, whose famous Oath still finds a place in modern medical ethics. After a long period in which quacks and mavericks flourished, the 19th century saw the beginning of the formal regulation of what had become a recognised and distinctive profession of physicians and surgeons which, in turn, laid the foundations of the Health Service that we know today. Inevitably, the law played an increasingly significant role in this regulation and, in parallel with this, a new culture of medical ethics has grown up to supplement the legal requirements.

While both the organisation and the capacities of the profession evolved fairly steadily until, say, the Second World War, since then there has been an exponential increase in medicine's ability to alleviate symptoms and to cure underlying disease. At the same time, medicine has changed from what was essentially an art into a discipline increasingly grounded in science. We have become so used to progress in treatment that it is sometimes forgotten how recently many of modern medicine's 'miracles' were developed. The modern face of medicine is dominated – at least in the eyes of the media and perhaps the public – by the astonishing range of options that are now available, while more recent techniques such as assisted reproduction, developments in genetic diagnosis and treatment, organ transplantation and, for the future, the potential of stem cell research, have combined to keep medicine and its practitioners in the limelight. The down side of this is that public attention is drawn more and more to medicine's mistakes and mishaps and the number of these seems to grow in tandem with the introduction of increasingly complex techniques.

Along with this, we have witnessed the growth of a community in which the professions are no longer seen as being immune to challenge – and this includes the medical profession. The widespread acceptance of 'human rights' as the primary basis on which to build a civilised society has encouraged people to demand respect for themselves and their decisions, and to expect these demands to be met and vindicated. This does not deny medical practitioners the right to use their expertise, but it does allow individuals to take a central place in decisions about themselves and about their own healthcare.

The resulting combination of increasingly effective – and expensive – medical capability distributed among a public that is more than ever aware of its rights, has generated both partnership and tension in the doctor/patient relationship. The management of a patient who is actively involved in his or her treatment decisions is likely to be more successful than is one that is dominated by medical paternalism. On the other hand, the armoury of treatments at the disposal of the modern doctor may make him or her frustrated when optimal medical advice is ignored or rejected by patients.

A body of law has also grown up around medical practice, teasing out the complex and often sensitive issues which arise when patients or their families cannot agree with their doctors. This law both reflects and delineates the doctor/patient relationship. It is to this that we turn in this book. If rights are to be exercised effectively, it is important that we know what they are. If challenges are to be mounted, they should be based on firm grounds. What we attempt to do in this manuscript is to explain and discuss the way in which the law tries to ensure that these criteria are met. It will become obvious to the reader, however, that the law, of itself, is often inadequately equipped to achieve this end. We will also ask, and try to answer, some difficult ethical questions. Although many tend to see law and ethics as entirely distinct entities, we do not believe this always to be true, and we hope that this position will be vindicated in the pages of this book.

Along with all other communal activities, modern medicine is now subject to the terms of the Human Rights Act 1998, which brings the European Convention on Human Rights into UK Law. For the moment, it remains unclear just how profound the impact of this legislation will be on medical practice. A number of rights, now specifically available in the UK, seem to have obvious importance in this field – for example the 'right to life', the 'right to respect for private life' and the 'right to marry and to found a family'. It must be said that British courts have been aware of these rights for many years – the United Kingdom was amongst the first signatories of the Convention in 1951 – and it might be expected that they have been adopted in the United Kingdom as a matter of course. However, delay in the complete effectuation of the Convention has resulted in the UK being challenged in the Court of Human Rights in Strasbourg on a number of occasions. The major impact of the 1998 Act will be that decisions of the Strasbourg court will now have the same persuasive effect as if they were decisions of a UK court. Similarly, all bodies, and individuals, that provide a public service will be accountable to the principles laid down by the European court. As these include Ministers, Health Authorities, Health Boards and individual doctors, it seems likely, not so much that medical decisions will be challenged more frequently but, rather, that the basis on which such challenges are adjudicated will be altered so as to reflect the European dimension.

Whether or not this will actually change medical practice remains to be seen. Doctors will likely argue that best practice would have taken these rights into consideration in any event. Even so, novel challenges – of which that contesting the refusal of the Human Fertilisation and Embryology Authority to permit sex selection of embryos produced by way of assisted reproduction is an excellent example – are likely to show that individual citizens now have an additional resource at their disposal should they attempt to vindicate their rights in respect of their own treatment or healthcare.

The modern doctor/patient relationship can, and often does, raise difficult problems and requires reasoned judgements to be made. Equally, the nature of this relationship cannot be separated from the values espoused by society as a whole. This is at its most obvious when matters such as the medical termination of pregnancy, or end of life decisions, are being considered. Equally, the impact of government on clinical decisions is evident when issues such as the allocation of resources are under review. Stirring all of these disparate issues into one large pot makes for interesting differences of opinion. It is these which we hope to expose and elucidate here. We do not attempt to influence the reader, nor are we able to come up with ready made answers, for what is ethically appropriate is largely a matter of evaluation by the individual; people will not always agree. This is, to an extent, exemplified by the authors of this book, who on the face of things, could hardly be more dissimilar. One of us is a lawyer and the other a doctor; one could be accused of male chauvinism while the other is a strong supporter of women's rights; one was practising medicine before the advent of the National Health Service while the other was not born until long after 1948. Thus, it is, in many ways, remarkable that we have been able to reach such a measure of agreement. In writing this book we hope to provide food for thought and some greater insight into the many problems that healthcare providers and patients face today and may be expected to face in the future. Second, and perhaps more explicitly, we have tried to outline what the current law is, why it is the way it is, and what it may be in the future.

Finally, it should be said that this book is not intended to be an academic text-book and, accordingly, we have not cluttered the text with large numbers of references to which access is limited. Rather we have tried to introduce the reader to the important legal and ethical issues raised by the topics under consideration. We have, however, added a selected bibliography to which those who want to delve further can refer.

However, we do think it is important to list some of the cases that we think are significant, not only to substantiate what we say but also to give the reader a further opportunity to get to the heart of things. Few people outside the legal profession will, however, understand 'case citation' and the following note is intended to clarify the matter.

All the important court decisions are reported – that is, the judgements, and the reasons for the judgements, are printed and published. Just as a news item is reported in many different papers, so are the reports of cases published in several different series depending, to a large extent, on the 'specialist' area of interest. Thus, a given case may be reported in several places. In order to avoid confusion we have tried to standardise our references and we have referred to the *All England Reports* whenever a case was published there. We have used the best alternative when this is not so and have added a list of abbreviations at the end so as to assist the healthcare professional who is unfamiliar with legal sources.

S A M McLean,
J K Mason,
March 2003

A NOTE ON ABBREVIATIONS

As stated in the Preface, we have, for the sake of simplicity, used the case reference to the All England Reports wherever possible. Other abbreviations used include:

AC	Appeal Cases
BMLR	Butterworths Medicolegal Reports
CMLR	Common Market Law Reports
DLR	Dominion Law Reports (Canada)
EHRR	European Human Rights Reports
FLR	Family Law Reports
ICR	Industrial Court Reports
IRLR	Industrial Relations Law Reports
Lloyd's Rep Med	Lloyd's Reports (Medical)
Med LR	Medical Law Reports
SC	Session Cases
SLT	Scots Law Times

For US cases:

A	Atlantic Reporter
NE	North Eastern Reporter
P	Pacific Reporter
S Ct	Supreme Court Reports
US	United States Supreme Court Reports

Bracketing the year

For clarification: In citing English cases, the year is in [ ] when the actual year is needed to locate the reference. ( ) brackets are used when there is also a continuing volume number to assist in location. No brackets are used in the citation of Scottish cases.

ABOUT MEDICINE AND THE LAW

It is, in many ways, a pity that we start this book off with this chapter. There is nothing demanding or contentious about it and much of it will be common knowledge to many readers. Nevertheless, we feel that there are many good reasons for what is essentially an introductory chapter. In the first place, many healthcare practitioners, confronted by an ever-increasingly litigious public, tend to see the medico-legal relationship as one of uncompromising conflict and we feel under something of an obligation to try to put the position in perspective. Secondly, political control of the healthcaring professions is extending rapidly and, as a direct consequence, the means and direction of professional control are being profoundly affected. The National Health Service Reform and Healthcare Professions Act of 2002, coupled with the massive changes to the Medical Act imposed by the Medical Act 1983 (Amendment) Order which is still in the draft stage, are likely to alter the legal ambience within which the healthcare professions work to an extent of which even the professionals themselves may be unaware. We think, therefore, that it would be helpful to outline some of the changes which are in the development stage. Finally, if, as we must, we are going to quote case law by way of illustration of our theme, we think it is essential that the medical reader is given some idea of issues such as the relative importance of these decisions – in short, we feel that a simple guide to the legal system will not be out of place. We will take a brief look at these issues in turn.

In doing so, we will concentrate on the medical profession itself but this is due only to considerations of space and to a desire to avoid unnecessary repetition. We have not lost sight of the fact that the doctor is only one of the many persons who make up the category of healthcare professionals. We are well aware that, in most instances, it is the doctor who makes the decisions but it is the nurses who carry them out – and in many situations, from the crèche to the hospice, this can involve both emotional pain and ethical distress. A patient's treatment in hospital may be *designed* by the doctors but it will be *provided* by the nurses and by many others in ancillary professions. In the nature of things, however, case law, in particular, tends to concentrate on the principals – and, in the hospital setting, these will commonly be the hospital authority and the doctor in charge of the case. Thus, if an individual is to be named in a case, it will be the doctor – and this will certainly be so in respect of general practice. The responsibilities of employees of a hospital are, however, subsumed under the umbrella of the employer's vicarious liability. As a result, nurses and other healthcare staff are rarely the primary focus of litigation, and there is, therefore, little to be gained by discussing the law as it relates to specific streams of healthcare – specialist books are available in nearly all instances for those who wish to probe deeper.

LEGAL INTERVENTION IN MEDICINE

It is a truism to say that the outstanding characteristic of modern medicine lies in its rapidly expanding technology founded on research. At the same time, it operates within a society that demands correspondingly expanding – and more esoteric – methodologies and which is encouraged to, and does, demonstrate an increasing personal involvement in assessing the quality of the medical treatment it is offered. Thus, no matter how hard everyone tries, there is bound to be scope for argument and, often, dissatisfaction. A major function of the courts is to resolve such disputes and a volume of case law is derived from the decisions reached.

Such law is, inevitably, retroactive and most people would agree that prevention is better than cure. For this purpose, we must be forewarned – and this is the function of statute law which is to be found in the Acts of Parliament. Insofar as it represents the will of the people, it is the most binding form of law. Very little that is written can be absolutely clear and unambiguous and, as a result, the courts may – and often do – interpret the meaning of a statute and, in doing so, they can go back to the Parliamentary debates so as to clarify the members' intentions at the time. The courts cannot, however, alter a statute – that is the prerogative of Parliament.

A statute is also described as primary legislation. It may be fairly wide-ranging and broadly descriptive – in effect, giving an outline of what Parliament wanted at the time. Somewhere or other, however, it will say that the responsible Minister can make Regulations which will explain just *how* these ideas are to be put into practice. The production of this so-called secondary legislation falls to the civil service and the result is usually published in the form of a 'Statutory Instrument' or 'Order' – which may, and almost always does, contain far more detailed law than does the Act itself. Keeping abreast of these developments is one of the more difficult aspects of obeying the law, but it is essential. This is, perhaps, particularly so in relation to the healthcare professions as, in the Healthcare Act of 1999, the Minister is empowered to modify their regulation by way of an Order in Council, rather than by Act of Parliament, whenever it seems expedient to do so – a power which, to some, seems to open the door to control by way of Ministerial decree. The very extensive changes to the Medical Act of 1983 which are now under consideration, and to which we refer below, are being effected by just such an Order.

The rationale behind this strategy is that, as everyone will admit, statute is a cumbersome instrument by which to keep the law and modern practice in step. An alternative device, and one that is increasingly used, is for the statute to establish an Authority or 'quango'[1] which will, in turn, produce a Code of Practice that indicates

---

[1] Meaning Quasi-autonomous Governmental Organisation.

how the statute is to be effected. Depending on the wording of the Act, the Code of Practice may or may not have the force of law. Most often, it will not do so but, at the same time, it may be influential to the point of being directive. An example of this, which we discuss in Chapter 8, is found in the Human Fertilisation and Embryology Act of 1990 which established the Human Fertilisation and Embryology Authority. Anyone who practises reproductive medicine within the terms of the Act *must* do so in accordance with the Authority's Code; otherwise, the Authority may well withdraw that person's licence to practise.

However, while statute can, and does, give us a broad-brush view of the law as it applies to the community, it cannot, as we have already intimated, deal with individual conflicts, each of which has its own individual characteristics which will dictate its interpretation and its outcome. This is the function of the courts which, in coming to a conclusion, will draw on any existing statute law, any previous judicial opinions in previous cases and, very importantly, a consideration of what would be regarded as right and proper behaviour in society as it is currently disposed. In this way, we build up what is known as the common law – and it is the common law that most noticeably controls behaviour between individuals and, hence, the doctor/patient relationship. Thus, statute and common law are, to an extent, complementary and each serves its own purpose. English law depends far more on statute than does Scots law but that is because the two systems are based on different premises that a book such as this cannot hope to describe.

One last aspect is worth considering. We all know that ignorance of the law is no excuse for breaking it. Statute law has the advantage that it is there for anyone to read, which seems rather fairer than asking someone to consult the crystal ball – which is what the common law often requires. This is why doctors are so often, these days, forced to consult the courts before taking treatment decisions.

Which leads us to emphasise that the courts can also work proactively – and, as we have just suggested, this will often be at the request of the doctors themselves. Thus, taking common examples from the medico-legal field, the court may be asked to deliver an injunction or, in Scotland, an interdict, which, effectively, prevents a party from taking a proposed course of action. A newspaper might, for example be intending to publish an article which the subject of the article or the hospital/primary care trust believes should be kept confidential; they can then apply for an injunction to prevent it happening. Alternatively, the court may be asked to invoke its inherent jurisdiction as protector of the vulnerable – that is, children or the mentally incompetent – and to make a declaration as to whether or not a proposed course of action in respect of that person would or would not be lawful. Here we see evidence of the amalgam of medical law and medical ethics, for many of the decisions made as to lawfulness are, in fact, resolutions of the doctors' ethical dilemmas. As one of our most senior judges once put it, the courts are being asked to function as a form of third opinion – an appropriate analogy in that, although it is not always so, the process is, perhaps, most often invoked when there is conflict between the healthcare team and an incompetent's next of kin. We will also see this happening when the current law is uncertain. Doctors might, for example seek a declaration as to whether or not it would be lawful to sterilise a woman who was at risk of pregnancy but who was unable, by reason of mental disability, to consent or refuse on her own behalf.

By and large, the court will always decide such matters on the basis of the patient's 'best interests' and, as will be noted at several points in the book, a distinction is drawn between 'medical best interests', which are within the purview of the medical profession, and 'overall best interests', which it is the court's function to adjudge. Should the doctor be in doubt as to his or her position, it is better to err on the side of caution and to invite a legal opinion. Indeed, currently there are two circumstances in England and Wales – removal of nutrition and hydration from a person in the permanent vegetative state and sterilisation of an incompetent woman – in which a judicial opinion *must* be sought. We discuss both of these circumstances in later chapters.

Thus far, we have been discussing the legal/medical interface in terms of private law, or controversies between individuals. An individual may, however, feel that he or she has been or will be wronged by the State or by an administrative body; such a person may then apply for judicial review of the authority's decision. The actions of *any* administrative body are subject to judicial review; the only criterion is that the body ultimately derives its power from a Ministry. Thus, in a typical case, a Health Authority or Board may decide to close an old persons' home – the residents affected can apply for a judicial review of the decision which would be halted if it was found to be unreasonable or unlawful. A Ms Coughlan was spectacularly successful in just such a case in 1999. Other examples include the case of Mrs Blood, who questioned the reasonableness of the refusal of the Human Fertilisation and Embryology Authority to allow her to use her dead husband's sperm, and that of Dr Colman who, unsuccessfully, challenged the right of the GMC to control his 'right' to advertise his particular expertise.

Divisions of the legal system

The majority of court cases which are of interest to healthcarers are first heard – hence, the court 'of first instance' – by a single judge who, like anyone else, cannot be immune to human error. The legal system has, therefore built up a hierarchal system that is designed to protect against this possibility. The following very simple notes are appended only so that the reader who has no training in the law can understand the terminology used in the rest of the book.

The civil law – that is, the law other than that associated with criminality and punishment by society – is administered in England and Wales by different branches of the court structure according to the nature of the case and the consequent need for specialist knowledge on the part of the judge. From the point of view of medicine and the law, the two most important divisions are the Family Division which deals, in particular, with matters concerning the welfare of children and the Queen's Bench Division which is responsible for civil litigation. Civil litigation, as implied above, is simply a matter of argument between two individual parties. When one of these claims to have been wronged by the other, the process is known as an action in tort or, in Scotland, delict. The action is raised by one 'side' – the claimant or, in Scotland, the pursuer. In the event of it being decided that he or she has suffered an 'injury' in the legal sense, the court will assess the damages payable in reparation in monetary terms. This is the process adopted in the great majority of claims for medical negligence – an important subject that we address in Chapter 6.

The Supreme Court of England and Wales consists of the High Court, the Crown Court and the Court of Appeal. Curiously, the term excludes the House of Lords which is, in practice, the highest court in the land. Civil cases are heard first in the High Court – which constitutes the court of first instance and in which a single judge sits without a jury save in exceptional cases. In the event that one side cannot accept his or her ruling, the case may go to the Court of Appeal (Civil Division). Three judges sit here and the court's decision is based on a majority. In the event that there is still dispute, the case can, once permission has been granted, go to the House of Lords where it will normally be heard by five judges or Lords of Appeal.

The Judicial Committee of the Privy Council is something of an anachronism in that its original purpose was to advise the Sovereign when the Sovereign wielded extensive executive power. It then became a form of 'Empire' Court which the Dominions and Colonies could use as a Court of Appeal – but that function is now vestigial. Apart from the fact that it is called upon to decide 'devolution issues' as between the Parliaments of Westminster and Holyrood, its main importance in the present context lies in it being the Court of Appeal from decisions of the General Medical Council but, again, this function is soon to be ended (see below).

The vast majority of criminal cases are heard in the Magistrates' Courts but important, serious cases are heard by a single judge sitting with a jury; appeal is to the Court of Appeal (Criminal Division). A further appeal is available, with the leave of the court, to the House of Lords.

Apart from those many cases that are decided in the Sheriff Court, civil cases in Scotland are heard in the Court of Session – which also serves as a court of appeal from the Sheriff Court. The court of first instance is known as the Outer House where a single judge sits. Appeal from there is to the Inner House where a bench of three judges usually sits although this can be extended to five or more if the case is of major importance. A further appeal is available to the House of Lords in Westminster where a varied number of Lords of Appeal are from Scotland – though there is no obligatory national bias as to which judges hear English and Scottish cases. The great majority of criminal cases in Scotland are dealt with in the Sheriff Court, the Sheriff sitting either alone or with a jury. Serious cases are heard in the High Court of Judiciary which also sits as a Court of Appeal. No appeal to the House of Lords is available in criminal cases.

The importance of this hierarchal structure does not depend only on the seniority and experience of the judges – on which basis, the courts should, theoretically, give a better opinion as the scale is ascended. More importantly, the courts are constrained by what is known as the principle of binding precedent – that is to say, that a lower court must follow the findings of a higher court when dealing with the same facts. Quite how 'binding' a precedent is when the courts are on the same level depends, largely, on how elevated is the level. But such delicate points are of little interest to us here. What matters is, that as a result of this combination, a decision from the House of Lords is more important – and the case is consequently of greater interest – than is a ruling by the Court of Appeal or the Court of Session; at the other end of the scale, a decision at first instance – for example, in the High Court – is liable to be overturned at any time.

PROFESSIONAL DISCIPLINE

It may seem unnecessary to discuss professional discipline in the healthcaring service in a book intended for healthcarers themselves – it could be seen as taking coals to Newcastle. The subject is, however, currently under intensive review and major changes are in train. Many healthcarers will be unaware of what is intended – and, indeed, we cannot be certain that intentions will be turned into deeds. For all these reasons, we thought it would be useful to set out the likely position, largely by way of a recapitulation of the currently drafted Medical Act 1983 (Amendment) Order of 2002.

The General Medical Council

A major function of the General Medical Council is to keep the register of registered medical practitioners. Since a person cannot practice medicine in the National Health Service or in the armed forces unless he or she is registered, and since only the GMC can register or de-register a practitioner, it follows that the disciplinary function of the GMC is the most basic form of control of a doctor's actions. It is, therefore, convenient to concentrate on this aspect of professional discipline although, as will be seen later, there are other mechanisms available which can have a profound influence on a practitioner's standing. It is to be emphasised, however, that, in future, registration will be something of a preliminary step to a career; continuing in practice will depend upon possession of a licence to practice which, in turn, will depend upon a (probably) quinquennial system of revalidation.

The GMC now consists of 107 members, but it is relatively certain that this will be reduced to 35 of whom 19 will be elected by the profession and 14 will be lay members – the numbers necessary for performing its varied functions will be made up by way of co-option.

It is unfortunate that the Medical Acts up to 1983 virtually prohibited the GMC from deciding whether or not a practitioner was a 'good doctor'; the disciplinary test was essentially whether or not he or she was a 'good member of the medical profession' and, as a corollary, the only competent charge against a doctor before his or her peers was that of being guilty of 'serious professional misconduct'. As a consequence, the GMC's control of a doctor's competence was effectively limited to his or her *education* and it was not until 1995, with the passing of the Medical (Professional Performance) Act, that it was empowered to control a doctor's *technical* incompetence.

Sweeping changes are now afoot as to the way in which the GMC controls doctors. The overriding disciplinary benchmark will be a doctor's fitness to practice, which can be challenged on five grounds:

- Misconduct – which, effectively, covers the old 'serious professional misconduct';
- Deficient professional performance – which will subsume the provisions of the 1995 Act;
- Conviction or caution following criminal offences – something that was specifically covered under the previous professional misconduct;
- Impaired physical or mental health; and
- A determination by any other body responsible for the regulation of health or social care professions that his or her fitness to practice is impaired.

Hearings will be before the relevant Fitness to Practice Panel and, in the event of his or her fitness to practice being found to be impaired, the doctor's name can, except in a 'health case', be erased from the register – in which case restoration to the register will not be available for 5 years. Alternatively, he or she may be suspended for up to 12 months or conditional registration – the conditions being specified by the Panel – may be imposed for up to 3 years. Any of these restrictions can be re-imposed when the original suspension order is reviewed. Finally, in the event of misconduct, criminal conviction or determination by another body, the doctor can be reprimanded.

An appeal against a decision of the Fitness to Practice Panel will, in future, be available to the High Court in England and Wales, to the Court of Session in Scotland and to the High Court of Northern Ireland. Hitherto, appeal has been direct to the Privy Council which, at one time, was disinclined to interfere with the purely professional aspects of the GMC's work (see the case of *Libman v General Medical Council* heard in 1972). Later appeals have, however, indicated a relaxation of this rule – it was held, for example, that the erasure of a Dr Bijl's name from the register was an unreasonably draconian punishment for making errors of judgment, while the performance of a Dr Kripendorf had been tested against the wrong standards. A significantly higher number of appeals have been successful since the passing of the Human Rights Act 1998, and it may well be that the High Court and the Court of Session, being closer to the coalface, will be even more prepared to take issue with the GMC than was the Privy Council. It is also to be noted, in passing, that the actions of the GMC and its Panels are subject to judicial review as described above.

Controlling bodies for other healthcare professions

We have already noted that doctors form only a part of the healthcare team. All those professions involved in that team have their own regulatory bodies that are prescribed either by statute or, more recently, by Orders in Council.

The most important of these from the point of view of medical practice is the Nursing and Midwifery Council, which replaces the United Kingdom Central Council for Nursing, Midwifery and Health Visiting.[2] The function of the NMC is to establish and improve standards of training and professional conduct for the professions of Nursing, Midwifery and Health Visiting and, in common with the modern approach to healthcare, its main objective in exercising its functions is to 'safeguard the health and well-being of persons using or needing the services of registrants'. The pattern of the Order establishing the Council closely follows that relating to medicine – including regulation under the overall umbrella of 'fitness to practise'. There are significant differences as to detail but we do not think that it is appropriate to expand on these here.

A number of other healthcare professions are covered by individual statutes – and, in some cases, these extend to what is popularly known as 'alternative medicine'. Thus, we have the Pharmacy Act 1954, the Hearing Aid Council Acts 1968 and 1969, the Opticians Act 1989, the Osteopaths Act 1993 and the Chiropractors

---

[2] The General Dental Council is established under the Dentists Act 1984 but we are, here, concerned with the delivery of general medical care.

Act 1994 – and no doubt the list will enlarge as practises such as acupuncture become more organised and acceptable.

Finally, we should mention the Health Professions Council which stems from the Professions Supplementary to Medicine Act 1960, and which establishes a central Council for the control of a number of essential, though smaller, professions including chiropodists, dieticians, medical laboratory technicians, occupational therapists, physiotherapists, radiographers, orthoptists, speech therapists and remedial gymnasts. Again, a register of each specialty is maintained and, again, the avowed purpose of the Council is the protection of those who require their services.

The Council for the Regulation of Healthcare Professionals

Perhaps the most far-reaching innovation has been the creation of the Council for the Regulation of Healthcare Professionals, the function of which is just what it says; to oversee and to regulate the existing Councils – the so-called regulatory bodies. The Council was established under the National Health Service Reform and Healthcare Professions Act of 2002 with the aim of promoting the interests of patients and other members of the public in relation to the performance of their functions by the regulatory bodies. It also has the positive duty of formulating principles relating to good professional self-regulation and encouraging regulatory bodies to conform to them – and, to this end, it can investigate and report on the performance of the individual Councils. Significantly, it can direct the regulatory bodies to change their rules and these directions must be obeyed. It will also be able to investigate complaints made against them. In addition, the Council can refer any disciplinary decision of a regulatory body to the High Court in England or the Court of Session in Scotland if it considers the penalty to have been too lenient – effectively, it can appeal to the courts on behalf of the public. Professional members of the Council must be in a minority. There is, as yet, no experience of the Council's work, although it does look as though self regulation by the healthcaring professions will no longer be absolute.

Statutory control of the healthcaring professions

As to the maintenance of standards in general, two major statutory bodies have been established. The first of these is the National Institute of Clinical Excellence or NICE which is designated a special health authority.[3] NICE's primary function is to advise the other Health Authorities as to what are the most useful and cost-effective treatments available. We return to NICE in the next chapter. Of greater importance in the present context is the Commission for Health Improvement (or CHIMP) which was set up under the Health Act of 1999 as a type of 'enforcement agency'. CHIMP's officers can visit the various NHS Trusts and will ensure that the arrangements made are in tune with the national standards – including those recommended by NICE[4] but also involving administrative and professional standards of efficiency on a broad scale.

---

[3] The equivalent organisation in Scotland is known as the Health Technology Board for Scotland.
[4] The authority of CHIMP does not extend to Scotland where similar functions are undertaken by the Clinical Standards Board, which is now part of NHS Quality Improvement Scotland.

The functions of CHIMP have been extended recently to allow the Commission to instigate the collection and analysis of data and to report on the results obtained by others.[5]

Other systems of 'quango control' of the professions are in or coming into place
as we write. Among these must be mentioned the National Clinical Assessment
Authority, the main function of which is to provide assistance to NHS bodies that are
concerned at the performance of individual doctors. On the face of things, this seems
to overlap with the anticipated functions of the GMC through its Fitness to Practise
Panel which is charged with investigating deficient professional performance. The
relationship between the two bodies is, however, currently somewhat uncertain.

We must also note the increasing authority granted by statute to involvement by
the public in the provision of their healthcare. The most important body from this
aspect is the Commission for Patient and Public Involvement in Health which has,
among others, three main functions. First, it must advise the Secretary of State about
arrangements for public involvement in, and consultation on, matters relating to the
Health Service in England; second, it must advise as to the provision of independent
advocacy services for patients wishing to make complaints; third, it must provide
assistance to Patients' Forums and Patients' Councils and set quality standards for these
organisations. A Patients' Forum, designed to monitor and review the operation of the
services provided, must be established for each NHS Trust and Primary Care Trust in
England. Patients' Councils must, essentially, be established in the area of each local
authority that has the power to overview the health and social services provided. The
basic function of the Councils is to co-ordinate the activities of the Patients' Forums
in the area and to ensure that the directions of the Commission are followed through.
At the time of writing, Patients' Forums have not been established in Scotland where
their function continues to be served by the current-style Community Health
Councils.

THE DOCTOR AND THE NATIONAL HEALTH SERVICE

The doctor's relationship with the National Health Service varies according to
whether he or she is working in a hospital or in primary care. In the former, doctors
are direct employees of the Hospital Trust. Accordingly, the hospital authorities are
responsible for their conduct in the same way as are any employers – they must, therefore, have an internal system for enforcing discipline and for satisfying the, now, several
inspecting organisations. How this is arranged depends on various factors including the
seniority of the doctor and whether a complaint against him or her relates to professional conduct or to technical competence. There is no need here to delve into the ins
and outs of the disciplinary process, which is remarkably complicated. Suffice it to say
that it allows for immediate suspension from duty as a precautionary measure if that is
warranted by the primary evidence. Once this is found to be sufficient, the case is heard
by an independent and specially selected panel – and it may go so far as to be reviewed
by a professional panel set up to advise the Secretary of State, who has the final word
as to the doctor's suitability for continued employment.

---

[5] CHIMP may, in fact, be merged with part of the Audit Commission to form a new Commission for
Healthcare Audit and Inspection.

By contrast, the doctor in general practice provides his or her services by way of a contract with the Primary Care Trust to provide services for patients. Allegations of breach of responsibility in respect of that contract can be brought by the administration or by patients or their representatives, and every Health Authority or Health Board must now establish a disciplinary committee, the basic function of which is to investigate complaints that a practitioner is failing to comply with his or her terms of service. If it is shown that there is a case to be answered, the matter is referred to the disciplinary committee of another Health Authority which may recommend that no action be taken or that a fine be imposed on the practitioner.

Alternatively, and depending on the nature of the allegation, the Health Authority can refer the case to the GMC, or to the police authority or it can take action itself to remove a practitioner from its list of those who are providing a service. This last sanction can be employed if it appears that the continued inclusion of a practitioner's name on the list of those under contract is prejudicial to the efficiency of the services provided; in other words that he or she is frankly inefficient, or that the practitioner has been guilty of fraud or that he or she is 'unsuitable to be included in the list'. In addition, the Authority can remove the practitioner contingently in an efficiency or fraud case. Alternatively, the Authority can suspend a practitioner when it feels that this is necessary in the public interest – and this happens very often when inquiries in respect of removal from the list are in progress. All of this will now be subject to appeal to the Family Health Services Appeal Authority; likewise, the Health Authority may ask the FHSAA to extend a period of suspension beyond their limit of 6 months. The FHSAA can, as a last resort, impose disqualification on the doctor – or any other NHS professional such as a dentist or pharmacist – on a national scale which is, effectively, saying that the person concerned is unfit to practice.

There are, it seems, so many committees, commissions and authorities devoted, in the end, to maintaining a good and efficient health service that one is entitled to wonder if they may not, so to speak, get in each other's way to such a degree as to be counter-productive. It is true to say that, at the time of writing, many of the new organisations have had little or no time to find their feet and their proliferation may be something of a knee-jerk reaction to fears that the standards of both the medical profession and the National Health Service were falling short of what was to be expected. Two black sheep do not make a black flock.

Nonetheless, there was an arguably good basis for such doubts and this is very well illustrated by the well-known case of Dr Shipman.

Dr Shipman, it will be recalled, was convicted of murder but not until he had killed a minimum of 15 of his patients. How, one wonders, could this have come to pass? At any point, the relatives of a victim could have complained to the Health Authority about what was, on the face of things, at least inefficient treatment. They could, although it would have been less easy, have reported their misgivings to the GMC. They could have raised an action against Dr Shipman for providing negligent treatment. They could, in addition, have asked the Coroner, through the police, to intervene in what appeared to be a suspicious death. But there are two major difficulties here. Firstly, an individual death has got to be *very* untoward before it is recognised as suspicious and it is bound to take some time before the fact that there are a number of similar deaths becomes common knowledge in the community. In fact, the breakdown in the system in this case was not so much within the ambit of healthcare as within the system involving the registration of deaths and the regulation of cremation – matters which are not within the remit of the Department of Health. We discuss these more fully in Chapter 16. Secondly, the relatives have got to know how to make a complaint before they can do so – and, if there is one good thing to have come out of the spate of sensational 'medical' cases that arose at the turn of the century, it is the rule that general practitioners must now set up a 'practice based' complaints procedure and must inform their patients of its existence. This is in addition to the general requirements of this nature which were established by the Hospital Complaints Procedure Act of 1995.

At the end of the day, this is the feature that is central to the problem of the 'bad' doctor – *all* the safeguards are reactive and depend upon the provision of information or the lodging of complaints. Dr Shipman's case is now the subject of an official inquiry which we must not pre-judge. It does seem, however, that the reason he escaped detection for so long can probably be attributed to his having been a single-handed practice; in other words, there was no professional colleague to identify problems and lodge a complaint. Although, therefore, it is of no relevance to that precise case, it is still encouraging to note that the employment status of healthcare workers who report their colleagues' faults is now protected by the Public Interest Disclosure Act of 1998 – in essence, provided the approved procedures are followed, and provided disclosure is initiated on a 'need to know' basis, a healthcare worker cannot, now, be discharged for 'blowing the whistle'.

Could a 'Shipman case' occur again? Nothing is ever entirely foolproof but, at least, and as a direct result of that disaster, any doctor applying for a position must now declare his or her criminal history; and a Health Authority must remove from its list any doctor they know to have been sentenced to more than 6 months' imprisonment.

THE LEGAL SYSTEM IN PRACTICE

This book is about healthcare workers and the law. In the last few pages we have laid out the basic ground rules which apply to the former and, since we are repeatedly referring to the courts and to 'cases' in what follows, we should do the same for the law and lawyers. We can, however, be far more brief – while most of us will, inevitably, visit the doctor periodically, we would hope that we could count our personal contacts with the law in a lifetime on the fingers of one hand.

But who will be involved on those less than five occasions? The legal profession is partitioned in rather the same way as is the medical profession where we have physicians, surgeons, anaesthetists, paediatricians and the like. Very few doctors would want to step out of their specialty – and it is unlikely that they will be able to do so once the system of licensing to practise is in place. Similarly, there are specialist divisions within the law. We have the fundamental distinction between barristers – or, in Scotland, advocates – who plead cases in court and solicitors who prepare them in their offices – a distinction which is, in fact, being whittled away. It is of far more importance in the present context that, in much the same way as in medicine, a specialist in commercial law would not want to dabble in, say, the criminal law. Again in the same way, the 'family solicitor' might not feel competent to undertake a complex case and would refer the client to a specialist in that particular branch of the law.

Indeed, this might be essential; a legally aided case concerning medical negligence, for instance, can now be undertaken in England only by a solicitor who is 'franchised' to do so.[6] Beyond that, there are some significant differences between the two systems. In the first place, specialisation in the legal profession is largely by way of practice and reputation – the specialist lawyer cannot be identified by the letters after his or her name. Secondly, whereas the medical specialist can *only* be approached through the primary carer, there is no such filter mechanism in the case of the solicitor – it is simply a matter of whether or not a case will be accepted.

The courts in practice

Most readers will be well aware that a criminal trial in the United Kingdom can be before a single judge or before a bench of magistrates and this is the common set up when the permissible penalties are set at relatively low level. Alternatively, for more serious offences, the case can be heard by a judge sitting with a jury – in which case the judge is there not to settle the case but, rather, to instruct the jury in the law so that they can come to their verdict.

Here, however, we are concerned almost exclusively with the civil law where, as we have already pointed out, it is now very uncommon for a jury to be called. The judge 'at first instance' sits alone, makes his or her decision and apportions recompense, or damages, if that is the nature of the case. There are, thus, great differences between civil litigation in this country and that in, say the United States where civil juries are commonplace. First, it is one thing to convince a jury, that is composed of men and women 'in the street', of the rightness of your case; it may be quite another to satisfy an experienced judge who has, so to speak, 'heard it all before'. Second, and running hand in hand with this, while the American jury can apportion massive damages, the British judge is constrained by what is known as 'quantum' – the way in which damages are assessed, and their extent, is more or less laid down. As a result, civil cases are far less dramatic in Britain than they are in America but, by and large, they result in a more predictable and evenly spread system of compensation.

Of more importance, perhaps, is the way in which evidence is presented and, by and large, there are two main processes – the inquisitorial and the adversarial. In the former, the 'judge' calls his or her own witnesses and examines them personally. Lawyers representing interested parties are there to insert points of importance for the judge to consider. The coroner's court is almost the only court in England and Wales that proceeds in this way – though it obviously has a specially important place in medical jurisprudence.[7]

The adversarial system is used in virtually every other type of court we are concerned with in this book. Here, both sides present their own evidence and can test each other's evidence in cross-examination, the objective being to convince the tribunal that one's argument is better than that of one's opponent. This system has aspects that are clearly open to criticism. One 'side' may, in fact, be wrong, yet their

---

[6] For the present, no such restrictions apply in Scotland.
[7] There is nothing similar to the coroner's court in Scotland. The nearest approach is the Fatal Accident Inquiry in which the proceedings are adversarial.

argument is better presented; similarly, the 'experts' who are giving evidence as to their opinion in the matter may, again, be wrong but may be far more experienced in expressing their views and, thus, be more convincing. There are very good reasons to suggest that, as a result, the adversarial system is not the best way to decide, say, whether or not an operation was properly performed. In fact, there are, now, many safeguards built in to correct the more obvious imbalances of the scales of justice. This is no place to go into detail but, for example, all of the relevant documents must be exchanged before trial and many aspects of the case will be agreed beforehand. Moreover, an overhaul of the whole system has been introduced recently under what is referred to as the Woolf Report. Most importantly, it is proposed that the greater part of the evidence will be given in written rather than verbal form and, although there are exceptions in cases involving medical negligence, experts will be called at the instance of the court rather than of the individual parties to the action. By and large, the days of the 'professional expert witness' have gone and the person who takes his or her case to court is increasingly likely to obtain a fair hearing and a just result.

And who pays for it?

An incidental objective of the Woolf Report was to cut down the cost of, and the time taken over, civil litigation. The Report recommends many changes to established practice – and there has not yet been time to decide whether these are, on the whole, good or bad – but the issue that anyone involved will want to know about most is the cost.

Here, the significant change is that legal aid has been withdrawn from cases involving alleged medical negligence. Instead, lawyers will accept cases on a so-called contingency fee basis. In other words, they will be remunerated from a proportion of the damages awarded – or, to put it in the vernacular, 'no win, no fee'. How this will affect the claimants/pursuers will depend very much on the nature of the individual case. It does not mean that many more cases will be accepted – lawyers will have to insure against having to pay the expenses of the other side should they lose, and their insurance premiums are likely to depend on their success or failure rate. The effect on the damages actually received is also likely to vary. The proportion retained by the lawyers may be more or may be less than their fees would have been under the old system – it all depends. Some of these problems are covered by the 'franchising' – and professional audit – of legal firms engaged in cases involving medical negligence to which we have already referred; the scale and quality of assistance are likely to be that much more smoothly distributed. We shall see over the coming years how all this will affect the healthcaring professions. One thing, however, that contingency fees will certainly do is to remove the previous unfairness by which the middle income group were denied legal aid but, at the same time, were quite unable to meet the costs involved in an action. In short, access to the courts will no longer be means tested.

CASES REFERRED TO IN THE TEXT

Bijl v General Medical Council (2001) 65 BMLR 10.

Kripendorf v General Medical Council (2001) 59 BMLR 81.

Libman v General Medical Council [1972] 1 All ER 798.

R v General Medical Council, ex parte Colman (1989) 4 BMLR 33.

R v Human Fertilisation and Embryology Authority, ex parte Blood [1997] 2 All ER 687.

R v North and East Devon Health Authority, ex parte Coughlan [2000] 3 All ER 850.

FURTHER READING

Finlayson B. 'Dealing with poor clinical performance', *British Medical Journal* 2001; 322: 66.

Montgomery J. *Healthcare Law* (2nd edn), 2003.

Silver MHW. 'Patients' rights in England and the United States of America', *Journal of Medical Ethics* 1997; 23: 213.

Walshe K. 'The rise of regulation in the NHS', *British Medical Journal* 2002; 324: 967.

Woolf, Lord. *Access to Justice: Final Report to the Lord Chancellor on the Civil Justice System in England and Wales*, 1996.

Woolf, Lord. 'Are the courts excessively deferential to the medical profession?', *Medical Law Review* 2001; 9: 1.

2

RESOURCES – WHO DECIDES?

It is very easy to say that the National Health Service should offer all treatments to all persons on a demand basis. Rationing, it might be argued, has no place in a healthcare system the aim of which is to provide universal healthcare free at the point of delivery. The question, however, is whether or not this is possible in the medical environment of the twenty-first century?

Consider the doctor who goes out to do an urgent home visit while patients are still in his or her surgery. He or she is responding to a need but, meantime, others are being deprived of a service they expected to receive. This is rationing, but it begins with a conscious decision to choose to do what is considered best in the given circumstances. It would be nice if the doctor did not have to make such a choice, but practical realities mean that this, or equivalent, choices will be made on a daily basis throughout the healthcare system. By the same token, if a general practice spends one thousand pounds on a particular patient's treatment, that thousand pounds has gone; it cannot be recycled or allocated to other patients, irrespective of need. Effectively, decisions as to the allocation of resources which are all of the same general nature – although not of the same significance – are being made routinely at every level of the service from the general practitioner's surgery to the desk of the Minister of Health.

Of course, if the doctor had started with two thousand rather than one thousand pounds, then he or she would still have money left over to use for other patients. In other words, rationing, or resource allocation, would disappear should more money be provided in the first place. Obviously, this is true to a limited extent, but it is not clear that the proposition could be extended indefinitely. Insofar as, arguably, the primary functional remit of the medical profession is to save lives, it is the one profession that has a 100% failure rate – for it is certain that all of us are going to die. Looked at in this way, pouring money indiscriminately into the system is doing little more than resisting the irresistible and there comes a point when the effort becomes unsustainable on both economic and logical grounds. Certainly, with extensive resources the inevitability of death can often be postponed and people may achieve increased lifespans of varying quality. However, it is also true that, in the absence of a bottomless crock of gold, decisions will still need to be taken about what lives to prolong and what quality of life to sustain. This takes us back to the original question; is rationing – and the concomitant discrimination entailed – an inevitable part of healthcare in the twenty-first century?

The difficulty, then, is that it is very nearly impossible to achieve universal agreement as to what constitutes acceptable discrimination. If the Government scraps our nuclear submarines and hands the money saved to the health service, we must still ask what will we spend it on? A great many people would consider the money well spent if it saved them a 4 hour wait in the casualty department, or reduced the waiting time for their routine hernia operation. Others, however, would opt for the provision of those services that postpone the time of death significantly, such as heart replacement surgery but, despite its attractions, options such as this raise their own, new, sets of problems. In the first place, the policy is cumulative – the more we concentrate on postponing death, the more patients there are demanding such treatment. Moreover, we cannot stop the brain deteriorating during an extended life-span. Thus, we must also consider the quality of life we are prolonging and its effect, not only on the individual, but also on society as a whole.

In essence, a major part of medical ethics falls into the philosophical category of utilitarian ethics, within which, the 'rightness' of a decision is judged by the amount of happiness it provides for the greatest number of people. It is this underlying principle which drives the government and the Health Authorities[1] in their unenviable task of allocating resources at community level.

DUTIES OF THE SECRETARY OF STATE

The National Health Service Act of 1977, which, with its many amendments, is still the current basic legislation governing the organisation of the NHS,[2] starts off by defining the duties of the Secretary of State (SoS). These are: 'to continue the promotion in England and Wales of a comprehensive health service ... and, for that purpose, to provide or secure the effective provision of services in accordance with this Act'. To this end, the SoS is given power to provide such services as he or she considers appropriate for the purpose of discharging his or her duties under the Act and to do anything: 'which is calculated to facilitate, or is conducive or incidental to, the discharge of such a duty'.

Thus, the Act does not guarantee a boundless provision of services for all – it foresees no more than the *effective* provision of services. Moreover, there is no bottomless financial pit – the SoS is empowered to provide such services as he or she regards as *appropriate* to the task and, clearly, this carries with it collateral powers of discretion as to what is appropriate given the overall facilities at his or her disposal. On the other side of the coin, the Act goes on to say that it is the SoS's duty to provide hospital accommodation and other services: 'to such an extent as he considers necessary to meet all reasonable requirements'. Again, we can see the latitude allowed – what is *necessary* and what is *reasonable* are matters for the SoS to decide and, at least in theory, there are no further constraints on what he or she can refuse or recommend. But this does not

---

[1] The comparable administrative tier in Scotland is known as the Health Board.
[2] The National Health Service (Scotland) Act of 1972 serves the same purpose in Scotland but, for the sake of simplicity, we will refer only to the English/Welsh Act.

give the SoS *arbitrary* powers – as with any administrative body, decisions are subject to the process of judicial review under which, as we have seen in Chapter 1, the High Court in England and Wales or the Court of Session in Scotland can consider the merits of an administrative decision if it is asked to do so by a properly interested party. This means of protecting the public interest is being used increasingly often. In the context of the provision of health services, the early case brought by Mr Hincks and his associates in 1979 is still as illustrative as any of both of the kinds of decisions which might be made and of the manner in which they will be dealt by the courts.

In this case, plans had been approved for the provision of an orthopaedic wing for the local hospital but the scheme was put off for 10 years because insufficient money was available. Members of the public, supported by the medical consultants in the area, sought a declaration from the courts that the SoS was in breach of his duty under the Act in doing so. This was refused in the High Court and the judge's decision was upheld in the Court of Appeal. It was held that the discretion given to the Secretary of State included the need to evaluate the financial resources available – the health service has to do the best it can within its total Parliamentary allocation of money. Moreover, it could not be said that services must be provided because a particular hospital is deficient in a particular service – it is the conditions in the region as a whole that matter. In short, the words of the Act: 'necessary to meet all reasonable requirements' should be read as being qualified to read: '… all reasonable requirements *such as can be provided within the resources available*'. The courts have consistently maintained this attitude and have, in fact, refined it.

The case bought by Mrs Walker in 1987 highlights the very personal nature of the problems that are potentially associated with allocation decisions. Mrs Walker's son was born with a heart defect which required surgical intervention; the baby was kept in hospital but was not in intensive care. Intensive care and individual nursing would, however, be needed for the operation. However, there were six beds but only four nurses. Mrs Walker protested that, every time a bed became available, a more urgent case was admitted – a consideration to which we will return later. She applied for judicial review of these decisions on the grounds that they were arrived at unlawfully and unreasonably. The trial judge viewed the application as being, at least in part, an attack on decisions as to the staffing within, and the financing of, the NHS and reiterated that the court was unable to investigate any case where the balance, distribution and use of any available money were concerned. The Court of Appeal then laid down the law in a way that is worth repeating verbatim:

> It is not for any court to substitute its own judgement for the judgement of those who are responsible for the allocation of resources. This court could only intervene where it was satisfied that there was a prima facie case, not only of failing to allocate resources in the way in which others would think that resources should be allocated, but of failure to allocate resources to an extent which was *Wednesbury* unreasonable

– and *Wednesbury* unreasonableness is legal shorthand for unreasonableness which no public authority could justify.

Thus, the gateway to taking the Secretary of State, or the Heath Authorities acting as his or her responsible delegates, to court on the grounds of misallocation of health services seemed to all intents and purposes, to be firmly closed. However, one ray of light from the perspective of the disaffected patient has emerged following the absorption into UK law of the European Convention on Human Rights by the Human Rights Act 1998. The impact of the 1998 Act is broadly speaking that courts will need to take direct account of decisions of the Court of Human Rights when interpreting UK law; in terms of judicial review this may be highly significant.

It has been suggested by many commentators that judicial review as an administrative (public) law remedy is ill-suited to the vindication of individual (private law) rights. In addition, the *Wednesbury* test sets a very high hurdle for claimants to meet, thus rendering this action of limited value. In the case of *Smith and Grady v UK*, however, the Court of Human Rights indicated that the *Wednesbury* test could be considered to set too high a standard where matters of human rights were concerned, leaving open the possibility that subsequent challenges may be more likely to succeed.

The cases so far described have dealt with what is essentially a matter of a conscious choice as to the deployment of resources within a clinical setting. It is far less certain that the Secretary of State can deny that choice on purely economic grounds. Many will remember the confusion that surrounded the introduction of the anti-impotency drug sildenafil (Viagra). Here, the SoS issued an interim circular advising doctors not to prescribe the drug and inviting Health Authorities not to support its provision at NHS expense. Although this advice was based on a preliminary opinion given by the Standing Medical Advisory Committee, the circular, at the time, contained no evidence of adequate medical appraisal and was clearly motivated by economic considerations. On being challenged in the High Court by the manufacturers (Pfizer Ltd) in 1999, it was adjudged to be unlawful in that it interfered with the duty of a doctor to give such treatment as was considered necessary and appropriate for an individual patient. Regulations were already in force which 'blacklisted' certain drugs or substances that have no therapeutic effect, or for which there are cheaper alternatives, or which may only be prescribed for particular conditions. By issuing this circular, the Minister had, effectively, circumvented the conditions designed to prevent abuse of those powers. A later circular, which limited the prescription of Viagra to those whose impotence resulted from specific conditions – and which was clearly the result of extensive professional consultation – has not, however, been challenged. Again, it will be seen that the courts will only intervene when a Minister has exercised his powers in what is regarded as an unreasonable manner (albeit with the caveat that the impact of the decision in *Smith and Grady* is as yet unknown). The courts' willingness to support the individual patient's right to individual consideration is important and we return to the subject below.

It scarcely needs emphasis that central funding is not allocated arbitrarily. Currently, the financial distribution is based on a formula elaborated by the Resource Allocation Working Party (RAWP) which, in a complex and, admittedly, fairly empirical way, derives from combining the population of each region with the standardised mortality rate for those aged less than 75. This may or may not be an entirely satisfactory measurement – to an extent, that depends on one's personal viewpoint – but it does mean that the Health Authorities know how much they have to spend and can, within limits, decide on how to do this.[3]

---

[3] The Scottish Executive Health Department has issued a document: *Fair Shares for All: The Final Report* (2000) which would put in place a weighted capitation formula, along with a proposed 'inequalities adjustment', in order to provide a distribution of resources more sensitive to local need.

Health Authorities and Health Boards

Whether the provider of services is a Primary Care Trust or a NHS Trust, the relevant body has to keep within its Ministerial budget and the service has to be run on business lines – this applies also to the Strategic Health Authorities themselves.[4] Thus, any decision which compels a Trust to spend beyond its means is, in fact, forcing that Trust into an unlawful position – and this is sufficient in itself to explain the reluctance of the courts to dictate on clinico-managerial matters within the health service.

OVERSEEING THE AUTHORITIES' DECISIONS

To an extent, then, the Health Authorities can stipulate what services they will fund and what they will not, but this licence has been monitored since 1974 when Community Health Councils (CHCs) were introduced. The Councils were established in relation to individual Health Authorities, essentially to be the patients' mouthpieces in respect of health promotion, the provision of services and of complaints by members of the public. Health Authorities were bound to consult the local CHC whenever they intended a 'substantial development' of the services provided. CHCs seem never to have been a great success. Their remit was relatively undefined and their power very limited. Moreover, it appears that even the regulations governing the use of CHCs could be ignored without fear of major retribution. In 1993, a London Health Authority closed a children's bone marrow transfusion unit without consulting the relevant CHC. A Mr Daniels challenged the legality of the procedure, but the court found its hands virtually tied when confronted with a *fait accompli* and made no declaration. As a result of the general dissatisfaction, CHCs are shortly to be abandoned and 'consumer interests' will be represented by a central Commission for Patient and Public Involvement in Health and by peripheral Patients' Forums, one of which must be established for each NHS Trust and Primary Care Trust. The function of the Patients' Forum will be 'to monitor and review the range and operation of services provided by the Trust to which they relate'. Thus, the views of the consumers as to the services which should be provided at general practitioner and hospital level are likely to be increasingly canvassed although, at present, it is difficult to see what will be the effect if the Trust is unable or unwilling to accommodate them.

An American experiment

Allocation of scarce resources by way of patient choice has, in fact, been introduced in the State of Oregon where, as a result of extensive public debate, the authorities have evolved a list of treatments which will, and will not, be available to those dependent on Medicaid. This sounds admirable in theory, but it has had its fair share of difficulties – not the least of which lies in the constantly changing list of priorities and the resulting incremental extension of the resources that are made available. Moreover, any system which depends upon the popular vote tends to marginalise the

---

[4] Which are accountable to the SoS for the overall co-ordination of the PCT's and NHS Trusts within their control.

minorities in the population; thus, say, treatments for conditions peculiar to an ethnic minority may never become readily available. We should think very carefully before setting off on the Oregon trail and, interestingly, the formula has been rejected in New Zealand where the nature of the Health Service and its inherent difficulties are very comparable to those in the United Kingdom.

GOVERNANCE

The Health Act of 1999 has also promised new and improved systems of surveillance or governance that are intended, firstly, to maintain and improve the general standards of healthcare provision and, secondly, to ensure its uniformity throughout the NHS – in short, to eliminate the variations of healthcare delivery from area to area that has become known as 'treatment by postcode'. Top of the tree, so to speak, is the introduction of Healthcare Frameworks, which will be developed by the Ministry of Health itself. Individual frameworks will be tailored to major care areas and groups of diseases. They will recommend patterns of service to be supplied in each area and the recommendations will be based on both the services' clinical value and their cost effectiveness. It will be seen throughout that the need to contain the costs of the NHS is recognised at all administrative levels and by all the main political parties.

As part of the process, the Government has established the National Institute for Clinical Excellence for England and Wales while, at the same time, a Health Technology Board, which has responsibilities and powers very similar to those of NICE, has been set up in Scotland. NICE and the Scottish Health Technology Board continue to address problems of inequality in the delivery of healthcare but their main functions are clinical – especially in relation to the management of the introduction of new techniques and new drugs into the NHS. As with any innovation, these bodies are having to establish their true niche within the health service and are not being given an easy ride. For example, one of NICE's first acts was to advise against the prescription of the anti-flu drug Zanamivir. Needless to say, this provoked a storm of protest from the manufacturers and there is, at present, no legislative power to enforce such advice. The words of the Chairman indicating NICE's mission deserve repetition:

> The most important criterion is the clinical need of patients but this must be considered in relation to the severity of the disease or condition, the benefits and costs of existing treatment, and the incremental benefits and costs of the new treatment under consideration.

In other words, some form of 'quality' rationing in the NHS is inevitable – as is the fact that it will rest on a powerful element of financial control. This particular example, however, serves to show that few things in this life are immutable; after much reconsideration, it has now been decided that Zanamivir will be available through general practitioners.

It is clear that effective 'rationing' depends on cost/benefit analyses and the moral dilemma besetting the distributor lies in the assessment of the weight to be given to each variable. There can be no doubt when the anticipated clinical benefit is clearly great, the paramountcy of the patient's clinical need must be accepted. Judgement is, however, less easy when the benefit may be low or doubtful of itself or when it may be low in comparison to that likely to accrue to those seeking another resource that has also been declared 'scarce' on economic grounds. The case of Mrs Seale, which will be referred to again in Chapter 8, is a good illustration of this latter situation. Here, the Health Authority was prepared to offer in vitro fertilisation services to infertile women, but could only allocate a total of £200,000 for the purpose. Accordingly, the decision was taken to limit the availability of treatment based on the criterion of age – it was decreed that it would be available only to those below the age of 36. Mrs Seale, who was aged 37 and who was refused treatment, sought judicial review of that decision. In this case, there was no doubt that treatment for Mrs Seale *might* have been effective; however, the live birth rate following IVF using the woman's own eggs falls significantly from the age of 35.[5] The judge could not say that it was unreasonable to take that as an appropriate criterion: 'when balancing the need for such a provision against [the Authority's] ability to provide it and all the other services imposed upon it under the legislation'. The Authority, it was said, was not bound to provide a service on demand to any individual patient for whom it might work, regardless of financial and other constraints, simply because it had undertaken to provide such a service. Rather it was justifiable to take into account the *comparative* benefits of the available services. It is of interest to note the several conditions governing the provision of assisted reproductive treatment – including an age limit of 38 – that have been proposed recently by the Expert Advisory Group on Infertility Services in Scotland.

By far the most significant example of the inherently low benefit type of case is that which was widely publicised as 'The case of Child B' in 1995. In this case, a 10 year-old child who suffered from leukaemia had undergone a course of chemotherapy in 1990. She relapsed in 1993 and was given a further course of chemotherapy combined with whole body irradiation – a treatment which the majority of experts would regard as unrepeatable. She received a bone marrow transplant in 1994 but relapsed again in 1995, at which point her doctors considered that no further treatment could be usefully given. Meantime, her father had been advised of an essentially experimental treatment that had a potential success rate estimated at between 2 and 10 per cent. The Authority declined to fund this further treatment which was estimated as likely to cost £75,000. B's father sought judicial review of the decision.

The judge in the trial court interpreted the conditions as transcending a simple test of the 'reasonableness' of the decision such as we have seen in other cases involving judicial review. Rather, he saw it as a matter of human rights and, particularly, of the right to life – and it was this right that, in his view, the decision offended. He was further of the opinion that the child's best interests were not to be measured in medical terms alone but should also take account of the father's assessment of the position; the Authority, he held, had failed in this respect. Finally, he said that: 'where the question is whether the life of a 10 year-old child might be saved, the responsible Authority must do more than toll the bell of tight resources'. In his view, the Authority had not adequately explained its priorities. He ordered that the Authority reconsider its decision in the light of his judgement and the Authority appealed against his finding.

---

[5] In 1994, the year of Mrs Seale's case, the live birth rate was 17.2% for those in the age group 25–29 and 12.3% for those aged 35–39.

The Appeal Court began by stressing that the courts had only one function in such cases – that is, to rule on the lawfulness of administrative decisions. It was held that the nature of the case was such that, despite the judge's strictures, the wishes of the family *must* have been considered; that the treatment requested was, at best, at the frontier of medical science; and, most significantly, that difficult and agonising judgements have to be made as to how a limited budget is best allocated to the maximum advantage of the maximum number of patients – 'and that is not a judgement that the court can make'. The Court found itself 'unable to say that the Authority acted in a way that exceeded its powers or which was unreasonable in the legal sense', and therefore allowed the appeal.

So we can see that the Court of Appeal has not changed its stance on major administrative decisions concerning the provision of healthcare since the case of Mr Hincks which was discussed above. There have, however, been at least two decisions which suggest that the law is not actually standing still in this area. The first concerns the prescription of the drug beta-interferon which was under trial for the treatment of multiple sclerosis at a cost of some £10,000 per patient per year. The NHS Executive had, in fact, issued a circular asking all health authorities to help with the introduction of the drug into the NHS, but the North Derbyshire HA, having overspent its overall budget, declined to do so on the grounds of insufficient resources. Mr Fisher, who was, thereby, denied treatment, took his case to court where it was held that, although compliance with the circular was not mandatory, the Authority's action was unreasonable in that, by restricting provision of the drug to those involved in the trial, it had failed to give serious consideration to the advice given in the circular. The Authority was ordered to adjust its policy accordingly.

The second case concerned three transsexuals who lived in an area where the Health Authority's policy included gender reassignment among the healthcare services that either would not be commissioned or would be commissioned only with restrictions. Specifically, it would not commission drug treatment or surgery that is intended to give patients the physical characteristics of the opposite gender. The patients sought judicial review of the decision, which the trial court held to be unreasonable. The Authority appealed but lost on several grounds; namely that it did not, in truth, regard transsexualism as an illness; that it did not specify the conditions under which treatment *would* be given; and that it did not require each request for treatment to be considered on its individual merits.

How, then, are these two cases to be harmonised with those that have gone before? Effectively, they say that an Authority is at liberty to allocate its resources in such a way as it decides will be for the overall good of the population it serves. That is a matter for the Health Authority and not for the Courts. But, in so doing, it must set out its reasons clearly and those reasons must be based on reasonable medical grounds. Unless these conditions are met, the policy becomes *unreasonable* and, therefore, unlawful. And, as a corollary to this, a restrictive policy must not involve a 'blanket prohibition'; there must be some way in which the individual can demonstrate his or her need for treatment. In short, the welfare of the individual patient remains paramount; but the individual patient cannot demand treatment if the Authority has reasonable grounds for withholding it in the prevailing circumstances.

AT THE COAL-FACE: THE PATIENT AND THE DOCTOR

This brings the discussion to the individual patient and his or her close contact with the actual healthcare providers. Here, the game-plan has changed. We are no longer concerned with the impersonal availability of medical and surgical treatment within a population; the distribution of these resources is now driven by *need* and its provision depends on how that need is interpreted within the doctor/patient relationship.

The extent to which both the patient and the doctor can be legally driven is very clear at its limits. At one extreme, it is now firmly established that a doctor cannot impose a treatment on an unwilling patient even although he or she is convinced it is the right treatment and even although the patient's refusal may result in his or her death. We return to the subject in Chapter 5. Meantime, the case that Ms S brought against St George's Hospital in London is a very good example. Ms S was 36 weeks' pregnant and was suffering from pre-eclampsia in a serious form. She was strongly urged to have an early delivery and, when she refused, her doctors applied the regulations made under the Mental Health Act of 1983 (for further discussion of which, see Chapter 15). An application for a declaration that urgent treatment given against the patient's wishes would not be unlawful was granted by the trial judge in emergency session, and the baby was successfully delivered by caesarian section. Ms S then appealed retrospectively against the judge's ruling and sought judicial review of the lawfulness of her detention under the Mental Health Act. We are concerned at this stage only with the first of these complaints. The Court of Appeal was at pains to acknowledge the existence of *some* foetal rights – 'whatever else [the foetus] may be,' said the Court, 'it is certainly not nothing', and its analysis deserves repetition in full:

> If it has not already done so, medical science will no doubt one day advance to the stage when a very minor procedure undergone by an adult would save the life of his or her child, or perhaps the life of a child of a complete stranger. The refusal would rightly be described as unreasonable, the benefit to another human life would be beyond value, and the motives of the doctors admirable. If, however, the adult were compelled to agree, or rendered helpless to resist, the principle of autonomy would be extinguished.

In other words, the right to self-determination, or the autonomy, that is possessed by a competent adult is paramount and there is little doubt that the courts will uphold this view for the foreseeable future. Then, what about the other side of the coin? Does 'patient autonomy' include the right to demand a form of treatment that the doctor is unwilling to provide?

Once again, at the opposite end of the spectrum, we have an unequivocal answer. In one of the several similar cases that are, rather confusingly, all known as *Re J* (this one reported in 1992), a mother demanded a form of treatment for her infant son that the doctors regarded as being medically futile. The senior judge of the civil court, the Master of the Rolls, saw the fundamental issue of the case to be whether a court, when exercising its power to protect the interests of minors, should ever require a doctor to adopt a course of treatment that the doctor considered was not in the best interests of the patient. He went on to say:

> I cannot at present conceive of any circumstances in which this would be other than an abuse of power … The doctor's fundamental duty is to treat the patient in accordance with his own best clinical judgement, notwithstanding that other practitioners who are

not called upon to treat the patient may have formed a quite different judgement or that the court, acting on expert evidence, may disagree with him.

Thus, again, there is clear support for the overriding importance of the principle of autonomy – but, in this case, the autonomy is that of the doctor. This seems not unreasonable, although not uncontroversial. Some, for example, may feel that this is a hostage to fortune as the doctor may exercise his or her autonomy wrongly, either by reason of ignorance or perversity. What protection does the patient have against this possibility? This, and similar questions, will arise throughout this book and will, we hope, be answered in the appropriate places. For the present, suffice it to say that it would take a very exceptional man or woman not to be aware of such potential criticism, yet every case will almost certainly have been fully considered – and, generally, in consultation with colleagues at several levels in the health-caring hierarchy. Secondly, as we will see in Chapter 6, the doctor's clinical freedom does not extend to making choices which would be unsupported by other doctors of reasonable competence. And, finally, we have seen in Chapter 1 that clinical audit is now a feature of hospital and primary care trusts – that, coupled with the extensive powers of the General Medical Council, is probably the patient's main protection against the maverick practitioner.

Even so, doctors are constantly making decisions, many of which will be painful to at least one interested party, as to the needs of their patients and, in doing so, they are entitled to – and, indeed, should – bear in mind the competition for scarce resources which arises even at the individual level. Thus, in the same case of *Re J*, another judge said:

> I would also stress the absolute undesirability of the court making an order which may have the effect of compelling a doctor to make available scarce resources (both human and material) to a particular child, without knowing whether or not there are other patients to whom these resources might more advantageously be devoted. The effect of such an order might have been to require J to be put on a ventilator in an intensive care unit, and thereby possibly to deny the benefit of those limited resources to a child who was more likely than J to benefit from them.

In other words, the doctor is entitled to consider the best interests of all those in his or her care in addition to those of the immediate patient; how this conflict is to be resolved with justice to all remains one of the major unsolved problems of modern medical ethics. It is unsolved largely because it is insoluble – given that two children are competing, say, for a single bed in the intensive care unit, the parents of the one who loses are *never* going to accept with equanimity that the decision was taken correctly. We have already seen how this affected Mrs Walker. Doctors faced with emergency decisions are, effectively, left on their own and, by and large, will choose intuitively – this is the sort of situation that serves to distinguish the 'good' from the 'average' doctor. Deeper analysis is, however, needed in less urgent situations and it is within these that some of the doctors' most serious ethical dilemmas are posed.

There are some factors which we believe should *not* be fed into an equation that seeks a 'just' solution to competition for a single resource. Here, we are talking about individual *patients'* interests. Tempting as it might be to do so, community interests – e.g. the relative values of the competing patients to the community – should not be taken into consideration when deciding who to treat. Many will attempt to introduce discrimination by age – but we argue determinedly against this in Chapter 16. We discuss the place of parents and relatives in treatment decisions in Chapter 4 but, for present purposes, it is clear that near-kin can have no decision-making powers on behalf of adult patients. As we have seen, a doctor cannot be compelled to provide treatment against his or her clinical judgement and, strictly speaking, the family is entitled to no more than a sympathetic hearing and thoughtful explanation of the problems involved in a one-to-one competition for a resource. What about the 'just deserts' of the competitors? Do we send the heavy smoker to the bottom of the queue for urgent cardio-vascular surgery or do we deny the alcoholic a chance to bid for the only available transplantable liver? Almost certainly not, although the majority of readers would probably regard this particular argument as being far more finely balanced than the other possible bases for discrimination we have outlined.

For the moment, then, we are left with the principle that resources of this degree of scarcity should be allotted on the basis of medical benefit alone – and, to some, this may be stating the obvious. But is it much more than a trite remark? It may be possible to distinguish the relative benefit to two individuals in extreme circumstances. But, in the vast majority, the prognosis of treatment is bound to be uncertain and to hold otherwise would be little more than a deception. Moreover, the case of *Re J* makes it clear that the courts would not condone *removing* a patient from, say, a ventilator in order to make room for a more deserving case; the pressure to leave one apparatus available so as to cater for such an eventuality is, therefore, ever-present.

Even so, all health economists will attempt a 'scientific' analysis of medical benefit and most will do this by applying the principle of QALYs – or quality adjusted life years. The idea behind this is to estimate the number of years of good quality that a given treatment will provide for a patient. The QALY can, therefore, be used in different ways. Theoretically it can distinguish the best of two or more possible treatments for a given patient and, here, it has a definite value – particularly when the cost of each treatment is added to the balancing pan. QALYs may, however, also be used to decide which of two patients will benefit more from a scarce treatment – and this is a far less acceptable application. To begin with, it clearly operates against the interests of the aged who, put simply, have fewer years to gain. Moreover, assessing the relative quality of two different persons' lives is a subjective exercise which the individual doctor is scarcely qualified to undertake.

For these and other reasons, many medical ethicists will maintain that the only just and honest way of relieving the contest for an irreplaceable resource is on the basis of 'first come, first served'. Although this minimises the clinical expertise involved, it has the philosophical merits of clarity and impartiality. It also has the pragmatic advantages that the *reasoning* behind the choice cannot be challenged and that the great majority of patients and their proxies would appreciate its fairness and integrity. Practices differ but we hazard a guess that this is the policy that is followed most widely in intensive care units.

CONCLUSION

None of this will be particularly satisfying to the reader who wants an answer to the problem of 'post-code treatment' – yet it may be that none is to be found. Probably the major tangible advantage of introducing ideas such as we have discussed has been that the subject of rational healthcare allocation has been well aired within the healthcare professions and is being increasingly argued in public and in the popular media. As a result, people are beginning to appreciate that, try as one might, the healthcare budget cannot be infinite nor can it meet every demand. The current drive towards improving the delivery of what we *have* got is, however, to be applauded.

CASES REFERRED TO IN THE TEXT

Associated Provincial Picture Houses Ltd v Wednesbury Corporation [1947] 2 All ER 680.

J (a minor), Re [1992] 4 All ER 614.

R v Cambridge Health Authority, ex parte B [1995] 2 All ER 129.

R v Central Birmingham Health Authority, ex parte Walker (1987) 3 BMLR 32.

R v North Derbyshire Health Authority, ex parte Fisher (1997) 38 BMLR 76.

R v North West Lancashire Health Authority, ex parte A, D and G (2000) 53 BMLR 148.

R v North West Thames Regional Health Authority, ex parte Daniels (1993) 19 BMLR 67.

R v Secretary of State for Health, ex parte Pfizer Ltd (2000) 51 BMLR 189.

R v Secretary of State for Social Services, ex parte Hincks (1980) 1 BMLR 93.

R v Sheffield Health Authority, ex parte Seale (1994) 25 BMLR 1.

Smith and Grady v UK (2000) 29 EHRR 493.

St George's Healthcare NHS Trust v S [1998] 3 All ER 673.

FURTHER READING

Cubbon J. 'The principle of QALY maximisation as the basis for allocating healthcare resources', *Journal of Medical Ethics* 1991; 17: 181.

Feek CM. 'Rationing healthcare in New Zealand: The use of clinical guidelines', *Medical Journal of Australia* 2000; 173: 423.

Frankel S, Ebrahim S, Smith GD. 'The limits to demand for healthcare', *British Medical Journal* 2000; 321: 40.

Ham C. 'Retracing the Oregon trail: The experience of rationing and the Oregon health plan', *British Medical Journal* 1998; 316: 1965.

Harris J. 'What is the good of healthcare?', *Bioethics* 1996; 10: 269.

Hurley J. 'Ethics, economics, and public funding of healthcare', *Journal of Medical Ethics* 2001; 27: 234.

Klein R. 'Dimensions of rationing: Who should do what?', *British Medical Journal* 1993; 307: 309.

Newdick C. 'Rights to NHS resources after the 1990 Act', *Medical Law Review* 1993; 1: 53.

Smith R. 'The failings of NICE', *British Medical Journal* 2000; 321: 1363.

Stewart. C. 'Tragic cases and the role of administrative law', *British Medical Journal* 2000; 321: 105.

3

THE CONFIDENTIAL RELATIONSHIP

Confidentiality is one of the most cherished aspects of the relationship between doctor and patient. The basis for medical confidentiality and its limits are, however, seldom explored – and, when they are examined it seems that there are surprisingly few hard and fast rules we can rely on. Nevertheless, there are a number of principles on which to draw – including those based on ethics, the law and professional conduct. These will be discussed in turn.

MEDICAL ETHICS

This is a field in which it is particularly difficult to separate a legal from a moral obligation. Put at its simplest, there are some relationships where the *need* for trust in confidence is so obvious that the parties to that relationship *expect* their confidences to be respected or, looked at another way, the expectation of *trust* establishes what is known as a fiduciary duty owed by the doctor to his or her patient.

The reasons underlying the need for confidentiality are complementary. First, if those who are sick do not trust doctors to maintain the information they disclose in confidence, they will not – it is argued – come forward for treatment. This is considered so important that, for example, compulsory notification of an infectious disease may be waived in selected conditions – notably, at present, in the case of infection with the human immunodeficiency virus (HIV). Second, doctors must be able to trust their patients to give them the *whole* story of their condition, otherwise, they risk working in partial darkness and, as a result, potentially reaching a wrong diagnosis and prescribing the wrong treatment.

CONFIDENTIALITY AND THE LAW

All of which is, on the face of things, so obvious that one would expect the law to be equally clear. But, in fact, this is far from so. Breach of medical confidentiality is a criminal offence in some countries – notably, from our point of view as members of the European Union, in France and Belgium. However, it is hard to think of a case which would be assessed as being of such public importance that it would be prosecuted in the criminal courts of the United Kingdom. Equally, its status as a civil offence is not wholly clear. It is nearly 20 years since the Law Commission, which advises the Government on desirable up-dates in legal policy, recommended that there should be a statutory offence of breach of confidence, which would include medical cases. Nothing has, however, been done and the current situation must therefore be judged by some rather unsatisfactory case law.

That there *is* a general duty on the doctor to respect the confidences of his patients was established, albeit indirectly, in a case in 1988 known as *Stephens v Avery*. This was not a case involving a doctor/patient relationship but, during the course of it, the court clearly accepted that the doctor/patient relationship was one which established an enforceable duty of confidentiality. Equally, the widely publicised *Spycatcher* case, which concerned the publication of the memoirs of a secret agent (and is known officially as *Attorney-General v Guardian Newspapers Ltd*) has relevance to medicine, in that it clarified the public interest in the legal protection of confidences which were imparted in an atmosphere of confidence. It also confirmed the circumstances in which the obligation would arise. First, the information divulged must have the *quality* of confidential information; second, the information must have been given in circumstances which indicated that an obligation of confidence was intended; and, third, there must have been unauthorised use of that information which resulted in detriment to the person providing it. The first two are clearly relevant to medical practice; the third, which may not, in fact, be essential in all cases, is built into the doctor/patient relationship insofar as disclosure of medical information automatically constitutes an invasion of personal privacy. Thus, a legal duty always exists in the healthcare environment, in addition to the professional or ethical duty.

The legal duty is not, however, absolute and is subject to modification. An analysis of the cases which have shaped and delimited the law in this area shows that major importance is laid on the public interest – the individuals' private interest is given comparatively little prominence. This is demonstrated particularly well by the case known as *W v Egdell*.

W's case is not easy to explain in a few lines but, essentially, he was a patient in a special hospital to which he had been admitted following conviction for the manslaughter of five persons and the wounding of several others. He wanted to be transferred to the less rigorous conditions of a regional secure hospital and, through his legal advisers, he invited Dr Egdell to examine him and to provide a report to support his application. In the event, Dr Egdell's opinion was unfavourable – he thought that W was still dangerous – and W withdrew his application, intending, instead, to depend on the periodic review of his circumstances by the Mental Health Review Tribunal which was due shortly. Dr Egdell, however, feared that this might be decided without his opinion being considered and, accordingly, he forwarded a copy of his report to the hospital authorities and to the Tribunal. W brought an action for breach of confidentiality on the grounds that confidentiality was an integral part of his contract with his doctor.

No-one involved doubted that Dr Egdell did owe W a duty of confidence but, even so, a balancing act had to be undertaken between, on the one hand, that duty and, on the other, the duty to protect the public from potential danger. In other words, whether or not an actionable breach of confidence had occurred depended not on general principles but on the precise nature of that breach. The trial judge chose to balance W's private right to confidentiality against the public's right to disclosure – and came down in favour of the public. The Court of Appeal, however, held that the correct balance against which to pit the public interest in disclosing a potentially dangerous situation was the public interest in being able to count on the confidential nature of the doctor/patient relationship. Admittedly, they came to the same conclusion, but the Court of Appeal's approach has greater importance since it confirms that the single most important feature in such cases is the question of danger to the public. As a result, each case will be judged by that standard, and the extent of the doctor's legal duty of confidentiality depends not on an abstract imperative but on how it affects the public. The law of Scotland has now been altered by way of the Mental Health (Public Safety and Appeals) (Scotland) Act 1999 so as to give effect to this conclusion and, despite the apparent change of interests, it has been shown to be compliant with the Human Rights Act 1998 in a case brought by a Mr Anderson and others.

The case of *X v Y*, heard in 1988, illustrates this principle from another perspective. In this case, the names of two general practitioners, who were hospitalised because of their positive HIV status, were leaked to a newspaper which wished to publicise them on the grounds of public interest and safety. An injunction was sought to prevent them doing so. The court granted the injunction on the grounds that the public interest in preserving the confidentiality of those with a serious medical condition greatly outweighed the danger to the public as potential contacts. Two points arise from this decision. First, it can be concluded that the *degree* of danger is an important feature. In this case, the doctors were general practitioners whose chance of transmitting the condition to their patients was, at worst, minimal. Second, conditions change with the times – and the law changes with them. Since the case of *X v Y*, the names of several doctors have been published in the newspapers in similar circumstances and no action has been taken against the editors. It may be that in these cases, unlike the case of *X v Y*, the information was not communicated to the press in circumstances which indicated the expectation of confidence and, although current policy is to limit the procedure, the use of 'look-back' techniques to identify those patients at risk may make the identification of an infected healthcare worker inevitable. However, the effect of other factors, such as the changing attitudes to HIV infection and the status of the doctors, or other practitioners concerned, must also be considered. There is an undoubted difference between, for example, the potential dangerousness of a general practitioner and an abdominal surgeon. By the same token, it could well be that different attitudes would be adopted towards conditions of greater infectivity, such as carriage of the virus for hepatitis B or C.

The courts' concern for the security of hospital records, and their parallel distrust of the healthcare 'mole', have been further emphasised in a recent case involving the murderer Ian Brady. In *Ashworth Hospital Authority v MGN Ltd*, a newspaper published items quoted from Brady's hospital notes verbatim. The hospital obtained an order to require the newspaper to explain how they obtained their information and to identify the employee who provided it. The newspaper appealed to the House of Lords on the grounds that security of their sources is of paramount importance to the press. Notwithstanding this, the House of Lords held that the security of hospital records was of such importance that it was essential that the source be identified and punished – if only as a deterrent for the future. The significance of the case in the present context lies in the clear implication that the duty of confidentiality extends to *all* of those working in a healthcare ambience (for which, see below).

CONFIDENTIALITY AND THE HEALTHCARE PROFESSIONS

As we have already noted, a general duty of confidentiality exists between members of the general public in circumstances where the relationship is such that they anticipate that the rule will be observed. That rule is formalised in the case of members of the healthcare professions through their controlling professional bodies.[1] We have seen in Chapter 1 that each of the specialties within, and ancillary to, the Health Service has such governance but, for the sake of brevity and ease of understanding, we will refer here to the General Medical Council (GMC) as a representative template for all of them.

Looking back through history, the Hippocratic Oath is widely regarded as the basis of the constitution of the medical profession. Hence, the policy that drives the GMC derives from it. The Oath still binds the doctor – at least theoretically – even although it is now seldom sworn in practice. It includes this statement:

> All that may come to my knowledge in the exercise of my profession or outside of my profession or in my daily commerce with men, which ought not to be spread abroad, I will keep secret and never reveal.

The Oath has been updated in the so-called Declaration of Geneva which says:

> I will respect the secrets which are confided in me, even after the patient has died.

The GMC lays very great stress on professional secrecy but, before considering this in more detail, it is worth noting two conditions of the Hippocratic Oath that are interesting in the present context. First, the confidential relationship is not confined to what passes between patient and doctor in the surgery or the hospital ward. The doctor is equally bound to confidence if he or she learns medical details during a casual conversation in the bar – irrespective of the source of the information. This is of practical importance. A member of the public – which includes a doctor – would not be subject to legal action if he or she publicised information obtained in this way; the fact that it was common knowledge would mean that there was no imported element of confidentiality about the disclosure. The doctor who did so, however, would still have to run the gauntlet of the GMC – the implication being that he or she might well not have been given the information if he or she were not a doctor.

Second, the qualification 'which ought not to be spread abroad' is of major significance. At one extreme, it could be taken to indicate that there are some matters which will not attract sanction for disclosure. On the other, it could be read as implying that there are some matters which are so serious that they *ought* to be disclosed – whether it be in the private or the public interest. This will be returned to later but, for the

---

[1] It will, of course, be noted that this applies to *all* professions that deal with the confidential aspects of their clients' lives. Thus, your solicitor, your accountant etc. are equally controlled – but we are concentrating on the healthcare professions in this book.

present, it is suggested that the prudent doctor will be very wary before relying on such interpretations. This is well illustrated by the case of Winston Churchill who led the country for the greater part of the Second World War. After his death, it transpired that he had been seriously ill for much of the time and his physician, Lord Moran, was criticised for not having publicised this at the time, in the national interest. This, then, is the doctor's dilemma at its highest level. Some might say that he has a duty to publicise his belief that conditions are ripe for wrong decision-making by a national leader; others would hold – and did hold – that we would very probably have lost the war in Churchill's absence.

In passing, it is notable that the Declaration of Geneva is firm in holding that the duty of confidentiality survives the patient's death and here we have a further example of how legal and professional standards can differ. You cannot, in law, defame the dead and, although the courts might well step in to defend the interests of a surviving spouse or children against those of a public eager for knowledge, no action for breach of confidence after death would be available on behalf of the deceased. The GMC might well take a different view, however, and has, for example, taken the very unusual step of censuring the Editor of the *British Medical Journal* for publicising details of the mental health of a dead celebrity in what he considered to be the interests of history.

To return to the main theme, the wording of the Declaration of Geneva is rather different from that of the Hippocratic Oath insofar as the former refers to 'respect' for the secrets confided in the doctor. Respect is an indefinite word, which leaves open the *degree* of respect to be paid – and this will depend on the circumstances of the individual case. Thus, it will be seen that the professional code as to patient confidentiality does not offer an absolute imperative – there is room for discretion. Added to this is the fact that the GMC itself has always regarded its code of conduct as being subject to interpretation in the light of prevailing public standards. Thus, the rules of the GMC, while considerably stronger than those of the law and, at the same time, carrying what may be more severe penalties, are such that not every technical breach of confidence will attract a penalty. It is important to be aware of what are the accepted exceptions that provide the basis for derogation from the general rule. These can be briefly described as follows:

The patient consents

Few people would quarrel with the concept that the consent of the patient to disclosure of information absolves the doctor from his or her duty of confidentiality. In this context, however, it must be emphasised that, to be valid, the consent would have to be specific – that is, the patient would be entitled to know just what, and how much, was being disclosed and, more particularly, to whom it was being disclosed. Proper consent must also be based on adequate information. The doctor who asks: 'Do you mind if I inform your employer about what you have told me?' is not entitled to assume that the patient understands that this might well involve him or her in some limitation of opportunities for advancement. In other words, the consenting patient must know why the doctor wishes to break confidence and the consequences of his doing so – there is little doubt that the GMC would interpret 'good medical practice' in this way.

Sharing information within the healthcare team

Most medicine is now practiced as a team effort and, in general, the 'team' has to be regarded as a single person who is represented by, say, the hospital consultant or the general practitioner. It would be absurd to suggest that the physician should obtain specific consent every time he wanted to discuss a case with, for example, the radiologist or the ward sister. The patient will probably understand this intuitively – and his or her understanding will be based on trust that the principal person has instructed his or her staff on 'hospital' or 'practice' professional ethics. This trust is backed up by the knowledge that the medical and nursing staff, together with members of the professions allied to medicine, are governed by professional councils who, at the end of the day, retain disciplinary powers over their members. Where this is not so, it is incumbent on the hospital or practice authorities to ensure that their employees are instructed in the duty of medical confidence and that obedience to that duty is included in their terms of contract. Thus, say, a secretary in the hospital who breached confidence would be subject to the discipline of fair dismissal.

But, what of the 'second opinion' – the doctor whose advice would be appreciated but who is not a member of the team with whom the patient is at ease and who may not even be associated with the hospital? It is doubtful if the doctor who mentions concern about a patient to a colleague is guilty of breach of confidence because it is, effectively, a recognisable aspect of patient care. Of course, much would depend on the circumstances of the disclosure and the extent of information provided; that is, any such conversation would have to be conducted privately and only necessary information should be disclosed. Equally, such disclosure may be deemed to be in the patient's best interests. In the latter instance, however, it is perfectly possible that the patient may not wish his or her medical details to be noised abroad, either in a specific or a general sense. For these reasons, ideally such a consultation ought to be subject to the patient's consent. The same would apply in the event of the patient's case being the subject of a 'staff case conference', which is, after all, as much for the education of the staff as for advantage to the patient, and the preservation of anonymity in such a situation would be difficult if not impossible to achieve.

Although it is, perhaps, not strictly to the present point, those who are not part of the team, but who play an essential part in hospital life, must be mentioned. What, for example, of the charity worker who brings round the mobile library and who breaks confidence as a result of what he or she has seen or heard in the wards? Would such a breach be actionable on the part of the offended patient? Much would, again, depend on the nature of the breach but, in general, the matter would be decided on the basis of whether or not the *reasonable person* in that situation would appreciate that the information carried with it a natural element of confidentiality. The person or persons who breached confidentiality in the important case of *X v Y*, which was mentioned above, were probably not 'healthcarers' as such and, after much reflection, the judge decided against publishing their names. Nevertheless, he said:

> The person who betrayed, for money, the trust imposed on him or her by [the hospital] should clearly understand that, although he or she may escape detection on this occasion, such luck a second time is wholly unlikely and, if caught, prison is the probable consequence

and we have seen in the Ashworth Hospital case, above, that this was no idle threat.

Disclosure to insurance companies and employers

Not infrequently a doctor will be asked for confidential information as to a patient's health for the purposes of employment or insurance. This will nearly always be at the patient's request but, even so – or if not – as we have already pointed out, the doctor should ensure that he or she understands the nature and purpose of the request and the likely purpose to which that information is to be put. It is true that the case of Ms Kapfunde, heard in the Court of Appeal in 1998, establishes that an employment medical officer is subject to a contract for services to the employer and has no duty of care to the employee. But the wise doctor will always obtain written consent to disclosure, which may after all have a profound effect on the examinee's future.

Disclosure in the patient's best interests

As we discuss in the next chapter, there may be times when the patient is unable to give a valid consent to disclosure of his or her health status, yet the doctor has good grounds for feeling that it would be in his or her best interests to do so. The most common situations of this type involve patients who are comatose or who are incompetent to do so because of either mental disorder or age. In such circumstances, the doctor can call on the legal doctrine of necessity which, put simply, means that it is permissible to take an action that is technically unlawful, provided that it is immediately necessary to safeguard the life or health of the patient or to prevent serious deterioration in his or her condition. Clearly, to invoke 'necessity' successfully implies that the action must be capable of subsequent legal justification and, in the present context, of vindication before the GMC.

There will often be little concern as to the application of the necessity doctrine in the case of the comatose patient. It might reasonably be assumed that he or she would almost certainly *want* his or her nearest and dearest to know the likely diagnosis or prognosis. There may, however, be times when disclosure of certain kinds of information would be a matter requiring further justification – this being, still, subject to the rule of necessity.

The question of competence is discussed at greater length in Chapter 15. For present purposes, it is only necessary to note that competence to consent to, in this case disclosure of confidential information, depends on the capacity to understand its implications and the ability to weigh these in the balance. Whether or not a patient is to be regarded as competent depends upon an assessment of his or her capacity – an assessment which must be made independently of both the particular form of mental disorder and (except in the case of the very young) of the age of the patient. This leads to consideration of the quality and extent of confidentiality which is owed to children.

CONFIDENTIALITY AND THE CHILD

It is not necessary to consider this in great depth here, however, as the child's right to confidentiality is but one aspect of the wider problem of his or her right to consent to medical treatment as a whole and this is addressed in Chapter 4. Both consent and confidentiality in respect of children are still defined by the important case raised by Mrs Victoria Gillick as long ago as 1983. The Department of Health had issued a directive that empowered doctors, in limited circumstances, to provide contraceptive assistance to minors below the age of 16 without the knowledge of their parents. Put at its simplest, Mrs Gillick sought a court ruling to the effect that this was wrong in law. The judge who first heard the case considered the child's capacity to understand the issues to be the most important factor and held that, provided that capacity was present, doctors acting in this way were acting lawfully. The Court of Appeal, however, concentrated on the duties of parents to look after their children's welfare and their parallel rights to be informed of activities which threatened that welfare. On these grounds, they decided unanimously in favour of Mrs Gillick. The House of Lords then reverted to reliance on the importance of the autonomy – or right to self-determination – of the 'mature minor' and found in favour of the Department of Health by a bare majority. As something of a side-issue, it was also decided that the doctor who advised the minor in this way was not aiding or abetting the criminal offence of having under-age sexual relations.[2]

There are a number of interesting observations to be made on the *Gillick* case. First, the extreme delicacy of the problem is illustrated in the fact that, although Mrs Gillick lost her case, more judges (5) voted for her than against her (4). It will be seen later, however, that the repercussions of the *Gillick* case have been so far-reaching that it is very unlikely that the issue would be so closely contested were it to be re-heard to-day. Nevertheless, as the court itself declared, the decision was not to be taken as 'a licence for doctors to disregard the wishes of parents whenever they found it convenient to do so' and the House of Lords laid down five criteria which had to be met before the doctor was not in danger of breaching the law. We return to these later but, from the point of view of confidentiality, the most important was that, in addition to being assured of the child's full understanding, the doctor must make every effort to persuade him or her to inform his or her parents of what was happening, or to allow him or her to do so, before undertaking his or her medical management in the face of his or her parents' ignorance – otherwise, the doctor laid him or her self open to disciplinary action by the GMC.

At the same time, the doctor has his or her own conscience to satisfy. He or she could, for example, consider the treatment involved to be so serious that he or she could not treat the minor in the absence of parental consent and, at the same time, live within his or her own ethical limits; occasionally, as when controlling or assisting pregnancy, he or she is protected by a statutory 'conscience clause'. In such circumstances, the doctor has no open mandate to breach confidentiality but should refer his or her patient to a professional colleague. All in all, it can only be said that the confidential nature of the treatment of minors below the age of 16 is, at present, unsatisfactorily vague. The child cannot be certain that his or her parents will not be consulted, while the parents may be unsure of the medical advice or treatment that the child, for whom they are responsible, is receiving. The answer lies solely in the doctor's assessment of the child's mental capacity.

---

[2] Though, lest there be any doubt, the under-age girl who has sexual intercourse commits no offence; criminality is confined to the man involved.

CONFIDENTIALITY WITHIN THE FAMILY

Situations often arise in which the doctor must decide whether he or she is treating the individual or the family as a whole. Decisions taken by or on behalf of the former will nearly always have a wider effect, and the question then arises as to how far these should be taken into consideration when managing the patient.

What, say, of the wife who seeks a termination of pregnancy without her husband's knowledge? Here, there can be little doubt that the doctor is firmly bound by his duty of confidentiality to his or her patient. Both legally and ethically, pregnancy is regarded as being such an intimate matter for the pregnant woman that her husband or partner has no intrinsic right to interfere in its management – despite the fact that he has an equal genetic relationship to the child within the uterus. But what if the wife seeks sterilisation on the same terms? A conscientious practitioner may well feel that this is not a decision that should be taken unilaterally. The doctor's first responsibility may well be to attempt to convince his or her patient that this should be a joint decision. This having failed, however, the answer does not lie in breach of confidentiality which, in the absence of danger, could seldom, if ever, be justified. Rather, the doctor may fall back on the well-accepted principle that there is no compulsion to provide treatment that he or she cannot approve – and, sometimes, as we have already noted, such 'opting out' has the backing of statute. Nevertheless, as the duty to refer the patient to another practitioner still remains, 'opting out' then becomes something very like 'passing the buck'. This is a less than ideal moral ploy – but it may be the only alternative to a deeply held conscientious or professional objection to providing a specific form of treatment under the veil of secrecy.

Conditions may, however, be different if secrecy creates real danger for other members of the family. For example, what if one spouse or partner is suffering from a sexually transmissible disease which he or she is unwilling to disclose to the other? Clearly, the first step is a frank discussion with the affected person, which might include seeking consent to disclosure. Should this turn out unsatisfactorily, however, and should there remain a serious and identifiable risk to a specific person, the GMC would almost certainly support the practitioner who took steps to ensure that that individual was informed of the risk. This would apply whether or not the individual at risk was also the doctor's patient.

Perhaps the most intractable problem associated with confidentiality within the family lies in the management of genetic information that comes to the doctor's notice. The significance of such information extends beyond the individual, and very careful thought must be given to how it is distributed. For example, a deleterious gene may express itself with varying and unpredictable severity; it may only cause damage if associated with another specific gene or with certain environmental factors; it may predict the possibility or the certainty of disease; it may display itself early or late in life; a treatment may or may not be available for the resultant condition – and so on. Moreover, genetic knowledge may have a completely different significance for those who already have a family as opposed to those who are considering embarking on parenthood. Add to this, the fact that some persons may not want to be given genetic information despite the importance it might have for them and it will be seen that genetic confidentiality has such unique features that it merits separate consideration. Accordingly, we return to the subject in Chapters 9 and 11.

THE PATIENT IN DANGER

The circumstances surrounding the discovery of violence within the family provide a scenario that is, effectively, unique. It is, for example, easy to say that the propriety of disclosure of such violence depends on the consent of the victim and that this should always be sought. But many victims of family violence are unable to consent by virtue of incapacity insofar as they will be either children or aged. The situation may be unclear even between these two extremes; valid consent or refusal of consent depends on the exercise of a free choice and the abused wife, say, may well be too frightened to exercise such a choice. The doctor's dilemma is, then, very real.

It might well be contended that enough children and old people have died or have sustained severe lasting damage for it to be self-evident that every case of suspected child or elder abuse should be reported to the appropriate authorities. But, like it or not, children *do* fall off swings and *do* spill hot water on themselves – and many readers will remember the disastrous consequences of well-intentioned but over-zealous searches for child abuse that were seen in Cleveland in England in 1987 and in the Orkney Isles in 1991. An old woman may, indeed, be subject to abuse but who is to say she is wrong when she maintains that she gets more benefits from contact with her grandchildren than she would obtain in an 'old peoples' home'. And the 'battered wife' may genuinely prefer to accept her situation rather than see the break-up of her family and the removal of her children into care. None of which is to say that breach of confidentiality should never occur absent the consent of the victim – rather, the balance may well be in favour of disclosure and may involve a *duty* in the case of young children. The overriding conditions are that, first, consent should be sought if it can be given and, second, that disclosure must be to an appropriate authority. It should be noted that, while the concept of confidentiality does not, of itself, establish a privileged position for informants, the case of *D v N S P C C* established that the public interest dictates that those authorities with 'a right to know' are entitled to protect their sources and to refuse to disclose their identities.

DISCLOSURE BEYOND THE HEALTHCARE ENVIRONMENT

Disclosure to the police

The doctor's first duty must always be due to his or her patients but, as we will see in many places in this book, there is a strong element of public interest in the practice of medicine. The doctor will very often come into contact with violent crime as a natural part of his or her work. One patient may be the victim of an assault; equally, another may have been injured during the actual perpetration of a crime. What, then, is the doctor to do if all the evidence indicates that the patient under care is, for example, a rapist who is being sought by the police? Certainly, there is no legal duty to inform the police (with limited statutory exceptions) although, in common with the rest of the public, the doctor must not give false or misleading information when approached. Negative advice of this type is, however, relatively useless; we must look for some more positive direction – and this is not easy to identify.

As we have indicated above, occasionally, the answer to the doctor/police relationship is made clear by statute. Thus, 'a person' who has knowledge of acts or anticipated acts of terrorism must inform the police and for these purposes 'a person' includes a doctor. Similarly, and on a rather more mundane scale, the case of *Hunter v Mann* confirmed that the same applies to 'any person' who, when asked, must provide information that can help to identify the driver of a vehicle that has been involved in a serious accident. But such examples are few and far between. More important in the present context are those statutory provisions that are designed to protect the patient and his or her records from examination by the police – which is, in practice, yet more direction of a 'negative' type. The main authority here is the Police and Criminal Evidence Act of 1984[3] which classifies medical records as 'excluded material' to which, as a general rule, the police have no access. The police involved in the investigation of a 'serious arrestable offence' must obtain an order from a circuit judge if they wish to search for such confidential documents and, even then, the provision of the order is subject to restriction. Moreover, the definition of medical records – that is, documents relating to the physical or mental health of an identifiable person – can be stretched. In one instance, the police searching for a brutal murderer sought to examine a record of patients' absences from a psychiatric hospital. The consultant's protests that these related to confidential medical matters were upheld by the Divisional Court and the police were denied access.

Interestingly, the court in this case expressed 'considerable reluctance' to apply the letter of the law, and it has to be noted that, while the police cannot command access to confidential documents, the doctor may disclose their contents voluntarily – subject, of course, to being able to justify doing so. Once again, then, we are back to a balancing act – this time between the nature of the confidential information and the importance to the public of the police enquiry and the administration of justice. There is little doubt that the GMC would support the doctor whenever the imbalance was sufficient to justify his or her action.

MEDICAL CONFIDENTIALITY AND THE LEGAL PROCESS

The confidentiality of communications between solicitor and client is protected by what is known as professional privilege. That is, such communications as are related to the conduct of the client's case are, in general, protected from disclosure to outside parties. Confidential communications between the solicitor and an expert witness acting on his or her instructions – who, for present purposes, will be a doctor – are included under such an umbrella of secrecy. But, for reasons that may seem obscure to the non-lawyer, it does not apply to the independent opinion of the expert him or her self nor, more understandably, to the documents or other evidence on which that opinion was based. Thus, W (see above) got little sympathy from the court when he alleged that Dr Egdell's report was a privileged document in legal terms, despite the fact that the Mental Health Act 1983 specifies that a restricted patient is free to seek advice from a doctor outside of the secure hospital system who may see all the relevant documents and who can undertake the examination in private. It is, however, fair to note that at least one of the judges in the Court of Appeal saw 'great force' in W's viewpoint – and it is possible that he might have won his case had he not been

---

[3] This does not apply to Scotland where the comparable situation is covered by the Criminal Procedure. (Scotland) Act 1995.

confined for a particularly violent crime and was thought to present a continuing threat to the public.

Medical records which have accumulated in the course of ordinary management and treatment must also be disclosed in the event of their being the subject of court proceedings. The claimant (or, in Scotland, the pursuer) – that is, the person who raises an action in a case of personal injury – can obtain medical records from the defendant even before proceedings have begun. Once the case has started, either side can demand a sight of a doctor's or a hospital's relevant records even if neither record is directly concerned in the action. In such circumstances, the court can stipulate that the documents must be produced to the applicant, his or her legal advisers or to his or her medical advisers. The court order is most important here because only a court order can provide absolute justification for disclosure; many an inexperienced doctor has had cause to regret acting merely because a solicitor has asked him or her to do so.

Once in court, the judge in the United Kingdom – although not in several States of the European Union – can order a breach of medical confidentiality whenever it is seen as being necessary in the interests of justice. The doctor who complies with the order is, then, protected absolutely from any action for breach of confidence. He or she may, and often does, answer a delicate medical question by way of a written note to the judge; but he or she must answer publicly if the judge decides that it is right for him or her to do so.

The public interest

Throughout this discussion it has been clear that the concept of the public interest presents one of the more difficult aspects of the legitimate disclosure of medical confidences. Time after time, it must be asked whether the public interest in disclosure of a person's medical status is of greater or lesser importance than is the public interest in preserving medical confidentiality, and it can seldom be absolutely clear that the right decision has been reached. No final firm rule can be laid down because every case will differ as to detail; in the end, the solution of the problem depends on a subjective balancing of interests by the individual doctor. Anomalous decisions are bound to occur.

Having said that, it has to be admitted that, in many cases, the balancing of interests in favour of the public is so obvious that the law *compels* the doctor to disclose what would otherwise be confidential medical information. The most obvious example is to be found in the reporting of cases of infectious disease. There are, admittedly, some who regard even this as being unnecessary in twenty-first century conditions. The great majority, however, would most probably feel that it would be a derogation of duty for an authority to allow, say, a person carrying the organism responsible for typhoid fever to be employed in a restaurant's kitchen. Similarly, most of us would sympathise with the legal obligation to report cases of industrial poisoning in support of safety at work. Some compulsory disclosures are, however, less easy to justify. The statutory reporting of, for example, cases of drug addiction or termination of pregnancy can have little or no impact on public health and is imposed, in the main, for administrative reasons. And we have already seen that there are some occasions on which a doctor must disclose medical information simply because he or she is 'a member of the public'. Yet there are other instances where the public health interest is very strong but reporting is not demanded by law – take, for example, the car driver with uncontrolled epilepsy who refuses to report the matter, as required by regulation, or to give up driving. Here, the doctor must perform his or her own 'balancing exercise' – although few, given this scenario, would debate the way the balance tips. In coming to a conclusion, the doctor will be guided by three major principles to which we have already alluded. First, disclosure must be limited either to the authority nominated by statute or otherwise 'with a need to know' – for instance, in the example above, the Drivers Vehicle Licensing Authority. Secondly, the doctor should have made a genuine attempt to persuade the patient to report the matter him or herself. And, finally, disclosure must be justifiable to the General Medical Council – a condition which, of itself, is sufficient to give rise to serious thought before taking action.

More interest may, however, attach to the problems associated with disclosure and criminality, problems which can be approached from two directions – first, where a person *has* committed a crime and, second, where he or she *may* do so.

The first is relatively uncontroversial. As has already been noted in connection with co-operation with the police, a doctor is not *bound* to assist in the apprehension of a criminal but few would question his or her moral duty to do so in the event of a serious offence. But, if he or she has a moral duty to assist, is there also a moral duty to promote the arrest of the patient? True, the public can expect positive activity towards the detection and punishment of serious crime. But, at the same time, cannot the criminal patient lay claim to a doctor/patient relationship of an ethical quality equal to that offered to his law-abiding counterpart? And, lest it be thought that the answer is easy, we can ask what *is* a serious offence? A doctor may think that his or her patient's injuries are compatible with his or her having fallen through a roof-light; but does that justify reporting that he or she believes the local housebreaker is in the surgery? It may be that any difference in the two examples lies in the fact that one involves an offence against the person and the other is against property. But, even then, one can talk in either case in terms of *relative* severity. Given that uncertainty, it is unlikely that all doctors would adopt the same moral stance.

The person who *may* commit a crime of violence is exemplified by one with a dangerous personality disorder who has, for one reason or another, been released from strict custody – and we revert to this topic in Chapter 15. Such a case arose in the United States case involving a Ms Tarasoff. Here, a psychopathic patient informed his psychotherapist that he intended to harm Ms Tarasoff. The therapist informed the University police of this but did not breach confidence to Ms Tarasoff who was later murdered. The family sued the University for the failure, through their employee, to protect Ms Tarasoff, and was successful. There has been no strictly comparable case in the United Kingdom. Similar actions for negligence, however, have indicated that there is no duty laid on a Health Authority to issue a *general* warning that a potentially dangerous person is at large but, as we go to press, the very recent case involving a murder by a dangerous immigrant (*Akenzua v Secretary of State for the Home Office* (2002)) raises some doubt – insofar as the police might be held, in the particular circumstances, to have been responsible for the death of a random individual.[4] There have been no

---

[4] The case was, however, taken in misfeasance of public duty rather than negligence. Misfeasance implies some form of wrongdoing on the part of an authority.

cases involving an identifiable potential target and it is equally difficult to predict the result should one arise. The probability is that there would be no legal obligation to warn the person at risk but that, should the doctor do so, the breach of confidentiality would be regarded as justified. In practice, however, confidentiality would probably represent no more than a lesser issue within the wider envelope of a duty to protect those at risk of physical harm.

THE PATIENT'S RIGHTS

Mention of patients' rights, however, raises a final question as to the confidential relationship between the two main parties – the doctor and the patient – as opposed to that related to third parties, which we have been discussing. In short, what right has the patient to knowledge of the doctor's attitude to his or her condition as expressed in the doctor's notes?

There is no doubt that ownership of the actual material on which the notes are written vests in the primary care or hospital trust and the patient cannot remove the relevant folder. Far more interest, however, lies in the confidential nature of the intellectual content. This is governed by the Data Protection Act of 1998 (as amended in 2000) which now applies to written and computerised medical records (save, to a minor extent, as to the notes of those who are deceased) and which, in general, protects the privacy rights of individuals' personal data. Data concerning health matters are classified as sensitive personal data and, as a simplification, we can say that the Act puts the principles as to third party involvement that are discussed above into statutory form. But what of the *patient's* right of access to his or her *own* notes?

There is no doubt that the Act provides a right to be given information as to any personal data held in note form but, at the same time, this is a qualified right. In practical terms, the right is only available following a request in writing. On a more professional level, among other exceptions, access need not be granted if, in the opinion of the Health Authority, disclosure would cause serious mental or physical harm to the patient or any other person – and this is a fairly open-ended and subjective condition. The major inference, however, is that a patient is not entitled to examine his or her own notes as held, for example, on the hospital ward for, to accept otherwise, would be to nullify that element of 'professional privilege' which the Act clearly identifies as an important part of patient care. It might be argued that, aside from the Act, there is a common law right to be able to see what has been written about oneself or, even, that it is subsumed under Article 8 of the European Convention on Human Rights, to the extent that to refuse access is to interfere with a person's private life. However, a Mr Martin raised such issues in a case heard by the Court of Appeal in 1994 when it was held that, even if there was such a right at common law, it would still be subject to the same conditions in respect of professional privilege and, thus, access would be similarly restricted.

Even so, it has to be remembered that Mr Martin's case was heard before the 1998 Act came into force and, while it is clear that a patient had no right to examine his or her hospital notes without supervision before that time, things may be changing – especially because the courts are now taking a progressively more positive attitude to privacy rights in general. We would have to say that matters are not entirely settled – particularly, say, in relation to a parental wish to examine a child's notes, and there are many who hold that the notes should actually *belong* to the patient. The practical answer is, perhaps, twofold. First, doctors should be diligent in refraining from making unprofessional notes that they would not want a patient to see and, second, they should, so far as is possible, ensure that any matters that came within the 'professional privilege' exception had already been aired within the context of a modern doctor/patient therapeutic partnership.

All of this applies, effectively, only to notes which are confined to the individual hospital's or doctor's use. Conditions change – and are regulated by the Access to Medical Reports Act of 1988 – when personal medical information is to be passed to an outsider such as an employer or an insurer. No such information can now be provided by a clinician without his or her patient's positively obtained consent. The patient can see the relevant report before it is delivered and, significantly, he or she can ask the doctor to alter anything that is considered inaccurate; the patient may add a note of dissent if this is refused. As usual, access can be restricted on the grounds of possible harm to the subject or others but, of course, the patient can always withdraw his or her consent if this clause is invoked.

CONCLUSION

A summary, such as we have given above, of the many ways in which breach of medical confidentiality can be justified has convinced some writers that the concept has only nugatory value. Nevertheless, it will be seen that many of the exceptions are, themselves, 'exceptional' and strict confidentiality remains the general rule in medical practice. It is recognised as such within the healthcare professions and by the law and it is expected by the public. It may be difficult to bring a successful action against a healthcarer based purely on breach of confidence, although arguably this may become easier given the increasing importance which is being attached to what are generally known as 'patients' rights' and, in particular, following the incorporation into UK law of the European Convention on Human Rights via the Human Rights Act of 1998. This would be particularly so were the patient to suffer tangible harm as a result of the breach. Even then, a successful action may be poor compensation for, say, the loss of reputation that has been sustained. As with most litigation, it is a matter of 'shutting the stable door after the horse has bolted' and, obviously, prevention would be far better than cure. In this respect, we re-emphasise the importance of the role of professional bodies such as the GMC. This, we believe, is one particular area where the standards of the GMC should be carefully monitored, for, at the end of the day, a powerful professional disciplinary mechanism is the public's most powerful weapon in defence of the confidential relationship.

CASES MENTIONED IN THE TEXT

A v The Scottish Ministers 2000 SLT 873.

Akenzua v Secretary of State for the Home Office [2003] 1 All ER 35.

Ashworth Hospital Authority v MGN Ltd [2002] 1 WLR 2033.

Attorney-General v Guardian Newspapers Ltd (No 2) [1988] 3 All ER 545.

D v National Society for the Prevention of Cruelty to Children [1977] 1 All ER 589.

Gillick v West Norfolk and Wisbech Area Health Authority [1985] 3 All ER 402.

Hunter v Mann [1974] 2 All ER 414.

Kapfunde v Abbey National plc (1998) 46 BMLR 176.

R v Cardiff Crown Court, ex parte Kellam (1994) 16 BMLR 76.

R v Mid Glamorgan FHSA, ex parte Martin (1995) 1 All ER 356.

Stephens v Avery [1988] 2 All ER 477.

Tarasoff v Regents of the University of California 551 P 2d 334 (Cal. 1976).

W v Egdell [1989] 1 All ER 1089.

X v Y [1988] 2 All ER 648.

FURTHER READING

Adler MW. 'HIV, confidentiality and a "delicate balance"', *Journal of Medical Ethics* 1991; 17: 196.

Boyd KM. 'HIV infection and AIDS: The ethics of medical confidentiality', *Journal of Medical Ethics'* 1992; 18: 173.

Brahams D. 'Medical confidentiality and expert evidence', *Lancet* 1991; 337: 1276.

British Medical Association. *Confidentiality and Disclosure of Health Information*, 1999.

Gilhooly MLM, McGhee SM. 'Medical records: Practicalities and principles of patient possession', *Journal of Medical Ethics* 1991; 17: 138.

Jacob JM. 'Confidentiality: The dangers of anything weaker than the medical ethic', *Journal of Medical Ethics* 1982; 8: 18.

Kottow MH. 'Medical confidentiality: An intransigent and absolute obligation', *Journal of Medical Ethics* 1986; 12: 117.

Ploem C. 'Medical confidentiality after a patient's death', *Medical Law* 2001; 2: 215.

4

THE THERAPEUTIC PARTNERSHIP

'Every human being of adult years and sound mind has a right to determine what shall be done with his own body ….'

This statement, drawn from an American case decided as long ago as 1914, sums up the conditions underlying both ethical and lawful medical intervention. When patients consult their doctors, they expect that decisions as to whether or not they will accept treatment rest with them. Indeed, they may also anticipate that they will be able to choose between different kinds of therapy. This is not to suggest that there is no role for the doctor; he or she is the person with the medical skills, and will, it is expected, act in a way which is of most benefit to their patients, including advising patients as to what he or she thinks is the best treatment. This is no different from consulting, say, a lawyer or an accountant – whenever we consult professional men or women, we invite them to exercise their training and skills. However, the fact that learned advice is sought does not inevitably mean that authority is handed over to the professional to make the final decision. The invitation to act is an invitation to provide advice and recommendations based on acquired skills – but it is for the individual to decide to what use that expertise will be put.

The issue of what doctors tell patients has always been rather more controversial than it has been in other professional interactions, reflecting perhaps both the significance of health itself and the complexity of this particular relationship. Although at first sight it might seem clear that people need the fullest possible information from which to 'determine what shall be done with their own bodies', other factors have traditionally been taken into account and arguments have been raised in favour of limiting the amount that is disclosed to patients. In addition, it will be noted from the opening quotation that its terms cover only the sane, adult patient. Different considerations, therefore, inevitably arise when the person is a child or is an adult who suffers from some learning or other mental disability. And, of course, there will be some times when discussion and patient decision-making are not feasible because, for example, the patient is unconscious.

THE COMPETENT ADULT PATIENT

We will return to the last three categories of patient later but, for the moment, it is important to establish what is the situation in the case of the normal adult. It is now widely recognised, both by the Department of Health and by the great majority of doctors, that involving patients in treatment decisions makes for better care, increased patient compliance with treatment and a better overall outcome. However, the creation of what has been called a 'therapeutic alliance' does not always mean that the ideal of the fullest possible disclosure will be reached in reality. As already noted, there are a number of arguments raised in favour of constraining the amount of information which it is thought necessary to pass on to patients – and the first part of this chapter will look at some of these.

Arguments against full disclosure

A number of commentators have referred to the arguments which would restrict information disclosure in the medical situation. One of the best of these commentaries comes from Allan Buchanan and we will use his analysis in what follows to provide relevant examples. Basically, he described three main kinds of argument. He called the first of these the prevention of harm argument.

Broadly speaking, this runs as follows: doctors are under an ethical and professional obligation not to injure their patients; some information, it is said, would cause harm to patients – for example by causing them distress or anxiety; the doctor is, therefore, entitled to withhold it. Buchanan goes on to question the significance and strength of this argument in the following way. There is no doubt that some kinds of knowledge may well cause harm – but is this a sufficient reason to withhold information if it is relevant to the patient? Doctors cannot *know* that knowing something will, in fact, cause harm unless they disclose it and the harm actually eventuates. In other words, the argument is inherently flawed.

The second argument, which is an extension of the first, suggests that the doctor/patient relationship is like a contract, with an implied warranty that doctors will act in the best interests of their patients, including doing no harm. As part of that contract, patients cede to the doctor the authority to make decisions on their behalf. However, although some may regard this as accurately describing the nature of the doctor/patient relationship, it is by no means universally accepted as the appropriate model and cannot, therefore, be generalised so as to include all patients and all such relationships – and, of course, this argument also suffers from the flaws described in relation to the first.

Buchanan's third example stems from what he calls the inability to understand. In this scenario, the doctor would be entitled to withhold information because disclosing it would serve no purpose since the patient would not, in any event, be able to understand what he or she was told. This can be criticised as being based on unwarranted and dubious evaluations of patients' capacities – evaluations which the doctor is neither equipped nor entitled to make. Of course, some medical information may be highly technical, but the patients' concerns are essentially human. What they want to know, for example, is whether a treatment will make them sick or leave a scar, not necessarily which pharmacological agent will make them sick or which instrument will cause the scarring. In short, it is possible to explain to patients what they both need and want to know without involving technical jargon. Equally, assumptions about the intellectual capacity of patients cannot stand unchallenged. Recently, for example, a research project funded by the Wellcome Trust found that the 'man in the street' was quite able – after explanation – to understand the complexities of genetics, that most difficult of sciences.

There is a fourth argument against disclosure which is essentially pragmatic. Simply put, this would say that it is impractical to tell a patient absolutely everything about the risks, benefits and alternatives involved in treatment because there just is not the time to do so – for example, with the average general practitioner's appointment lasting about 10 minutes, there is no possibility that everything which the patient might think is relevant can be covered. In addition, doctors point with horror to the situation in the United States where, it is claimed, patients are deluged with excessive information in order to safeguard the clinician from litigation. This is thought to be unhelpful in the long run and to be a policy that does nothing to enhance the doctor/patient relationship.

Arguments in favour of disclosure

Most obviously, the primary argument in favour of full disclosure of the pros, cons and alternatives to specific treatments is that patients have the right to make their own decisions about whether or not to accept recommended treatment, and indeed which treatment to accept. That is, patients have the right to determine their own destiny or to exercise their autonomy. They can do this only if they are given enough information to help them understand the consequences of their choice – and only the doctor has that information. Autonomy has become the trumping ethical value in the last 50 years or so, and is no less important in healthcare delivery. Indeed, autonomy rights dominate the European Convention on Human Rights, to which the United Kingdom courts and legislators are now bound following the enactment of the Human Rights Act 1998.

As we have already seen, there are also other arguments which favour disclosure. Not least, there is now evidence that the patient who is informed about his or her treatment is more likely to do well. The involvement of patients in treatment allows them to take a meaningful role in maintaining their health and enhances their relationship with the doctor and other healthcare workers. So, full involvement in therapeutic decisions goes beyond the goal of maximising patient autonomy and can lead to positive benefits for the individual's health.

However, the need to ensure that a sensible balance is reached must also be recognised. It would not necessarily be in the interests of patient care were doctors obliged to provide every piece of knowledge that they possess by virtue of their training. What patients need is information which is likely to be relevant to their own choices. The problem remains as to how this is to be assessed. The doctor who decides what information the patient might need or want will always be subject to allegations of paternalism and, indeed, may be wrong. If, however, the decision were to lie with the patients, they would need to have *all* of the information before they could decide what was useful and what was not. There is no easy answer to this conundrum that will satisfy everyone but, given what has been said about the importance of respect for autonomy, we must accept that the decision to withhold information which could be relevant needs to reflect the underlying assumption that the patient has a right to be fully informed.

PATIENT AUTONOMY, ETHICS AND THE LAW

Patients' expectations that they will be told everything about their illness and its proposed treatment are, as we have noted, grounded in the ethical concept of autonomy or self-determination. At the same time, of course, it is generally accepted that the right to behave autonomously may sometimes be overridden by or in the interests of others. For example, there is no autonomous right to kill someone else, even if making a rational, self-determined choice to do so, because the greater good of society demands that such behaviour should be outlawed. Equally, however, it can reasonably be expected that a decision whether or not to write a book will not be interfered with unless, say, the book is being used to defame someone – in which case, it might not be published.

In addition to being something to which individuals aspire, respect for autonomy is one of the cornerstones of the doctor/patient relationship. Doctors' professional ethics require them to use their expertise with the patient's right to self-determination firmly in mind and, by and large, doctors will take this obligation very seriously – even in cases where the capacity of the patient may be in doubt. Both ethically and practically, the self-determining patient is the ideal model from the points of view of doctors and patients alike.

However, before going on to consider how the law has approached this question, it is worth dealing with one type of patient who may seem to turn all of this talk of autonomy on its head – namely, the patient who doesn't want to know. Many doctors will say that there are some patients who simply want them to make all the decisions and who have no interest in receiving information. This could be taken to suggest that the patient is not acting autonomously and, therefore, to cast doubt on the propriety of any treatment which is offered. Certainly, it could present problems for the doctor who is committed to involving his or her patients in healthcare decisions for the reasons we have already identified. However, it is important to remember that one can act autonomously by *refusing* information just as much as one can be self-determining by *requesting* or *receiving* it. A choice not to know is no less an autonomous choice, and is no less worthy of respect, than is a wish to be informed. However frustrating, doctors must give equal respect to a refusal of information, provided that they are satisfied that the refusal is well informed.

If the notion of autonomy is taken seriously, it would be expected that respect for it would attract a more forceful commitment than that due to a simple ethical concept. It would, thus, be reasonable to suppose that it would also be strongly supported in law and that failure to respect it would be censured. To an extent, this is what happens. Touching others without their consent is an assault or battery – and this is so no matter the underlying intention of the touching nor, within limits, how serious the touching actually was. Thus, a doctor who, for example, operated on a patient, or examined one physically, without his or her agreement would be guilty of assault even although he or she was certain that the surgery or the examination would benefit the patient. No special exemptions apply to doctors in this respect.

However, the picture becomes complicated when the patients' grievance is not so much that they did not consent to the touching but, rather, that they were given insufficient information on which to make an informed and meaningful decision as to whether or not to agree. The patient may, then, feel that he or she is entitled to compensation because the doctor has assumed an unwarranted authority over his or her body.

It is now clear, at least in the United Kingdom, that the patient whose complaint relates to the extent and quality of information disclosure cannot seek compensation using the law of assault or battery, but must raise an action in negligence. As will be seen in Chapter 6, this has very real consequences for the patient's chance of a successful outcome. When an action is raised in assault/battery, it is only necessary to show that the intervention was made without consent and, as we have noted, it is technically unimportant whether or not any harm actually occurred for the action to succeed. In contrast, when an action is raised in negligence, the patient has to show that the doctor breached a duty of care which was owed to the patient and that harm occurred to the patient as a direct consequence of this. Thus, when an invasion of bodily privacy results from an alleged failure to provide enough information, the aggrieved patient has not only to show that the consent that they apparently gave was not based on sufficient information. They must also show that, had the allegedly missing information been provided, they would not have accepted the treatment and would, thus, have avoided the harm of which they complain.

There are a number of questions which the courts will have to address and reach a conclusion on when considering such a complaint. For the sake of clarity, these will be discussed in turn although, inevitably, there are overlaps.

How much information should have been disclosed?

It is self-evident that this question is absolutely critical to the decision. It is equally obvious, however, that it is very difficult to answer. Unless we opt for an extreme position – for example, either that *all* information should be disclosed or that *none* should – some kind of balance will require to be struck between the expectations of patients and the practices of doctors. The House of Lords considered this matter in some depth in an important case brought by a Mrs Sidaway. While each of their Lordships reached their decision in slightly different ways, some general conclusions can be drawn from the case.

Although at least one judge suggested that there might be some risks which it is self-evident should be disclosed, the general agreement of their Lordships was that disclosure of information was broadly covered by the test routinely applied in other cases involving medical negligence – that is, the so-called *Bolam* test. This holds that a doctor will not be negligent if he or she acts in accordance with a practice that is held to be reasonable by a responsible body of medical opinion. The test and its implications will be considered in more depth in the next chapter but, for present purposes, its importance lies in the extent of the defence that it makes available to an accused doctor. In short, it will generally be sufficient to satisfy the court that the non-disclosure was not negligent, and the patient's case will fail, if the doctor is able to find a 'responsible body of medical opinion' which would support the decision to withhold the information in question.

Thus, in a very real sense, the answer to the question: 'how much information should have been disclosed?' can be reached by evaluating what other doctors would have disclosed. It must also be remembered that, in terms of the *Bolam* test, it matters not that there is another school of medical thought which would have disclosed the information; the defence is satisfied so long as one responsible body of opinion agrees with the doctor concerned. Of course, as we have seen, it might well be thought that disclosure should be mandatory in some situations, no matter what other doctors say (the example used in Mrs Sidaway's case was if there was a 10% risk of, say, a stroke resulting from the operation). Certainly, as was later emphasised in the case of *Bolitho v City and Hackney Health Authority*, the courts reserve to themselves the right to decide that even a responsible body of medical opinion is wrong, although they seldom exercise this prerogative. Equally, however, they have also indicated that a risk of less than 1%, which was the risk in fact run by Mrs Sidaway, would not fall into the category of one which *must* be disclosed.

Patients may feel less than satisfied with this. Indeed, they might well argue that, if their autonomy is truly to be valued, it is for them, not the doctors or even the courts, to decide what information would affect their decision; medical choices are personal to the patient and they will be affected by matters which are non-clinical. For example, one might be prepared to take the risk of sickness following treatment in some situations but not if one hoped to attend one's son's wedding the next day. In other words, patients might reasonably feel that their personal circumstances are critical to the evaluation of what it was and was not proper to disclose in the circumstances.

What test is to be applied?

This leads directly to the second issue on which courts have to pronounce. The real issue for aggrieved patients is whether or not they, personally, would have wanted to receive information and to use it to come to a conclusion. This information may not, as we have suggested, relate only to the statistical probability of a risk arising but may be of concern to that particular patient only. However, as again we have already seen, this particular issue can only be addressed if *all* the available information is disclosed – and this may be neither feasible nor, in fact, beneficial. Thus, the courts have been reluctant to demand full disclosure based on what would in law be referred to as a subjective – or individual – patient test.

Rather, different positions have been adopted in different jurisdictions. In some of the States in the United States and, more recently, in Australia, the courts have moved away from the *Bolam* test and have chosen, rather, to ask the question: 'What would the prudent patient have wanted to know?' Broadly, this test would have us ask not what the individual patient concerned in the case would have wanted to know, but rather what a reasonable patient might have expected to be told in similar circumstances. The test is, therefore, still distanced from the person raising the action but, at the same time, it does attempt to place patients' rights at the forefront of the debate. However, it should also be noted that even the prudent patient standard allows for non-disclosure of certain information, based on what is known as therapeutic privilege. This allows doctors to withhold information which they believe might be harmful to the patient – echoing one of the arguments we outlined above.

Nonetheless, the United Kingdom courts have continued to endorse the principles of *Bolam* by adopting what has been called a prudent doctor or professional standard.

Many would say that this approach pays scant attention to the claims of individual, or even prudent, patients and serves merely to hand over to doctors the authority to decide what information should be disclosed, subject only to the constraint that the decision must be accepted as reasonable by 'a responsible body of medical opinion' and, ultimately, by the courts. Since doctors, like all professionals, are likely to be reluctant to criticise their colleagues – and in light of a residual adherence to the arguments attempting to justify non-disclosure that have been outlined above – it is likely that the patient will have a very difficult task in convincing a court that an alleged failure to disclose information was, in fact, negligent. Indeed, although it was hoped by some commentators that the decision in *Bolitho v City and Hackney Health Authority* - effectively, that the medical opinion relied on must also be capable of withstanding logical analysis – would dilute the power of the *Bolam* judgement, little evidence has as yet emerged to support that expectation.

Even so, doctors should be aware of a 'wind of change' that is beginning to blow. In *Lybert v Warrington Health Authority*, for example, the Court of Appeal held that, while it was possible that a warning – in respect of sterilisation – had been given, there was evidence that 'a sufficiently clear and comprehensible warning was never given', thus emphasising the importance of *understanding* as well as information. But, perhaps the strongest indication comes from the most senior judge at the time, Lord Woolf, in *Pearce v United Bristol Healthcare NHS Trust* who said:

> ... if there is a significant risk which would affect the judgement of a reasonable patient, then it is ... the responsibility of the doctor to inform the patient of that risk, if the information is needed so that the patient can determine for him or herself as to what course he or she would adopt.

Here, there is at least an inkling that the courts may consider the position of the prudent patient to be overtaking that of the prudent doctor – *Pearce* can, perhaps, best be seen as an amber rather than a red light.

Proving harm

Patients who allege that the information on which they based their decision to undergo treatment was inadequate clearly have a hard task in seeking to satisfy the courts that this was so. However, assuming that they get this far, they must still prove that it was the failure to give that information that caused the harm of which they are complaining. This is known in law as the element of causation.

Essentially, as we have seen, the complainer has to show that he or she would not have agreed to the treatment if the missing information had been passed on. This runs into the practical difficulty that people who have been harmed as a result of treatment are, inherently, likely to believe and say that they would not have accepted that particular risk if they had known about it and the courts are reluctant to proceed on the basis of what could be seen as hindsight. Thus, *proving* that this is the case is likely to be very difficult. Here again, courts have chosen to address this question in terms of what they believe the average or 'prudent' patient would have done. This entails weighing up the benefits of accepting the treatment and the risks inherent in it. However, such an exercise is clearly not necessarily the same as an evaluation of what the *actual* patient might or might not have wanted or, in fact, would or might have done. This is of major practical importance, in that it is always open to the defender to suggest that the patient would have gone ahead anyway even if given full information. One unfortunate result is that the outcome of this plea ultimately rests upon whether the patient is a good or a bad witness, insofar as only he or she *knows* the answer – and the evidence cannot be reheard in the Court of Appeal if the opportunity is lost in the trial court.

None of this should be taken as suggesting that it is impossible to succeed in such cases. However, it is obviously not easy to do so, and this will remain the case for so long as the courts in the United Kingdom adhere essentially to the *Bolam* test – a test that, as we have seen, has been abandoned in other parts of the Commonwealth, particularly in Australia, as being applicable in cases based on inadequate information disclosure.

CHILDREN AND YOUNG PERSONS

Generally speaking, the capacity to make decisions or to consent to medical treatment in a child is governed by common sense or common law – it is relatively obvious that someone must speak for a child, say, below primary school age and that the someone should be the person with parental responsibility. The law will uphold this principle in virtually every case subject to certain constraints. One of these, as we have seen, is that the parents cannot demand treatment which the doctor is unwilling to provide on the basis of a reasonable clinical opinion. The case of *Re C (a minor)* (1997), which involved Jewish parents requesting continued intensive care for their child who was suffering from spinal muscular atrophy, is in point; the court agreed with the doctors in considering further ventilatory treatment to be futile and not in C's best interests. This issue is considered in more depth in Chapter 6.

The mature minor

Rules become blurred, however, when we reach the limits of their application. Quite clearly, a child's actual capacity to make significant choices varies throughout childhood and does not perform a dramatic U-turn on his or her eighteenth birthday in England or sixteenth in Scotland. As a result, medical law, at least, has adopted the trans-Atlantic concept of the 'mature minor' and has done this through both statute and common law. The legal status of such children for present purposes differs in England and Wales and in Scotland and the two situations need to be dealt with separately.

England and Wales

The first indication of such differences is be found in the Family Law Reform Act 1969, section 8 of which says:

> The consent of a minor who has attained the age of 16 years to any medical treatment which, in the absence of consent, would constitute a trespass to the person, shall be as effective as it would be if he were of full age

and it then goes on to say that, once that is given, the consent of a parent or guardian need not be obtained. While this is clear enough, it still leaves an artificial cut-off point in respect of capacity – might not the 15-year-old be mentally capable of making his or her own health decisions?

This issue was addressed and settled in 1985, when the House of Lords concluded the case brought by Mrs Victoria Gillick, who sought to challenge the right of the Health Authority to disseminate information about the availability of contraceptive advice for girls under 16 years of age. The circular that had been issued indicated that, although an attempt should be made to obtain parental consent, doctors could, if this failed, nonetheless prescribe contraception for such minors. Mrs Gillick challenged this both in respect of her own children and also on a general basis, claiming that parental rights to decide what was in the best interests of their children were being eroded.

As we have seen in Chapter 3, the House of Lords ultimately rejected Mrs Gillick's argument – a decision that has come to be applied across the whole spectrum of minority decision making. The essence of the House of Lords decision was given by Lord Scarman who said that the parental right to control children's actions diminishes as the child's understanding increases and:

> terminates if and when the child achieves a significant understanding and intelligence to enable him or her to understand fully what is proposed.

In short, for the American 'mature minor' we can read in England 'the *Gillick*-competent minor'.

The difficulty as to understanding, however, lies in the definition of 'significant'. We can see that, in fact, there is no definition and that, both in England and Wales and in Scotland, the child's capacity to make independent decisions must be determined by the individual medical practitioner – in other words, what should be an objective standard is being set by subjective opinion to which either the child or his or her parents may object.

Scotland

The law has developed differently in Scotland. Traditionally – and well before the *Gillick* case was heard – Scots law recognised various levels of maturity accruing to children. Thus, at 12 (for girls) and 14 (for boys), children moved from the status of pupil to that of minor. This had significant, albeit ill-defined, consequences as to their legal capacity to enter into agreements. In 1991, however, the Age of Legal Capacity (Scotland) Act was passed in order to clarify the legal position of children. The legislation abolished the status of pupil and settled on 16 as the age at which young people were considered to be fully capable of attending to their own affairs. At the same time, the Act specifically introduced an exception to the rule, giving children *under* the age of 16 the right to agree to medical and surgical procedures – the requirement being that they can understand the nature and consequences of what they were doing.

THE INCOMPETENT ADULT

An adult person may be incompetent – or lack capacity – to make decisions as to accepting or refusing treatment by way of mental disorder or because of unconsciousness. Incapacity due to mental disorder in the adult is governed to a large extent by statute law. Accordingly, the relevant discussion is best left to Chapter 15. We are left, then, with consideration of the unconscious adult and, although the ethics of the management of such a person are by no means limited to those of information disclosure, this is not an inappropriate place in which to look briefly at those who are unable, for this reason, to make treatment decisions of any sort. The important issue is that someone will have to make a choice for them should the relevant situation arise.

This is a surprisingly complex subject. Legally speaking – and, perhaps, contrary to popular belief – the next of kin have no decision-making powers, although their opinion will, of course, be valuable in reaching a conclusion. Similarly, the courts in England and Wales (although not in Scotland) have no mandate to *consent* on behalf of an adult – though they can declare that providing treatment would not be unlawful, which comes to much the same thing. As we will see in Chapter 15, treatment of the incompetent patient in the *absence* of consent is authorised by statute only in respect of conditions associated with the mental condition that leads to incompetence. Surgeons who want to perform an operation on an adult who is incompetent from *any* cause are, therefore, in a cleft stick. They can go to the court for assurance that their action would not be unlawful – but this is a complex and expensive route to take, and one which would be adopted only in cases of special ethical significance where the medical profession was unsure of its ground. Alternatively, the individual doctor can shield behind the legal doctrine of 'necessity' which says, in essence, that, in well defined circumstances, one can do something that would otherwise be unlawful provided that the lawful benefits of so doing outweigh the consequences of the unlawful act itself. The benefits will be judged in terms of the patient's best interests. The doctor so acting is, in a way, second guessing the reaction of the law, but experience indicates that he or she will be supported if these conditions are met. Indeed, in a very famous case known as *Re F*, the House of Lords implied that the doctor might well have a *duty* to grasp the nettle. The opinion in a case known as *Re S* (heard in 2000) has, however, sounded a word of caution, suggesting that the courts are becoming less inclined to accept medical opinion as to such a patient's best interests at face value. The current thinking is that, whereas doctors may decide that a treatment is in the patient's best *medical* interests, it is for the court to decide whether it is in the patient's *overall* best interests.

Some qualification must also be made in respect of the adult who is only temporarily incapacitated. Clearly, it would be nonsense to suggest that treatment in such cases would *have* to be authorised by a court – amongst other things, it would probably take far too long in the conditions envisaged here. Once again, however, the doctrine of necessity comes to the rescue of doctor and patient alike. On the application of this doctrine, doctors can proceed to provide treatment which is urgent and necessary in the best interests of their patients. However, given that the patient is likely to recover capacity, the doctrine cannot be extended to include non-urgent treatment. The normal rules as to consent would then apply; the surgeon who was not prepared to await recovery could well be found guilty of assault – and, in passing, the same might apply to additional non-urgent surgery for a condition that was discovered for the first time when the patient was already under an anaesthetic.

CONCLUSION

The provision of information is a critical aspect of good medical care. It allows individuals to make decisions for themselves, decisions which may be informed by personal as well as medical considerations. No doctor, however well-meaning, can or should presume to know their patients so well that he or she can make decisions on their behalf without previous consultation and discussion – and few, if any, would do so nowadays.

However, the delicate problem of how much information should be and is given remains. On the one hand, it can be argued that only full disclosure of all aspects of treatment can be compatible with the notion of personal autonomy. On the other, we have seen that the UK courts have held to the *Bolam* principle – and continue to do so – with some tenacity. The result is that the law distances decision-making from the individual by requiring that, with a few exceptions, only that information which is deemed appropriate by the medical profession need be disclosed – and, consequently, often denies patients compensation when they feel aggrieved. As we have already mentioned, good arguments can be raised – and have been in the courts of Canada and Australia – to the effect that the *Bolam* test, which originated as a test of *technical* competence, has little or no place in the provision of information which is central to decision making on the patient's part. And there is, indeed, some evidence that the more recently appointed judges are moving towards that position.

Meantime, we must live with the law as it now stands, and this is well expressed in the summary given by Lord Templeman in Mrs Sidaway's case:

> Where the patient's health and future are at stake, the patient must make the final decision. The patient is free to decide whether or not to submit to treatment recommended by the doctor and therefore the doctor impliedly contracts to provide information which is adequate to enable the patient to make a balanced judgement.

The doctor who falls short of that standard is acting negligently.

CASES REFERRED TO IN THE TEXT

Bolam v Friern Hospital Management Committee [1957] 2 All ER 118.

Bolitho v City and Hackney Health Authority [1997] 4 All ER 771.

C (a minor: medical treatment), Re [1998] 1 FLR 384.

F, Re [1990] 2 AC 1.

Gillick v West Norfolk and Wisbech Area Health Authority [1985] 3 All ER 402.

Lybert v Warrington Health Authority (1995) 25 BMLR 91.

Pearce v United Bristol Healthcare NHS Trust (1999) 48 BMLR 118.

S (Adult patient: Sterilisation), In re [2000] 2 FCR 452.

Schloendorff v Society of New York Hospital (NY, 1914) 105 NE 92.

Sidaway v Board of Governors of the Bethlem Royal Hospital [1985] 1 All ER 643.

FURTHER READING

Brazier M. 'Patient autonomy and consent to treatment: The role of the law', *Legal Studies* 1987; 169.

Buchanan A. 'Medical paternalism', *Philosophy and Public Affairs* 1979; 7: 49.

Chalmers D, Schwartz R. '*Rogers v Whittaker* and informed consent in Australia: A fair dinkum duty of disclosure', *Medical Law Review* 1993; 1: 139.

Jones MA. 'Informed consent and other fairy stories', *Medical Law Review* 1999; 7: 103.

McLean SAM. *A Patient's Right to Know*, Aldershot, Dartmouth, 1989.

Stauch M. 'Rationality and the refusal of medical treatment: A critique of the recent approach of the English courts', *Journal of Medical Ethics* 1995; 21: 162.

5

REFUSAL OF CONSENT

It might seem surprising that our consideration of consent to treatment did not directly tackle the question of refusal of consent. After all, it might be said, these are merely opposite sides of the same coin. In many ways this is true, but – as will be seen – there are both ethical and legal complexities in respect of refusal of treatment that justify its separate consideration. In some cases, the consequences of failing to accept treatment may be no more than mildly disturbing. In many such cases, the patient's health will recover, albeit, perhaps, more slowly. In others, however, refusal of treatment may amount to a life-threatening decision which tests the doctor's dual commitments, on the one hand, to respect the autonomy of the patient and, on the other, to maximising his or her health.

The law on this subject appears to be clear, at least where the individual patient has the necessary legal capacity – a question that is discussed briefly below and in more detail in Chapter 15. A sane, adult patient can refuse even life-saving treatment on grounds that are rational, irrational or unknown. In other words, the *reason* for the decision is not open for scrutiny or debate; put simply, a competent decision once made must be respected. If, indeed, the law is so clear, then why does it require consideration? Thirty years ago, the court in the case of *S v McC: W v W*, cautioned that:

> English law goes to great lengths to protect a person of full age and capacity from inter-ference with his personal liberty. We have too often seen freedom disappear in other countries not only by coups d'état but by gradual erosion: and often it is the first step that counts. So, it would be unwise to make even minor concessions.

It might be thought, then, that the law would seldom be involved in such matters. Both historically and in the present, however, issues arise which need to be addressed, as even the most apparently straightforward statement of the law has, on occasion, proved itself to be neither uncontroversial nor always approved. Equally, one might imagine that very few people would wish to make such extreme decisions, but as we will see, particularly in Chapter 12, this assumption can be shown to be false. There are a number of situations in which individuals may wish to reject treatment, and the legal status of these choices will be considered below. For ease and clarity we have chosen to separate the kinds of decision into a number of different categories.

REFUSAL BASED ON PRINCIPLE

For some people, rejection of medical treatment is based on a principle, often derived from their religious faith. It might be anticipated that decisions based on faith would routinely be respected, not least because the European Convention on Human Rights (now incorporated into UK law by the Human Rights Act 1998) guarantees the right to freedom of religious expression, including presumably the right to live according to the tenets of one's faith, as well as guaranteeing respect for private and family life. There is little by way of hard authority on this subject in the case of adults – the situation in respect of children will be discussed below. The major case in this area, that of *Re T*, is, however, worthy of consideration.

In this case, Ms T had expressed her objection to receiving a blood transfusion which, should it become necessary, would be life-preserving. Her refusal followed a discussion with her mother who was a practising Jehovah's Witness, although Ms T, herself, was not practising that faith at the time. In the event, the Court refused to accept the validity of her decision, because it was felt that it had been reached as a result of pressure from her mother. At the same time, however, the court indicated in the strongest terms that a competent adult can legitimately refuse even life-saving treatment and the words of Lord Donaldson merit repetition:

> An adult patient who suffers from no mental incapacity has an absolute right to choose whether to consent to medical treatment, to refuse it or to choose one rather than another of the treatments being offered.

And again:

> It exists notwithstanding that the reasons for making the choice are rational, irrational, unknown or even non-existent.

What the outcome would have been had Ms T simply continued to object on the basis of religion alone can be surmised from this. Although this case was heard before the Human Rights Act came into force, presumably the guarantee of freedom of religion in that Act would, to-day, reinforce the law's commitment to respect for autonomy. However, it is clear from other judicial comments in *Re T*, and from later cases, that the law will not entirely absolve religion from the suspicion of coercion. The decision is additionally interesting in that it leaves clinicians with the difficult task of assessing whether or not any influence apparently exerted by a third party is sufficient to negate the person's capacity for autonomous behaviour; an extremely difficult decision to make.

The circumstances in *Centre for Reproductive Medicine v U* (2002), which is about consent to a procedure rather than to treatment, illustrate the dilemma vividly. Here, a woman wished to be inseminated with the sperm of her dead husband. The clinic clearly had moral objections to the procedure and maintained that the man had withdrawn his consent before he died. The question arose as to whether he had been subjected to undue pressure to do so. The court agonised at length over the distinction between advice and coercion and, eventually, concluded, 'with regret', that the pressure was such as an adult should have been capable of resisting had he so wanted.

In a different, but rather similar situation, a Canadian court upheld the validity of an advance directive by a Jehovah's Witness refusing life-saving blood transfusion. The doctor who ignored the terms of the directive was successfully sued by the woman concerned, even although her life had been saved by the unauthorised transfusion.

REFUSAL ON PERSONAL GROUNDS

Refusal of treatment also encompasses situations where it appears that the individual simply wishes to discontinue treatment, usually because they find their physical or mental condition intolerable. Interestingly, many religious groups would have considerable difficulty in supporting such a decision, even in the face of a distressingly poor quality of life, on the basis that life and death decisions are for God alone to make. Nonetheless, some unfortunate people may find themselves the victims, for example, of neurological disorders, which leave them alive but unable to do anything for themselves. Several of these cases are discussed in rather more detail in Chapter 12; for the present, we can note that, for many of them, the choice to refuse any further treatment may seem the logical and, indeed, the right option.

In the 1992 Canadian case of *Nancy B v Hôtel-Dieu de Québec*, a young woman suffering from the Guillain-Barré syndrome sought removal of the respirator which was keeping her alive. The court in this case was able to use her refusal of consent to the continuation of treatment as authority to remove the ventilation, as the general rule, discussed above in relation to the United Kingdom, that involuntary treatment is not lawful applies throughout the Western world. Although it was quite clear that her intention was to die, the court specifically declared that those closing down the respirator would not be guilty of murder or of assisting suicide – an issue that is, again, considered in more depth in Chapter 12.

The specific issue of refusal of life saving treatment came to public attention in the United Kingdom in the recent case of *Ms B v An NHS Hospital Trust*. This case was raised by a woman who had ultimately become ventilator-dependent having sustained a haemorrhage in her spinal column in 1999. As a further bleed was possible, Ms B executed an advance directive (for which, see below) at that time, stating the circumstances in which treatment would be unacceptable. She was readmitted to hospital in 2001; her condition had deteriorated to the point at which she was tetraplegic and entirely dependent on a ventilator. Staff were aware of the advance directive but decided that it was not sufficiently specific to apply to the circumstances in which Ms B found herself. Psychiatric advice was also sought, and although medical opinion varied, ultimately she was assessed as being competent to make decisions about her present and future healthcare.

Ms B remained steadfast in her clearly expressed wish to have the ventilator removed in order that she might end her life on her own terms. Her doctors were equally intransigent in their refusal to respect her wishes. Court involvement therefore became inevitable. In the event, Dame Elizabeth Butler-Sloss decided that Ms B did indeed have the competence to make such a decision. It followed, therefore, that in continuing to ventilate Ms B, her doctors were effectively committing an assault, and Ms B was awarded a nominal sum of damages to take account of this. Although it was clear that Ms B's doctors had found this an extremely distressing situation, they – and therefore all other doctors – were forcefully reminded by the court of the right of individuals to make such choices. Indeed, it was emphasised that, even in the face of severe physical disability, a person 'who is mentally competent has the same right to personal autonomy and to make decisions as any other person with mental capacity.' Moreover, the court reminded us that competence is assumed; it is its absence and not its presence that needs to be proved.

REFUSAL IN THE COURSE OF PREGNANCY

While the two situations outlined above will be comprehensible to many – even if not uncontroversial – this category of refusal will be the most difficult to come to terms with. Although the embryo or foetus has no legal standing, and therefore no legal rights, most people would regard it as being worthy of some form of respect and protection. Thus, while it is incorrect in law to talk of the foetus as having a right to life, it would normally be presumed that a pregnant woman would do everything in her power to ensure that her foetus has the best possible chance of life – indeed, the best possible chance of life of as good a quality as is possible. However, it is not always the case that pregnant women are prepared to undergo interventions themselves or undertake lifestyle changes in order to protect the foetus, and courts have struggled with this issue in the past.

The first case to bring this matter to public attention in the UK was that of *Re S* (1992). In this case, Ms S refused to agree to a caesarean section, even although it was clear that both she and the foetus risked death without it. She cited religious objections to the surgery as her reason for refusal. A court was hastily convened, and after less than 30 minutes, the Judge – impressed by the medical evidence as to the threat to pregnant woman and foetus – authorised the surgery to go ahead. It must be said that the reported judgement is, perhaps necessarily, extremely brief and cites in its support only one case: the US case of *Re AC*.

Unusually, the judge appears to have failed to note that this American decision had already been reversed on appeal. Its value as precedent then, was effectively nil. Briefly, the case involved a young woman, Angela Carder, who was terminally ill and pregnant. At about 26½ weeks into the pregnancy it was felt that her death was imminent. Her treating physicians, however, believed that it might be possible to save the foetus and proposed to carry out a caesarean section. Mrs Carder (and interestingly her husband and parents) was unwilling to accept a caesarean, but despite her protests the court authorised it to go ahead; the surgery was carried out. Neither Mrs Carder nor the child survived. As we have indicated, this decision was eventually reversed on appeal – too late for Mrs Carder. This was not the only US case in which women were forced into non-consensual surgery, but it probably represents the most acute example. Nor was *Re S* to be the only case to reach UK courts. Subsequent cases have also addressed this question, and these will be briefly discussed in what follows.

In *Tameside and Glossop Acute Health Services Trust v CH*, a schizophrenic patient was held to be incapable of understanding that, without intervention, the foetus (which she wanted to survive) would die. In *Norfolk and Norwich Healthcare (NHS) Trust v W*, a woman who presented at hospital in labour, but denying the fact of her pregnancy, was also deemed to be incompetent despite the fact that a psychiatrist gave advice that she was not suffering from a mental illness. It has been pointed out that the decision in *Tameside* was particularly strange, given that it was held that: 'the performance of a caesarean section on a schizophrenic woman could be 'treatment' of her mental disorder within the terms of the Mental Health Act 1983' (the implications of such treatment are discussed in Chapter 15).

Each of these cases demonstrates the – perhaps self-generated – dilemmas in which the early courts found themselves. Clearly they were considering the moral status of the foetus but, in so doing, were underestimating its lack of legal standing, and paying insufficient attention to the legal standing and rights of the woman. The cases also reveal a tendency to see refusal of life-saving treatment as being evidence of incompetence *per se*, even when the treatment was not life-preserving for the woman. However, we will see in Chapter 15 that, even were such a refusal to amount to a form of legal incompetence, it would not, of itself, justify overriding the expressed wishes of the person concerned.

Other cases, however, followed *Re S* and have clarified the legal approach. One of the most significant of these was the case of *Re MB*. In this case, the court laid down guidelines which make it clear that pregnant women have the same rights as any other person. The guidelines are, therefore, worth restating here:

1. Every person is presumed to have the competence to consent to or to refuse medical treatment unless and until that presumption is rebutted.
2. A competent woman who has the capacity to decide may for religious reasons, other reasons, for rational or irrational reasons or for no reason at all, choose not to have medical intervention, even although the consequences may be the death or serious handicap of the child she bears, or her own death. In that event the courts do not have the jurisdiction to declare medical intervention lawful and the question of her own best interests objectively considered, do not arise.
3. Irrationality is here used to connote a decision which is so outrageous in its defiance of logic or of accepted moral standards that no sensible person who has applied his mind to the question to be decided could have arrived at it.

Thus, it would seem at first sight that pregnant women were given absolute rights to decide for themselves whether or not to accept treatment or other interventions, irrespective of the impact these decisions might have on themselves or the foetus they were carrying. To that extent, therefore, the judgement was welcomed as a clarification of what was becoming doubtful law. However, the court also indicated that these guidelines might not apply in all cases and that 'the decision must inevitably depend on the particular facts before the court.' It is not clear in what circumstances this caveat might apply, but the fact that it exists presumably means that it was envisaged that it could, in certain circumstances, be used.

Following the decision in *Re MB* came the case of *St George's Healthcare N.H.S. Trust v S*. In this case, S strenuously objected to a caesarean section, and it seemed that she understood the consequences of this refusal of treatment. Thus, S was legally competent to make this decision. However, rather than respecting that choice, S was compulsorily admitted to hospital for assessment under the mental health legislation and the surgery proceeded. On appeal, it was held that the use of mental health legislation in this situation was inappropriate and that in any event, even if a person is detained under this legislation, it cannot simply be assumed that he or she is legally incompetent. This effectively restates the logic of the case of *Re C*, discussed in Chapter 15, in which a man suffering from paranoid schizophrenia was nonetheless deemed competent to make healthcare decisions; even, in fact, a decision which was life-threatening. However, the existence of the caveat in *Re MB* remains a potential source of conflict, and it will be of interest to see what impact, if any, the Human Rights Act 1998 will have in this area.

REFUSAL OF FOOD

It is open to argument whether refusal of food constitutes refusal of medical treatment – much depends on the circumstances. Feeding the tetraplegic who cannot do so him or herself can certainly be so described, and this was confirmed in the case of *Airedale NHS Trust v Bland* which is mentioned at several points in this book. Assuming the patient was declared competent to decide, but was unable to eat without medical assistance, refusal of further alimentation would, then, be subsumed under the general prerogative of competent adults to make their own choices. Such cases must be very rare but they have occurred and the principle has been upheld – at least in the courts of the United States.

We are more concerned with the physically capable person who refuses to eat. The ethical dilemma in such cases then assumes a new dimension – should that person's life be saved by forced feeding? Again, the conditions in which such a step may be taken are not uniform. On the one hand, we have the scenario of the 'hunger strike' where the decision to self-starve is, essentially, a form of protest, sometimes on personal grounds and sometimes with a political motive. On the other, we have self-starvation as an integral part of the psychotic condition of anorexia nervosa.

Hunger strikes

Insofar as this is a problem confined to the prison doctor, we will not deal with it in detail. It does, however, raise some interesting ethical problems. How, for example, is the balance to be set between respect for the individual's choice and the statutory duty of the prison authorities to preserve the health of the inmates? Is it logical to distinguish one's reaction to suicide by refusal of food from, say, suicide by hanging? Is it right to medicalise the problem when the success or failure of a hunger strike may have profound political repercussions?

The arguments have continued since the days of the suffragettes but now seem settled by the case of *Secretary of State for the Home Department v Robb* heard in 1995. Here, it was established that an individual's right to self-determination outweighed any countervailing interests of the state and that it was lawful to withhold nutrition and hydration should the prisoner so wish. The judgement was at first instance and was permissive, in that it did not prohibit the authorities from giving food by force if they thought it right to do so. It is also interesting that, in reaching his conclusion, the judge applied the principles of medical law despite the fact that the prisoner was of sound mind and understanding.

In fact, the courts will not be slow to grasp the medical straw when the opportunity arises. In 1999, the notorious murderer, Ian Brady, went on hunger strike in protest at the possibility of being removed to an ordinary prison. Brady was, at the time, held in a special hospital under the Mental Health Act 1983 with a diagnosis of psychopathic disorder, and the responsible medical officer instituted forced feeding. Brady applied for judicial review of that decision. Put very briefly, the judge hearing the case concluded that going on hunger strike was a manifestation of Brady's personality disorder which was such as to incapacitate him in relation to all of his decisions about food refusal and forced feeding. Accordingly, the decision to force feed was not unreasonable and was lawful. Considering the difficulties involved in the treatment of personality disorder which we discuss in Chapter 15, this conclusion might be seen as embodying an element of opportunism. The underlying sentiment can be assessed from the judge's words:

> It would be a matter of deep regret if the law had developed to a point in this area where the rights of a patient counted for everything and other ethical values and institutional integrity counted for nothing.

One wonders, again, what will be the effect of the Human Rights Act in such cases. Current evidence suggests that it will be increasingly hard to justify what are, irrespective of good intentions, violations of a person's bodily integrity.

Anorexia nervosa

Here we are on more solid medical ground. Yet, even so, the problems remain — how can we justify using force to treat a person who resists and who is not, apparently, incapacitated from making his or her own treatment decisions?

Possibly the most significant case in point has been that known as *Re W (a minor) (medical treatment)* (1992) — significant because the person involved was aged 16. The case, therefore, tested the English Family Law Reform Act, section 8 of which gives authority for such a minor to consent to treatment but, at the same time, fails to deal adequately with a minor's refusal of treatment or with any residual parental powers in such a situation (this is discussed further below). W suffered from anorexia nervosa; she refused all treatments and her health was deteriorating rapidly. In authorising treatment in a special unit, the court adopted a similar form of circular argument to that we have just noted. In essence, it was held that the disease was capable of destroying the ability to make an informed choice; as a result, the wishes of the minor constituted something which, of itself, required treatment. In addition, the court made it clear that, faced with such a clash of wills, it had full powers to make a special order; and this despite the provisions of the Children Act of 1989 which give a mature minor the right to refuse psychiatric or medical treatment in defined circumstances. Even more significantly, the court held:

> No minor of whatever age has power by refusing consent to treatment to override a consent to treatment by someone who has parental responsibility for the minor and a fortiori consent by the court.

This may be seen as muddying the waters, but it has been followed in other cases involving minors – indeed, in the 1997 case *Re C (detention: medical treatment)*, authorised the forcible detention of a 16-year old on the grounds that, if it was in her best interests to be treated, it was in her best interests to be detained so that the treatment could be given.

Similar attitudes have prevailed in adults where the problems associated with compulsory treatment of *physical* conditions under the Mental Health Acts – discussed in greater detail in Chapter 15 – have been highlighted. In short, is loss of weight a physical condition which lies outside the Act or is it classifiable as part of the mental disorder and, therefore, treatable without consent? In *Re KB* (1994) the judge argued that anorexia nervosa is an eating disorder and that relieving symptoms was just as much a part of treatment as was treating the underlying cause. It was clear, he thought, that forced feeding lay within the ambit of lawful compulsion in the circumstances of the case.

Finally, we should mention the case of *B v Croydon District Health Authority* (1995) which concerned a woman who had a compulsion to self-harm – and this included denying herself something that she enjoyed; namely, eating. The problem of the lawfulness of force feeding a psychopath was, again, raised. The case is particularly interesting in that it went to appeal. Again, the Court of Appeal supported the trial judge on much the same grounds, in holding that treatments designed to alleviate the consequences of the disorder can be seen as being ancillary to treatments calculated to alleviate an underlying psychopathic disorder. There was no conceptual vagueness about treating the symptoms or consequences of mental disorder as if they were treatments of mental disorder itself.

There is no doubt that, as we have intimated, some of these decisions may be seen as being sophistic. Alternatively, they could be regarded as representing the most sensible solutions. At the very least, they demonstrate the anxiety of the judiciary to save lives when that is possible and, when in doubt as to the competence of the decision-maker, to err on the side of taking what most people would see as the 'right' decision. But, as we have said, the influence of the Human Rights Act in this area has yet to be tested fully.

CHILDREN AND REFUSAL OF TREATMENT

Although the situation of the very young child seems clear – namely that parents have the right to make decisions on their behalf – this is not uncontroversial when the decision is to refuse rather than accept recommended treatment. The situation appears to be that parents cannot refuse treatment for a child if that refusal is regarded as unreasonable. Reasonableness is generally brought into question when there is a conflict between the doctor and the parent and such cases are frequently brought to the courts for adjudication. Perhaps the majority relate to refusal of blood transfusion on religious grounds, the courts' attitude to which can be summed up in the well known words of an American judge in 1952:

> Parents may be free to become martyrs themselves. But it does not follow that they are free, in identical circumstances, to make martyrs of their children before they have reached the age of full and legal discretion.

We know of no British case in which the courts have refused transfusion for a child and, indeed, we know of only one case where life saving treatment was refused at the request of the parents against medical advice. This case, known as *Re T (a minor)* (1997), was not based on religious belief and, admittedly, involved the very serious therapy of a liver transplant. Clearly the case had very special features, including the fact that the parents were described as 'health professionals'; nevertheless, we must regard it as a remarkable exception to the general rule.

Equally, the decision in the case of *Gillick v West Norfolk and Wisbech Area Health Authority* seemed to clarify the position for the mature child. As we have indicated in Chapter 4, a number of cases have arisen which indicate that the position is not quite so clear as might appear at first sight. A more subtle interpretation has begun to emerge, in England at least, which suggests that the children's 'rights' in this respect are limited. Indeed, as the law differs between Scotland and England and Wales they will be dealt with separately.

England and Wales

Although the *Gillick* case indicates that mature young people can accept medical treatment – that is that they are treated as autonomous – a series of judgements has shown that they may not necessarily be able to refuse it. When such a refusal occurs, parents or the courts may override it in what they see as the 'best interests' of the young person – although the doctors are, of course, not bound to provide the treatment and, in such circumstances, will consider the views of the mature child very seriously. At the end of the day, the persuasive conditions will be found in the balance between, on the one hand, the young person's ability to understand and, on the other, the significance of the decision.

Thus, the courts have been particularly reluctant to allow an apparently '*Gillick* competent' child's decision to stand when the child refuses treatment that is potentially life saving. In this way, a 15-year-old girl, R, who resisted treatment for her disturbed psychiatric state, was found to be incompetent because her mental state fluctuated widely from day to day. A refusal of blood transfusion by a similarly aged boy, E, on religious grounds was overturned on the grounds that the judge could not 'discount the possibility that he may in later years suffer some diminution in his convictions'. And, perhaps most surprisingly of all, we have M; an apparently competent girl of 15, whose refusal of a heart transplant – surely one of the hardest of antipathies to live with – was overruled on the grounds that, although she was quite clear in her intentions, she was overwhelmed by her circumstances. Interestingly, her subsequent acceptance of the therapy was deemed to be competent.

How, then, can we account for these apparently anomalous decisions? Probably the majority of people would regard consent and refusal as but different aspects of the same phenomenon. Others, while agreeing with this in general, might hold that the *degree* of understanding required to refuse professional advice is greater than that required to accept it. This is no place to continue the debate; suffice it to note that the English courts, being acutely aware of the consequences of allowing a young person to make a decision which might result in death, will generally adopt the latter view.

Scotland

We explained in the previous chapter when the child in Scotland acquires the capacity to agree to treatment both in common law and also by virtue of the Age of Legal Capacity (Scotland) Act. The Act does not specifically mention refusal of treatment but it has been inferred that the Scottish child, once deemed competent, would be authorised to refuse treatment as well as to consent to it. Although there have been no significant cases in which this was argued, this interpretation would certainly conform with the Scottish legal tradition. This conclusion also seems to be reinforced by the terms of the Children (Scotland) Act 1995, which makes it clear that – even in the case of a child under the age of 16 – the authority of parents or guardians to decide on his or her behalf subsists only for so long as the child is incapable of acting independently. It can, however, be definitely stated that, at the age of 16, the young person in Scotland is free to make whatever decision he or she chooses in respect of medical treatment. Nobody else, neither the parents nor the courts, can interfere in their choices – always assuming, of course, that they are not otherwise legally incapacitated.

MENTAL DISABILITY AND REFUSAL OF TREATMENT

We have already discussed the case of *Re C*, and it is, therefore, unnecessary to dwell on this matter. Suffice it to say that competence will be assumed to exist even in the presence of mental disorder, as in other cases concerning adults. It is for those seeking to overturn the decision of a person with a mental disability to establish that he or she is *not* competent. For a fuller discussion of competence, see Chapter 15.

ADVANCE DIRECTIVES

It is, of course, not only when treatment is imminent that patients may wish to control what happens to them. For many, an interest in determining what can and cannot be done to them also extends into the future. Thus, increasingly, individuals are recording their wishes about future treatment in documents variously referred to as 'living wills', advance directives or advance statements.[1] However, just as there is a considerable body of support for the use of advance directives, so too there are those who express considerable concern about them. Prominent amongst these commentators are John Robertson and Ronald Dworkin, both of whom argue that the person who makes the declaration or directive is not, in essence, the same as the person in respect of whom it comes into effect.

Thus, they suggest, I may – when well and competent – imagine that life would be intolerable should I suffer from a particular condition. Accordingly, I may compose a directive indicating to those caring for me that, at the time when this situation arises, and I am not longer able to express a view, I do not wish certain treatments to be given. However, when the condition actually transpires and I am legally incompetent, I may in fact be perfectly happy and, had I been able to express an opinion at that stage, it might well have differed from the one recorded in advance.

---

[1] This last terminology is that which is favoured by the British Medical Association.

For this and other reasons, some healthcare professionals are concerned about the legal position of such directives and many experience some reluctance in implementing them. Certainly, it does seem that doctors have a right to interpret advance directives so as to ensure that they are indeed applicable in the given circumstances. In the case of *Re T*, for example, Lord Donaldson put the situation as follows:

> ...what the doctors *cannot* do is to conclude that, if the patient still had the necessary capacity in the changed situation, he would have reversed his decision ... what they *can* do is to consider whether at the time the decision was made it was intended to apply in the changed situation.

Thus, the doctor is invited not to second guess the individual, but to second guess his or her intentions; either way, it is a difficult decision and one that is unlikely to be taken in a neutral manner, given that many people feel intensely about this subject. In a recent poll of 300 UK doctors, for example, although 96% accepted that a competent patient has a right to refuse treatment, only 61% were prepared to end a patient's treatment knowing that it would be fatal to do so.

Over the years, advance directives have, despite the objections to them, come to be regarded as essentially binding documents. In the case of *Airedale NHS Trust v Bland*, for example, Lords Keith and Goff both indicated that, had Anthony Bland signed an advance directive, this would have been given legal status. In 1994 a Practice Note was issued which stated that an advance directive 'will be a very important component in the decisions of the doctors and the courts.' Also, the British Medical Association has published a statement on advance directives indicating that they should be taken seriously by doctors, but stopping short of saying that they were in fact always binding.

However, two cases seem to have removed any doubt from the question of the status of advance directives. In the case of *Re C (adult: refusal of medical treatment)* a man was authorised to make what was clearly expected to be a binding decision about future healthcare should he lapse into incompetence. More recently, the case of *AK (adult patient)(medical treatment: consent)* confronted the legal standing of the advance directive head on. In this case, the patient in question was a 19-year-old man with motor neurone disease who had executed a directive requiring that all nutrition, hydration and ventilation should cease 2 weeks after he became incapable of communicating as his condition deteriorated. Although the court indicated that doctors should satisfy themselves that this still represented the patient's wish (see Lord Donaldson's remarks above) it also made it clear that an individual can indeed make such a statement and that it should be respected.

Thus far, we have spoken about advance directives in as much as they represent a refusal of treatment. Although this chapter is concerned with treatment refusal rather than consent to treatment, it would be remiss not to note that such directives may also be used to *authorise* treatment when competence is compromised. Thus, although a patient cannot compel doctors to provide treatment which is either unlawful or which offends their own consciences, patients can competently leave requests *for* treatment, which they can expect to be honoured. As one of the present authors has suggested elsewhere, the 'positive' advance directive might be a useful mechanism by which to render elective ventilation lawful (see Chapter 13 for discussion).

CONCLUSION

Although, therefore, it might at the outset seem as if respecting patients' autonomous decisions about treatment is the critical value which underpins the approach of the law to treatment decisions, this has in fact been uncontroversial only where the decision is to consent to medical treatment as recommended by doctors. When patients seek to exercise their right – now or in the future – to reject recommended therapy, they are more likely to face challenge. Yet logic suggests that respect for autonomy should ensure that it is the making of the decision rather than its content which is important. Equally, in the case of young people, the position in English law, at least, appears to require of the mature minor a level and quality of understanding of the consequences that would not be required of an adult. While this may be under-standable, it is arguably inconsistent with the rights attributable to young people when they acquire '*Gillick* competence'.

It is an article of professional faith that the 'good' medical outcome is cure or alleviation of symptoms. Understandably, doctors and other healthcare professionals see death as a failure, and it is therefore easier for them to accommodate a decision to accept therapy than it is to witness a refusal of treatment, especially when it is likely to result in deterioration of an existing condition, or even the death of their patient. Yet, a true commitment to respect for autonomy requires that such choices are also honoured. After some initial uncertainty, it appears that UK law is now firmly committed to respecting patient choice, even when it is made in advance of an illness arising or deteriorating, and even when it risks the life of the patient or a potential child, so long as the person making the choice is deemed legally competent to do so.

CASES REFERRED TO IN THE TEXT

Airedale NHS Trust v Bland [1993] 1 All ER 821.

AK (adult patient)(medical treatment: consent), Re (2001) 58 BMLR 151.

B v Croydon District Health Authority (1995) 1 All ER 683.

B (Nancy) v Hôtel-Dieu de Québec (1992) 15 BMLR 95.

C (adult: refusal of medical treatment), Re [1994] 1 All ER 819.

C (a minor) (detention for medical treatment), Re [1997] 2 FLR 180.

E (a minor), Re (1990) 9 BMLR 1.

KB (adult) (mental patient: medical treatment), Re (1994) 19 BMLR 144.

M (child: refusal of medical treatment), Re [1999] 2 FLR 1097.

Malette v Shulman [1991] 2 Med LR 162.

Practice Note [1994] 2 All ER 413.

Prince v Massachusetts (1944) 321 US 158.

R (a minor) (wardship: medical treatment), Re [1991] 4 All ER 177.

R v Collins, ex parte Brady (2000) 58 BMLR 173.

S v McC: W v W [1972] AC 25.

Secretary of State for the Home Department v Robb [1995] 1 All ER 677.

T (a minor) (wardship: medical treatment), Re [1997] 1 All ER 906.

T (adult: refusal of medical treatment), Re (1992) 9 BMLR 46.

W (a minor) (medical treatment), Re [1992] 4 All ER 627.

FURTHER READING

Annas G. 'She's going to die: The case of Angela C', *Hastings Center Report* 1988; 18(1): 23.

Draper H. 'Anorexia nervosa and respecting a refusal of life-prolonging therapy: A limited justification', *Bioethics* 2000; 14: 120.

Dworkin R. *Life's Dominion*, Harper Collins, 1993.

Elliston S. 'If you know what's good for you: Refusal of consent to medical treatment by children', in McLean SAM. (ed), *Contemporary Issues in Law, Medicine and Ethics*, Aldershot, Dartmouth, 29, 1996.

Lewis P. 'Feeding anorexic patients who refuse food', *Medical Law Review* 1999; 7: 21.

McLean SAM. 'Transplantation and the "Nearly Dead": The case of elective ventilation', in McLean SAM. (ed) *Contemporary Issues in Law, Medicine and Ethics*, Aldershot, Dartmouth, 1996.

McLean SAM, Ramsey J. 'Human rights, reproductive freedom, medicine and the law', *Medical Law International* 2002; 5(4): 239–258.

Mason JK, McCall Smith RA, Laurie GT. *Law and Medical Ethics* (6th edn), Butterworths, 2002.

Robertson J. 'Second thoughts on living wills', *Hastings Center Report* 199; 2(6): 6.

Somerville A. 'Are advance directives really the answer? And what was the question?' in McLean SAM. (ed), *Death, Dying and the Law*, Aldershot, Dartmouth, 1996.

6

MEDICAL NEGLIGENCE

Medicine is not only a science; it is also an art. Thus, there is scope for disagreement between doctors; things may be done differently by different doctors; doctors' personalities vary and they may approach their patients in different ways – and sometimes things will go wrong. The fact that something does go wrong does not necessarily mean that the doctor has been negligent and that patients either can or will sue their doctor; nor does it inevitably mean that the doctor will be disciplined (see Chapter 1). Much of the dissatisfaction that sometimes arises within the doctor/patient relationship results from the *way* in which doctors deal with their patients – by being rude or apparently uncaring – rather than from the *quality* of the treatment itself. Correspondingly, very often all that patients will be seeking is an honest, polite and speedy response to their complaint.

In some situations, however, it may be that the grievance concerns something more serious. The aggrieved patient then has, essentially, two options. Firstly, he or she can pursue the doctor through the disciplinary channels of either the National Health Service or of the doctor's governing body – that is, the General Medical Council (GMC). Both of these have been described in Chapter 1. For the present it need only be pointed out that, in taking this route, the patient is, in fact, seeking a combination of retribution and reform of the system. The Health Authority (Health Board in Scotland) can, and often does, offer an *ex gratia* payment when one of its employees has clearly failed in his or her duty but it is under no obligation to do so and the sum offered is unlikely to be substantial. The GMC, of course, has no such powers. Thus, the patient who feels that he or she has suffered a loss due to injury which ought to be compensated in monetary terms must take the second option – that is, pursuing litigation, or suing, in the courts. There is no reason why both courses should not be adopted, but it is important that patients fully understand which procedure is appropriate in any given situation.

THE COMPLAINTS PROCEDURE

The procedure whereby a patient can instigate a complaint about his or her doctor's behaviour was strengthened and revised in 1996, and is currently undergoing further scrutiny. All hospitals and general practices are obliged to have a complaints mechanism in place and patients must be made aware of how this can be accessed. Ideally, matters will be resolved by relatively informal discussion within the organisation and this should be arranged within 2 days. However, in the event that the patient is not satisfied with the response, it is also open to him or her to contact the local Health Authority/Board's complaints manager; following this, an independent review panel may be convened. The procedure is relatively straightforward and is designed for ease and informality. We need not discuss this further, save to point out that similar arrangements are in place to deal with complaints against other healthcare professionals, such as nurses. Employers other than hospitals or practices – for example, nursing homes – will, or should, have similar mechanisms in force.

All of this seems fairly straightforward. The second option, that of litigation, is far more complex and deserves rather more attention.

LITIGATION

Complaints mechanisms will not satisfy the demands that some patients may have. In these cases, they may then seek to sue. As we have seen, one reason for doing this is that, by litigating, the patient may receive compensation for any harm which arose as a result of clinical action or inaction. In short, litigation is the law's way of ensuring that people have a chance of restitution for any civil wrong that they have sustained.

No-one likes being sued and there are many reasons for this. Litigation is public and many feel that the mere fact of being sued is enough to blight a career, irrespective of whether or not they were actually at fault. Thus, the threat of litigation provokes real fear, and people will go to some lengths to avoid it. Those who deprecate the widespread use of the courts following medical mishap contend that it forces healthcare providers into practising what is called 'defensive medicine'. This means, for example, that, in order to insure against every eventuality, they will carry out investigations that may not be strictly necessary for the adequate management of the case. Others would argue that such intensive investigation is, in fact, 'best' rather than 'defensive' medicine as it seeks to find the absolute cause of a condition, for example, rather than relying on differential diagnosis. Equally, changing a practice because a colleague, behaving in the same way, has been found to be negligent is not 'defensive' – it is sensible and equates to good rather than defensive practice.

The law does not demand that unnecessary tests are undertaken – indeed, it might hold that undertaking unnecessary interventions would in itself be negligent. However, whether or not there is a real, as opposed to a perceived, need to practice defensively, it seems to be the case that some doctors will engage in such practices which, at best, constitute a financial drain on a straitened health service and at worst, put patients to increased inconvenience, or even risk, by exposing them to superfluous interventions. However, the problem of defensive medicine should not be overstated in the United Kingdom. In fact, it is very much a US phenomenon, substantially based, we believe, on the consumerist model of medical funding and care in that country.

Even so, litigation is undoubtedly increasing in the United Kingdom,[1] albeit for different reasons in a different healthcare system. It is certainly true that the historic deference to doctors has largely disappeared. Patients are more demanding – and are encouraged to be so, for example, by the institution of Patients' Forums. Equally, we live in a society in which people expect that legitimate demands will be met and are less afraid to challenge when they do not get what they want. It seems inevitable that this attitude should have spilled over into public perceptions of doctors and nurses. At the same time, the resulting so-called 'litigation explosion' has apparently had an impact – for better or worse – on the reaction of the healthcare professionals themselves and, rightly or wrongly, many aggrieved patients will see court action as the only recourse open to them. The previous chapters have, however, hinted that this may be by no means an easy option, and success by way of litigation is very difficult to achieve.

Three things have to be proved before a claim that a patient has been harmed by the actions of a medical or nursing practitioner can succeed. First, it must be shown that the practitioner owed a duty of care; second, that the duty was breached; and, third, that the breach of duty caused the harm complained of. We will consider each of these in turn briefly.

Duty of care

It is fairly obvious that an appropriate legal relationship must exist between the parties before injurious behaviour can form the basis of legal action; that is, there must be a relationship that generates the obligation or duty of care. The circumstances in which a duty of care arises are now absolutely clear – a duty is established between the healthcarer and the patient as soon as the former offers to treat. This arises even if the doctor or nurse stops to help in an accident or in another form of emergency, although the *extent* of the duty may be different in these circumstances. It would not, for example, be reasonable to expect the same high standards from a person tending to a victim at the roadside as could be expected in a hospital setting. Nonetheless, the duty does exist and it is worth remembering that it exists immediately when the professional extends an opinion or offers to treat. Existence of the necessary legal duty is not dependent on where or how it comes about; rather, it is established by the exercise of professional skills. Whether or not it has been later breached will depend on what could reasonably have been expected given the actual circumstances.

Breach of duty

This issue is considerably more complex. Patients, or prospective patients, might think it reasonable to expect the duty of care to include many things that are not specifically required by law. For example, doctors have no legal obligation to keep absolutely up-to-date with developments in their specialisms, although most would feel that they had a professional obligation to try to do so. It is also sometimes forgotten that a doctor has no obligation, and cannot be always expected, to *cure* a particular illness.

---

[1] All healthcarers, including nurses, are subject to the same constraints but, since doctors are the most common target, we will refer only to them for the sake of clarity.

In judging the nature of a duty of care, the law has developed standards which are general rather than specific. So, it might be negligent not to provide the most modern treatment in some cases, but it will not always be so. Equally, while it might not be a breach of duty not to cure some illnesses, it might well be so where cure is relatively straightforward. Doctors have, for example, been found negligent following a patient's death from malaria, a condition in which the diagnosis and treatment are standard.

In addition, doctors are not expected to perform at the level of the most experienced consultant in their area – rather, they are expected to achieve the standards of a reasonable doctor. This is something of a two-edged sword and is not easy to apply in a hospital setting. Thus, a patient can expect a reasonable standard of treatment from any 'registered medical practitioner' and junior doctors cannot excuse negligence simply by pleading that they *are* inexperienced. Nevertheless, they also cannot be expected to achieve the highest possible standard of care. This problem was given in-depth consideration in the important case known as *Wilsher*. In that case, it was maintained that a baby's eyesight had been damaged as a result of treatment given by comparatively junior doctors. Two important conclusions were reached. Firstly, that, harsh as it might sound, the standard set for the hospital doctor was that of a doctor holding a position in the team, irrespective of his or her actual status in the 'learning process'. Secondly, in some mitigation of this, it was held that the novice meets his or her required standard of care by consulting with more experienced colleagues when appropriate. Given this condition, the patient is, at least in theory, always under the care of senior staff.

The general rule by which courts will judge whether or not doctors have breached their duty of care was established in the cases of *Bolam* in England and *Hunter v Hanley* in Scotland. The effect of each is much the same, and as courts tend to combine them under the heading of the *Bolam* test, we will follow that convention in what follows. Although we have already discussed this test in the narrower field of doctor to patient communication, it is worth reconsidering its general application at this point.

The relevant conditions come in two parts. The first concerns the level of competence demanded of a doctor; this, in turn, informs the second, which deals with the definition of failure to practice within those terms. As to the former, it was laid down that the standard of competence:

> is that of the ordinary skilled man exercising and professing to have that special skill. A man need not possess the highest expert skill at the risk of being found negligent. It is a well-established law that it is sufficient if he exercises the ordinary skill of an ordinary man exercising that particular art.

To an extent, this answers the problem of the junior and senior doctor outside of the hospital environment. A senior partner in general practice is professing to have the skills of a senior partner and will be judged on that standard; a junior partner makes no such claim and, subject always to the fact that minimum competence is expected of a person who is 'registered as a medical practitioner', and to the fact that a junior can and, wherever possible should, seek advice when needed, his or her performance will be assessed at that level.

We have already seen that the second limb of the *Bolam* test requires of doctors that, within the envelope of the first, they act 'in accordance with a practice accepted as reasonable by a responsible body of medical opinion'. Except in certain circum-stances, to which we will return later, they will not be found negligent if they can show that this is what they have done. It is, therefore, worth analysing in a little more depth just what this test actually involves.

Perhaps unsurprisingly, there has been considerable criticism of the law for adopt-ing the approach encapsulated in the *Bolam* test, because it seems to indicate that, if some other doctors do X, then doing X is, by definition, not negligent. Many would suppose that the corollary – that, if some doctors would *not* do X, then X might well be regarded as malpractice or negligence – would also apply, but the *Bolam* test seems to rule out such a finding. It has, therefore, been suggested that the test does little more than hand over to fellow professionals the task which should be the prerogative of the law – in other words, that it is doctors themselves, rather than the law, who will decide as to what constitutes negligence. It would surely be strange if this conclusion were true since negligence is a legal concept and, as such, it should be for the law to put flesh on its bones. In addition, this interpretation more or less dashes the hopes of patients who think they have been wronged since, save in very obvious cases of malpractice, it should not be difficult to find 'a responsible body of medical opinion' that agrees with the doctor who is being sued.

What happens in court, however, is not a completely accurate picture either of the incidence or the management of alleged negligence. For example, indefensible cases will be settled out of court; that is, an arrangement will be reached before trial, although the likelihood is that the agreed damages in this situation will be less than might have been awarded by the court. Otherwise, the application of the *Bolam* test in the United Kingdom courts has meant that patients have been relatively unlikely to succeed in actions for negligence because, in the form that it has developed, the die is cast once a favourable body of opinion had been found. As we have pointed out, the legal test does not require that all, or even the best, doctors should agree with the practice of the doctor who is being sued. The law acknowledges that medical prac-tice may vary and the courts have, traditionally, shied away from intervening in clini-cal matters. As a result, the fact that one reasonable body of opinion would not criticise the action of the defendant doctor can be sufficient to cause the patient's action to fail – no matter that there are 99 other views on his or her practice.

It seems clear that, over the years – and depending very much on who are the senior judges in the civil division – doctors do appear to have been better protected against the results of litigation than have other professional groups. However, there have been noticeable, albeit not particularly radical, recent changes. For example, the senior judge of the civil division, the Master of the Rolls, has said that a 'responsible body of medical opinion' must also be respectable and, in an important case known as *Joyce,* it was held that clinical practice could only be acceptable if it could stand up to analysis – otherwise, it was said:

> … it leaves the decision of negligence or no negligence in the hands of the doctors, whereas that question must at the end of the day be one for the courts.

In what is, perhaps, the most significant recent judgment, the House of Lords in *Bolitho* restated the position that the court can decide whether or not a practice that is acceptable to a responsible body of medical opinion is, in fact, sufficiently based on logic as to ensure that a patient's claim should fail. In other words, the courts have repeated that they need not accept a practice as being reasonable just because other doctors say it is. It is arguable that they always had this discretion but had been reluctant to use it. Indeed, even before *Bolitho* it had been held in the case of *Smith v Tunbridge Wells Health Authority* that failure to warn of risks was negligent, despite expert evidence supporting the omission, since the court considered it to be neither reasonable nor responsible. Further evidence of a change of judicial attitudes may be gleaned from the more recent case of *Pearce v United Bristol Healthcare NHS Trust,* in which the court seemed to move some way towards recognising the needs of patients by holding that doctors should disclose information about significant risks that could be expected to affect the decision of a *reasonable person* whether or not to proceed with treatment. In addition, the General Medical Council recommends that full disclosure should be made wherever possible. Thus, it may be that both the medical profession and the law are moving towards setting a higher standard of information disclosure than has previously been the case.

Causation

Assuming that the patient can clear these first two hurdles, however, a further one still remains. As was seen in Chapter 4, it is still necessary to show that the breach of duty *caused* the harm complained of; this is known in law as proof of causation. We have already indicated how hard it is to establish causation in cases where information disclosure is under consideration, but it might be expected that it would be relatively easier to do so in the general field of negligence. One might suppose, for example, that, if a patient is worse after receiving treatment, then the causative link between medical treatment and the harm complained of is clear.

In fact, however, the issue is far from simple. For example, in one case, a casualty doctor made a mistaken diagnosis and sent a patient home who was, in fact, suffering from arsenic poisoning. The patient died later. However, although it was agreed that the misdiagnosis was negligent, it could not be said to have led to the harm (that is, the death) because no treatment was available which could have averted the harm. In the *Bolitho* case to which we have already referred, the doctor failed to respond to a call to examine and intubate a child suffering from respiratory distress. It was alleged that she was negligent both in failing to examine the child and in failing to intubate. However, she argued that she would not have intubated even if she had examined the child, and her position was supported by a 'responsible body of medical opinion'. Thus, her failure to attend may have been negligent, but the harm was not directly linked to this, as she would not have done anything even had she attended – and this inaction was supported by some of her professional colleagues.

There are many other examples. In the Scottish case of *Kay*, a boy was given a massive overdose of penicillin as treatment for meningitis. After his recovery, he was profoundly deaf. The doctor admitted negligence in the provision of the overdose but medical opinion was that this was unlikely to have caused the deafness which is a well-known side-effect of meningitis. Accordingly, the action failed. There is a certain logic behind these decisions, but the consequence is that it becomes virtually impossible for a patient to win a case when the *Bolam* test is applied to causation as well as to the question of whether or not a breach of duty has occurred.

Very rarely, however, the problem of causation does not arise. This occurs when the connection between cause and effect is so obvious that it speaks for itself – the Latin phrase *res ipsa loquitur* is then applied. This is particularly useful when the precise form of the negligence that caused the injury is not obvious, but the relationship between the medical intervention and the harm is self-evident. Although it might be anticipated that this doctrine would be regularly used, the courts are, in fact, extremely reluctant to allow the plea. This is largely because the defendant is forced into the position of having to rebut the evidence that he or she was negligent – and this offends against the general principle that a person is legally innocent of wrongdoing until proved culpable. The injured plaintiff would be unwise to rely upon the principle which, in reality, does very little to ease the problems involved in establishing a successful action against a doctor.

POLICY CONSIDERATIONS

The law is, to an extent, governed by policy considerations in all its branches and medical law is no exception. While it is true that the courts are reluctant to find that a highly qualified professional person has acted inappropriately, and that they are even more disinclined to interfere in clinical matters, analysis of decisions over the last 25 years suggests that the current policy in respect of medical negligence has been firmly rooted in the fear of encouraging defensive medicine, something on which we have already touched. Given what we have already said about defensive medicine, it could be argued that this is an inappropriate basis on which to establish legal policy. Equally, it appears to value the interests of the community of actual or potential patients over those of the individual aggrieved patient. Also underlying policy, for example, is a parallel fear of the financial costs to the National Health Service that would result from too many awards of substantial damages.

This last issue is one of considerable importance. The NHS (at least in England and Wales; less obviously in Scotland) is currently struggling with a potential liability in negligence which is so substantial that patient care may suffer as a result. In light of this, it is worth considering what remedial options might be available. In part, the pressure on the NHS was generated by changes to the system of professional indemnity of doctors. At one time, all doctors were required to carry indemnity from one of the three medical defence organisations which effectively insure doctors in the United Kingdom. However, as medicine became ever more interventionist and 'high-tech', the possibilities of something going wrong increased, leaving many more dissatisfied patients seeking to raise actions in the hope of obtaining compensation. Equally, while modern medicine can achieve enormous benefits, the results of a medical accident are, correspondingly, more serious and the sums awarded in compensation in successful cases must, inevitably follow upwards. The consequent escalation of insurance premiums began to place an excessive burden on junior doctors. At the same time, the costs involved by the introduction of differential premiums were discouraging doctors from entering the 'high risk' specialties – such as obstetrics – which were becoming seriously understaffed. As a result, the system of what has been called Crown indemnity was introduced in 1990. Under this scheme, the legal liabilities of all hospital doctors are now covered by their employers rather than by private insurance-type arrangements made with defence organisations. Thus, the burden of paying out when damages are awarded now falls squarely on the NHS – and the spiral of financial strain shows no signs of abating. A few years ago, it was estimated that the cost of negligence claims in England was in the region of £53 million annually. The problem is of such proportions that, although the individual NHS Trusts are still legally liable for the results of negligence, the management of cases is now centralised within the NHS Litigation Authority, which was established within the last decade.

WHO WILL BE SUED?

In certain limited circumstances, the hospital itself may be *directly* liable for things going wrong – people expect administrative efficiency when, for example, they attend an Accident and Emergency Department. The hospital cannot delegate responsibility for the organisation of such a department and must be held responsible if injury results from administrative inefficiency.

Such cases are, however, relatively rare. More often than not, an individual is apparently responsible for the harm done and intuition tells us that he or she should be held to account for it. However, we have just seen that, in the hospital setting, Crown indemnity ensures that the hospital, not the individual doctor, assumes responsibility for recompense. Thus, there is no practical point in suing the hospital doctor and the action will be brought against the hospital authority – that is, the National Health Service Trust.

It may be felt that this is wrong, given the potential effect on the Service as a whole. The effect may, however, not be so severe as might be supposed and, in purely practical terms, the situation may not be greatly different from that pertaining before 1990. Very often, and particularly when people are working as a team, it may be difficult if not impossible to identify a single person as being responsible for a given outcome – indeed, it may be that it is the *system* itself, rather than those working within the system, that is at fault. Thus, as we have already noted, the relevant Health Authority may be held to be directly liable for harm done. More significantly in the present context, the law has developed the principle of 'vicarious liability' under which an employer is responsible for the actions of the employees. Successive cases have shown that the law applies this principle right across the hospital hierarchy. The Trust has, therefore, always been liable for any negligence by a doctor authorised to work for it, and actions under the previous system were generally taken against both the hospital and the doctor. What has altered, however, is the proportion of the damages payable by the Trust itself and the doctor's defence organisation, something that was previously a matter of mutual agreement.[2] It should be noted, in passing, that Crown indemnity covers doctors only for the work that they do for the NHS. A doctor who, for example, undertakes private practice will be directly responsible to his or her patients. In the event of negligence, it would then be appropriate to sue him or her personally – and, for this reason, doctors are well advised to maintain some form of private insurance.

---

[2] The costs of settlement of individual claims are now spread throughout the NHS in that NHS Trusts must be members of and contribute to the centralised Clinical Negligence Scheme for Trusts. Accounting for costs is controlled by the NHS Litigation Authority.

The position in respect of general practitioners is different, in that they are not employees of the Service but, rather, are under contract to provide a service. An action in negligence taken against the individual doctor would, therefore, again be appropriate, subject always to the fact that the practice as a whole is liable for its individual partners. Once again, in order to ensure the recompense of patients who are negligently injured in general practice, all general practitioners must hold approved indemnity cover, but, strangely, this has been compulsory only since the passing of the Health Act of 1999. At the time of writing, general practice is being reorganised into major administrative bodies known as Primary Care Trusts. It remains to be seen whether vicarious liability will, in time, be extended to them.

CRIMINAL NEGLIGENCE

Although accusations of criminality in respect of therapeutic errors are extremely rare in the United Kingdom, the chapter would not be complete without a mention of the subject.

In essence, and to quote from the very old, albeit very significant, case of *R v Bateman*:

> In order to establish criminal liability, the facts must be such that ... the negligence went beyond a mere matter of compensation between subjects and showed such disregard for the life and safety of others as to amount to a crime against the State and conduct deserving punishment.

Thus, the test of criminality is a very severe one. The State is unlikely to intervene unless the patient dies and, although there have been a scatter of prosecutions in the last 30 years, there have been even fewer convictions. The classic case is that of *R v Adomako* which went all the way to the House of Lords. Here, an anaesthetist failed to notice that his patient was in distress when this was of a nature to be glaringly obvious to any competent practitioner. The criterion established was that of gross negligence – which is hard to define but which was described in the House of Lords as being limited to doing something that no reasonably skilled doctor should have done.

ALTERNATIVE SYSTEMS OF LIABILITY

Although not of direct relevance to the doctor in standard medical practice, there are other systems of liability which exist within the United Kingdom and which are worthy of brief consideration for the sake of both interest and completeness.

Vaccine damage

By the 1970s, considerable controversy surrounded the recommendation of routine vaccination against certain conditions. Particular attention focussed on the pertussis vaccine which was believed by some doctors to cause brain damage in certain children. Indeed, the United Kingdom was, unsuccessfully, challenged in the European Court of Human Rights where it was alleged that the promotion of vaccination programmes by

Government potentially breached Articles 2 (the right to life) and 8 (the right to respect for private and family life) of the Convention.

At that time, the situation was covered by common law, which required that any person who believed that harm had been caused by vaccination was required to establish all the elements considered above. However, following the report of the Royal Commission on Civil Liability and Compensation for Personal Injury (the Pearson Commission), it was conceded that those accepting vaccination were doing so on the basis of government advice and were performing a valuable public service. Accordingly, a new legal regime was proposed which came to fruition in the shape of the Vaccine Damage Payments Act 1979. Briefly, the Act permits a lump sum payment to be made in certain circumstances without the need to establish that the individual manufacturer or the doctor giving the vaccine was at fault. However, the necessary circumstances include that the claimant must establish severe disability and, having done so, the amount of money available is only £100,000 – which may seem inadequate given the severity of some forms of vaccine damage.

Although the Pearson Commission described this system as being one of strict liability (see below), it is probably better described as a no-fault system, in that, firstly, it is not necessary to establish negligence or fault and, secondly, the funding comes from central government. Decisions as to eligibility are under the overall responsibility of the Secretary of State, but the Act established independent medical tribunals to consider problems such as those relating to causation and the extent of the disablement suffered by the disabled person. The findings of these tribunals are final, although the Secretary of State can reconsider them in well defined circumstances.

Although there is evidence that the scheme is operated in a relatively restrictive way, the shift in liability is to be welcomed as it does, at least in theory, remove some of the problems identified in the fault based system which we have already discussed. Nonetheless, presumably in recognition of the fact that not every claim with some merit would succeed under the scheme, a residual right of an action in negligence remains, however unlikely it is to succeed.

Liability for defective products

Liability is described as strict if, like the no fault model described above, there is no need to prove fault. However, a significant difference between the two lies in the individual(s) who are liable to make recompense. As we have seen, in a true no fault scheme this will generally be the state whereas, in a strict liability scheme, it will be the person or organisation that generated the risk. This latter regime is most common in respect of medical or pharmaceutical products.

In the UK, these products are covered by a variety of statutes, most notably the Sale of Goods Act 1979 and the Consumer Protection Act 1987. The former legislation broadly requires that products must be fit for the purpose for which they were intended, and provides a right of action based on breach of contract. This differs from the negligence or fault based action in that a contract is generally constrained by standard (express or implied) conditions and, therefore, there is less room for interpretation. Thus, an action in contract may hold out a greater chance of success for the claimant.

The 1987 Act, on the other hand, establishes a strict liability scheme for producers (including producers of medical products). The legislation was a direct response to European law, contained in Council Directive No 85/374/EEC, but its roots probably go back to the tragedy associated with thalidomide in the late 1960s. It is estimated that about 400 children in the United Kingdom were born suffering from phocomelia linked to their mothers having taken thalidomide in the course of their pregnancy. Although no case against the UK distributors of the drug was ever successful, *ex gratia* payments were eventually made to these children, many of whom are now adults and still battling for what they see as adequate compensation.

There were a number of possible barriers to a successful action on behalf of these children – for example, it was unclear whether or not an action could be brought for damage sustained before birth – but the direct relevance here lies in the immense difficulties of establishing the necessary elements of an action based in fault. The move to strict liability would, it was anticipated, mean that any future victims of such a disaster would be presented with less difficulty in establishing their case and obtaining compensation. Article 6 of the Directive states that a product will be defective when it does not provide the safety which a person is entitled to expect taking all the circumstances into account, including:

a. the presentation of the product;
b. the use to which it could reasonably be expected that the product would be put;
c. the time when the product was put into circulation.

A product shall not be considered defective for the sole reason that a better product is subsequently put into circulation.

A number of criticisms have been levelled at the legislation, not least the inclusion of the so-called 'development risks' defence in UK law. Section 4(1)(e) of the Act provides that producers will not be liable where they can prove that:

> the state of scientific and technical knowledge at the relevant time was not such that a producer of products of the same description as the product in question might be expected to have discovered the defect if it had existed in his products while they were under his control.

This defence was included in the Directive as an option for member states, although not every member state has chosen to incorporate it into their domestic legislation. The problems that it introduces are self-evident in that it potentially provides manufacturers with a defence which is very like that which would be available under a fault based system; the anticipated value of the strict liability regime is, thereby, reduced, if not negated.

A detailed consideration of strict liability would be out of place here, but one last point of interest can be made. In the particular light of the fact that patients had been in the past infected with HIV and Hepatitis C following receipt of blood and blood products provided by the NHS, the law had to decide whether or not blood could, for these purposes, be considered to be a product, thus permitting victims to use the route of the Consumer Protection Act rather than being forced to rely on the fault based action. This matter was resolved affirmatively in the case of *A and others v National Blood Authority and another*, a case which has contemporary resonance given the recent highlighting of the risk of transmission of CJD through blood and blood products.

CONCLUSIONS

Such concerns are, however, for governments, not for us. We have seen in Chapter 1 that extensive changes in the management of medical negligence claims have been set in motion. These are aimed not only at achieving fairness between patients and the healthcarers in cases of dispute but also at limiting the costs of any resulting legal actions.

For the present, there is much evidence that efficient intervention through complaints procedures will often satisfy aggrieved patients. Indeed, many patient groups argue that, very often, people will only go to court when they have not been dealt with satisfactorily by one of the routes which avoids litigation. If doctors are encouraged to be open and honest with their patients when something goes wrong, as they increasingly are being encouraged to do, it may be that the rising tide of litigation will reduce itself to a small wave. However, for some people, compensation is both wanted and needed. The system must be able to accommodate this group in a manner which is fair, speedy and transparent.

CASES REFERRED TO IN THE TEXT

A and others v National Blood Authority and another [2001] 3 All ER 289.

Barnett v Chelsea and Kensington Hospital Management Committee [1968] 1 All ER 1068.

Bolam v Friern Hospital Management Committee [1957] 2 All ER 118.

Bolitho v City and Hackney Health Authority [1997] 4 All ER 771.

Commission v United Kingdom (Re the Product Liability Directive [1997] 3 CMLR 923.

Hunter v Hanley 1955 SC 200.

Kay v Ayrshire and Arran Health Board [1987] 2 All ER 417.

Joyce v Merton, Sutton and Wandsworth H A (1996) 7 Med LR 1.

Pearce v United Bristol Healthcare NHS Trust (1998) 48 BMLR 118.

R v Adomako [1994] 3 All ER 79.

R v Bateman [1925] All ER Rep 45.

Smith v Tunbridge Wells Health Authority [1994] 5 Med LR 334.

Wilsher v Essex Area Health Authority [1988] 1 All ER 871.

FURTHER READING

The Pearson Report. *Royal Commission on Compensation for Personal Injury*, 1970.

The Woolf Report. *Access to Justice: Final Report to the Lord Chancellor on the Civil Justice System in England and Wales*, 1996.

Brazier M, Miola J. 'Bye-bye Bolam: A medical litigation revolution?', *Medical Law Review* 2000; 8: 85.

Fenn P, Hermans D, Dingwall, R. 'Estimating the cost of compensating victims of medical negligence', *British Medical Journal* 1994; 309: 389.

Ferguson PR. *Drug Injuries and the Pursuit of Compensation*, 1996.

Ferner RE. 'Medication errors that have led to manslaughter charges', *British Medical Journal* 2000; 321: 1212.

Hoyte P. 'Unsound Practice: The epidemiology of medical negligence', *Medical Law Review* 1995; 3: 53.

Maclean A. 'Beyond Bolam and Bolitho', *Medical Law International* 2002; 5: 205.

Seeking Patients' Consent: the Ethical Considerations General Medical Council, 1999. The report is available at the GMC website: www.gmc-uk.org.

7

USING PEOPLE FOR RESEARCH

The use of human beings as experimental subjects has a long history. The art of modern medicine has been evolving steadily over the last few centuries and every time a doctor used an innovative treatment during that time, he or she was, effectively, conducting an experiment. Isolated experimentation of this type, however, was often ill considered both in terms of its appropriateness and its consequences – as was once said: '… we have a long history of human experimentation, and just as long a history of abusing it.'

Yet, it is widely accepted that research is an important part of modern medicine, not least because it is only as a result of research that medicine can advance, and it could be argued that a medical profession which did not seek to advance would be in dereliction of its duty. Scientific enquiry which results in developments which will benefit patients is conducted for the public good and the public, in its turn, *expects* that research will be carried out in the interests of improved patient care. Perhaps most significantly, medicine has become increasingly sophisticated in the last 50 years and its increasingly scientific nature has heralded the widespread development of organised experimentation, generally by way of clinical trials. The word 'organised' is important here, as it is the preparation of, and adherence to, a planned protocol that distinguishes true research from experimentation. This chapter will focus on the former although a brief mention of the latter will be made at the end.

The fact that findings from laboratory and animal models cannot be presumed to translate directly into human outcomes requires the use of human beings themselves in research, and the anticipated benefits to medical progress provide the basic rationale for the presumption that human research is generally a good thing. However, this simple logical link between the 'good' of progress and the 'rightness' of human research does not go completely unchallenged in contemporary society. The National Bioethics Advisory Commission of the United States put the dilemma this way:

A wide variety of important research studies using human subjects has long played an essential and irreplaceable role in advancing biomedical and behavioral science, thus enhancing our ability to treat illness and better understand human behavior. In recent decades, however, researchers and commentators alike have become increasingly sensitive to the ethical issues associated with such research studies, especially as they concern the rights and welfare of the subjects.

This sensitivity received its first major public airing during the War Crime trials following the Second World War, which exposed the extent to which Nazi Germany's disrespect for human rights was tied up with the callous and careless use of humans as research subjects – sometimes in pursuit of legitimate scientific knowledge, at other times, apparently, with no real expectation of learning anything of value. Two aspects of what was learned at Nuremberg led to a global outcry following the exposure of these appalling abuses of humanity. Concern was expressed, firstly, that the subjects had not consented to their involvement in such trials and, secondly, and significantly, that some 'research' was little more than a hideous exercise of power which could not be justified in terms of scientific or clinical progress.

Yet, despite the extent of the atrocities exposed at Nuremberg, the response of many legal systems was relatively casual. Almost as if it was to be assumed that Nazi doctors and scientists could be clearly differentiated from those of other nationalities, little legislation was put in place to control the possibility of excessive experimental zeal. Thus, in the absence of clear legal regulation, we have come to depend on a variety of other mechanisms to ensure some clinical and scientific conformity with the aspirational view of research that was expressed in the Nuremberg Code.

However, some might say that the commitment to the ideal of free, voluntary and knowledgeable consent that was expressed in that Code has become less firm as the distance between the demise of the Nazi regime and today's science lengthens. Close examination of the Nuremberg Code and its modern medical equivalent, the Declaration of Helsinki, shows that the latter has moved away from the absolute necessity for a free and voluntary consent towards permitting the use of proxy consent in some cases. We will return to this later.

THE DECLARATION OF HELSINKI

The Declaration of Helsinki was drawn up by the World Medical Association in 1964. It has been subject to frequent revision and was most recently revised in Edinburgh in 2000. Over the years, the Declaration has come to assume supremacy as the ethical code to which all research protocols must conform. Every research project undertaken in the United Kingdom now has to meet the terms of the Declaration, the terms of which are worthy of taking some time to analyse.

It begins with a restatement of the fundamental nature of medical practice, namely that its primary aim is to safeguard health, and – in the context of research – it insists that the well-being of the human subjects should take precedence over the interests of science and society. Recognising the potential contribution of human research in safeguarding and improving health, the Declaration also makes the point that research must 'conform to generally accepted scientific principles, be based on a thorough knowledge of the scientific literature and on adequate laboratory and, where appropriate, animal experimentation'.[1]

---

[1] It also insists that the welfare of animals used for research must be respected.

It also requires that each potential subject 'must be adequately informed of the aims, methods, … anticipated benefits and potential risks of the study and the discomfort it might entail'. There is no general mandate to undertake research into any and all interesting questions. Rather the Declaration, in its new format, insists that 'medical research involving human subjects should only be conducted if the importance of the objective outweighs the inherent risks and burdens to the subject.' In addition, the Council of Europe's 'Convention for the Protection of Human Rights and Dignity of the Human being with Regard to the Application of Biology and Medicine' makes the same point, stating that research may only be undertaken if 'the risks which may be incurred by [the subject] are not disproportionate to the potential benefits of the research'. Two fundamental constraints, therefore underpin and will shape the ethical research protocol. First, consent must be obtained, and secondly, a risks/benefits analysis must be undertaken. Although they are apparently distinct, in fact these two principles form a continuum – if risks/benefits analysis is not done, the requisite information to seek agreement to participation will not be available. For convenience and sense, therefore, they will be dealt with together under the broad umbrella of consent.

Consent

The aspirations contained in both the Nuremberg Code and the Declaration of Helsinki, focus on the importance of the voluntariness of a person's participation in research, emphasising the need to obtain a valid consent before a person becomes a research subject. It is taken as imperative that he or she must be informed of the risks and benefits which may result from participation; this is expected to provide sufficient safeguard to ensure that the participation of a competent adult is voluntary.

However, even the strong and basic presumption that consent is an essential prerequisite to research has not always been sufficient to prevent unethical practices. For example, scandal reared its head in New Zealand in the 1980s. A doctor working in an Auckland hospital held to the belief that cancerous changes in the individual cells of a woman's cervix (carcinoma *in situ*) did not necessarily mean that the tumour would spread and that women whose cervical smear results were abnormal need not, therefore, receive treatment. Whether or not this view was scientifically justified or justifiable, the fact remains that, over a period of 15–20 years, the doctor in question left women patients untreated, without their knowledge and without obtaining their consent to what was, at best, an unusual therapeutic regime. In other words, he did not tell them of his hypothesis nor of how it differed from those of others so as to give them the opportunity to reach their own decisions; essentially, he involved them, without their knowledge, in an indefensible research programme. He was severely disciplined, but many women were left ill and devastated.

Leaving aside maverick situations like this, there are reasons to doubt whether real consent is, in any event, ever *truly* available in the context of research. We have already discussed the extent of disclosure that is needed before treatment is given, and have concluded that it is less stringent than patients might have expected. However, the important Canadian case of *Halushka v University of Saskatchewan* emphasised the need for, if anything, a higher burden of disclosure when an individual is being invited to participate in research. The court said in that case:

> The duty imposed upon those who engage in medical research … to those who offer themselves as subjects for experimentation … is at least as great as, if not greater than, the duty owed by the ordinary physician or surgeon to his patient. There can be no exceptions to the ordinary requirements of disclosure in the case of research as there may well be in ordinary medical practice. The researcher does not have to balance the probable effect of lack of treatment against the risk involved in the treatment itself. The example of risks being properly hidden from a patient can have no application in the field of research. The subject of medical experimentation is entitled to a full and frank disclosure of all the facts, probabilities and options which a reasonable man might be expected to consider before giving his consent.

However stringent this requirement may be, it does not, and probably cannot, ensure that a valid consent is actually given. It is one thing to say that consent to research requires full disclosure, and, by implication, full knowledge of the associated risks and benefits, but it is quite another to say that this is in fact attainable. It is an essential requirement of research that the enterprise involves a question to which the answer is, as yet, unknown. That being the case, full information is *ex hypothesi* not available. Indeed, it would be unethical to conduct the research at all if full information were known and, as a result, there was no question to be answered. Inevitably, therefore, while consent to participation in research may require a uniquely high level of disclosure, it remains doubtful whether or not disclosure serves the same purpose that it does in routine treatment. What it *does* do is to give the subject the opportunity to appreciate both that there are uncertainties and that he or she may not, in fact, benefit from participation − or, worse, that it may be positively detrimental. Thus, the consent which is taken as validating involvement in research is different in kind from that which validates routine therapeutic intervention − it is more demanding in some ways and, arguably, less so in others.

Research and the legally incompetent

What has been said about consent so far is based on the model of the competent, adult patient. However, common sense tells us that there may be others whose involvement in research would be useful. For example, only the very young may be suitable test subjects for a new therapy or technique if the condition to be treated is one that only affects children. The dementing elderly may be the only group that would be useful to involve in trials of drugs for the treatment of Alzheimer's disease, and so on. Technically, strict adherence to the Nuremberg Code seems to rule out the participation of either group in research, as they manifestly cannot give an 'informed' consent.

Just as obviously, however, to prevent research in these areas would be to deprive many current − and, even more, future − patients of the possibility of improved treatment or cure. Thus, while it may not be in the best interests of the individual to be non-consensually involved in research (unless, of course, they benefit directly from it), it is not in the interests of society that they are precluded from involvement. It is in these cases that we see one critical difference between the Nuremberg Code and the Declaration of Helsinki. The former would probably prohibit such research, whilst the latter permits it.

The latest version of the Declaration of Helsinki indicates that substitute consent should be obtained from the legally authorised representative in accordance with applicable law. This would apply to those who are adult and incompetent, either permanently or temporarily. When we analyse the situation, however, we must reach the conclusion that, strictly speaking, a certain amount of research currently undertaken does not conform to the terms of the Declaration. Under the law in England and Wales, relatives have no authority to make medical decisions on behalf of their family members – other than in cases in which the courts are involved, an adult is deemed to be the only person empowered to speak for him or herself. In other words, there is no person legally authorised to consent on behalf of the incompetent adult. Despite this, and in the absence of any alternative, a practice has evolved by which the relatives are invited to authorise the research to proceed. The situation has recently been modified in Scotland, where the Adults with Incapacity (Scotland) Act of 2000 provides limited authority to involve an incompetent adult in research provided, and only provided, that it relates to the condition causing the incompetence – a condition that is, incidentally, also imposed by the Declaration of Helsinki itself. The Act also authorises the appointment of a guardian or a welfare attorney. Consent to participation in a research programme must be given by such a guardian if one has been appointed. If not, the Act specifically vests the power of decision in the subject's nearest relative. In either case, however, the decision to participate can be challenged in the courts by anyone having an interest in the welfare of the proposed research subject.

Parents will be asked to give consent when the research subject is a minor, and, therefore, not deemed to be legally competent. Even then, however, it must be noted that the exercise of parental authority to make medical decisions on behalf of a child is valid only where the decision taken is 'in the best interests' of that child. It might be thought that involvement, even in research designed to deliver benefit to the subjects themselves, may not be so clearly in the child's best interests as to meet the requirements placed on parents. And almost unarguably, parental authority is insufficient in law to permit of the child's involvement in non-therapeutic research (see below) that involves more than a negligible risk.

This conclusion generates an immediate tension between the interests of society in research going ahead and the interests of protecting the inviolability of the human person. Its resolution in practical terms seems to be a compromise between individual and collective values, with neither clearly predominating and neither completely satisfied.

THE NATURE OF RESEARCH

Research was traditionally referred to as being divided into two main categories – non-therapeutic research and research combined with clinical care (therapeutic research). In the latter, there is an intention/hope that benefit will accrue to, at least, some of the patients; there is no such expectation in the former. The most recent version of the Declaration of Helsinki drops this classification and speaks only of 'all medical research' and 'medical research combined with medical care', for which it lays down additional principles. Nonetheless, the therapeutic/non-therapeutic divide is a useful one and we will keep to it for ease of description.

Non-therapeutic research

This kind of research opens up a number of controversial issues. Three main groups may be involved. First, healthy volunteers may be recruited. The major question in this situation concerns the extent to which people should be permitted to run unknown risks in the possible interests of others. Given that a risks/benefits analysis will have been done, it seems to us to be generally acceptable for people to be permitted to act altruistically in the interests of society. However, it must not be forgotten that the voluntariness of participation remains a real issue, nor that there are limits to the risks people may be permitted to run with their own bodies, even if their consent has been freely given. This was made very clear in a case, unrelated to medicine but of conceptual significance, which eventually reached the European Court of Human Rights. In this case, known as *Laskey, Jaggard and Brown v UK*, the Court held that it was permissible for states to criminalise behaviour, even if it involved conduct which had been freely consented to by competent adults and was undertaken in private; in this case the behaviour in question involved sadomasochistic homosexual practices. Although medical interventions are generally deemed to form a separate category – after all, surgery is inherently an assault, but one which is legalised by consent – there is an analytical and practical message derived from this case which is relevant in medical research.

Secondly, 'captive populations', such as students, may be invited to participate in trials and it is clear that – with the best will in the world – there may be an element of duress here. Equally, some volunteers may be prepared to participate because of financial inducements. Although there are guidelines which suggest that payment should be limited so as not to amount effectively to coercion, there is little doubt that financial reward might well encourage some to come forward who would not otherwise have volunteered.

Finally, and perhaps most problematically, those who are extremely unwell may agree to participate in research even although they have been clearly informed that it is not anticipated that it will produce any benefit from them. Potentially, the pressure of their condition might lead them to ignore such advice, in the hope – however faint – that the researcher may be wrong and that there will indeed be a benefit. Concerns about this have led many commentators to question whether or not research into new (and sometimes controversial) therapies such as xenotransplantation could ever meet the requirements of a voluntary consent.

Therapeutic research

The Declaration of Helsinki holds that, subject to proven methods being non-existent or ineffective, the doctor must be 'free to use unproven or new diagnostic and therapeutic measures, if in the physician's judgement, it offers hope of saving life, re-establishing health or alleviating suffering.' This, of course, is set against the backdrop of the general provisions of the Declaration which have already been referred to. Thus, a risks/benefit analysis must be undertaken and free consent is a prerequisite to involvement – except in those certain circumstances where proxy consent may be sufficient.

The critical characteristic of this kind of research is that there is reason to believe that it may be of benefit to present – and future – patients or, as the Declaration has it, research is justified by its potential diagnostic or therapeutic value. Although the necessary elements of the design of clinical trials (see below) cannot guarantee that benefit will accrue to every patient involved in the research, no patient will be given less than the best treatment that is currently available. Thus, if the new product or technique proves to be better than the old, the groups receiving the old one will ultimately benefit but are, meantime, arguably being done no harm. Conversely, the group receiving the new treatment may be placed at some – albeit slight – risk, but will benefit if the new treatment does, in fact, prove to be more efficient or effective.

THE DESIGN OF RESEARCH

A number of scientific imperatives control the way in which a well-structured and potentially successful research project – be it therapeutic or non-therapeutic – is carried out. First, as we have already intimated, the researcher should be able to present a genuine null hypothesis – that is, there should be a question to which the answer is not known, and which cannot be known without the involvement of human subjects. Second, the group of people used in the research should share broadly similar characteristics; the results obtained will be of little or no use if this is not so. Third, the research subjects must be given different treatments in order to test the relative efficacy of one over the other. Thus, in therapeutic research, one group in the study will be given the existing treatment and one will be given the new treatment; at the end of the study, it will be possible to measure the extent to which one treatment is better than the other. This is what makes a 'controlled' trial – and the art of producing good research lies in the adequacy of the 'control'. Fourth, extraneous factors must not influence the outcome of the trial. It is well known for example that the mere provision of 'medical treatment' can have an apparently beneficial effect – this is known as the 'placebo' effect. Not only that, but doctors themselves may subconsciously influence the results and it is generally agreed that the best design for a trial is the randomised double blind trial. In this situation, groups are randomly allocated to the old and the new therapy and neither the doctors nor the patients know who is receiving which. In cases where there is no pre-existing 'best' treatment, researchers may have to use a placebo, an inert substance, on one side of the trial. To do so is not uncontroversial – it does, for example, involve an obvious deception – but the practice is permitted by the Declaration of Helsinki and it is sometimes the only practical way forward.

No matter what factors make up the requirements of the 'scientifically' optimal trial, some immediate problems emerge from the very nature of its design. Perhaps most significantly, researchers must end a trial if it becomes clear that harm – or disbenefit – is being caused to one or other of the research groups. However, the decision to halt a trial prematurely may be very difficult to make. It may be, for example, that the group doing well is those on the new treatment. It may, then, be perfectly clear to the person on the spot that it would be to the benefit of the control group to cut short the trial. Others, however, might say that the research has not progressed through the rigours of the process which are required before it is widely acceptable – in particular, it may not stand up to the statistical analysis which is needed in order to prove that the new treatment is effective. Halting the research means that it is, then, wasted and many patients will be denied its benefits. Not stopping the trial, on the other hand, might result in significant harm to some people; the requirement that potential harm should not be disproportionate to the benefits expected from the trial would, thus, be breached.

WHO CONTROLS RESEARCH?

We noted earlier that the rush to impose tight controls over research, which might have been expected in the aftermath of the Nazi war crimes trials, did not materialise. Certainly, the Nuremberg Code was promulgated, but adherence to it was essentially voluntary and its efficacy was, thereby, reduced.

It was not until the 1970s that systems were finally put in place in the United Kingdom by which clinical trials could be monitored. On a recommendation from the medical Royal Colleges, hospitals where research was being conducted were expected, from then on, to establish Local Research Ethics Committees (LRECs). These Committees – now extant in every health district – were intended to include a mixture of scientific/medical and 'lay' people, whose obligation was to scrutinise research protocols with a view to ensuring that they were, indeed, ethical. The research could go ahead only if the LREC approved the protocol.

The increasing use of multi-site research – using patients from a variety of hospitals and geographical areas – resulted in the creation in the 1990s of Multi-centre Research Ethics Committees (MRECs) who deal, on the same basis, with trials – generally of pharmaceutical products – which are conducted throughout a region or throughout the country. The MREC's recommendations cannot be overturned by an LREC unless the LREC can show some local reason for not permitting a trial to go ahead. In part at least, the MRECs were also designed to avoid the, not uncommon, situation in which a researcher obtained clearance from some of the LRECs to whom it was submitted but failed to get agreement from others. This problem was expected to disappear if only one body was involved. In addition, in Scotland, the MREC acts as the ethics committee for research conducted under the terms of the Adults with Incapacity (Scotland) Act 2000.

At one stage, considerable, and wide-ranging, doubt was expressed as to the efficacy of LRECs. Early investigations into their work showed that in some cases the 'lay' representation – thought to be of critical importance – could scarcely be described as 'lay' and there was little in the way of disinterested membership. Some committees never met, or did their business over the telephone, and their size ranged from a very small to a very large group.

Over the years, however, the research committee culture has become stronger, with relative uniformity now prevailing. In addition, the requirement for lay representation is taken very seriously. In part, this change may be due to a recognition of the potential value of research ethics committee scrutiny. In part also, it seems likely that it is the result of pressure from the medical profession itself. The endorsement of a research programme by a properly constituted ethics committee is now an indication of its value; few reputable medical journals will now publish work which does not bear this stamp of approval.

Criticism of RECs has not, however abated completely and it is, in many ways, surprising that the control of research involving humans was left for so long to a non-statutory, grace and favour system. It has not escaped notice that there may be a paradox in the fact that we have had legislation since the 19th century which controls, polices and monitors research using animals, yet, until the passing of the Adults with Incapacity (Scotland) Act 2000, no such system had been introduced to oversee any research involving human subjects in the United Kingdom. Hopefully, this problem is now to be eradicated. Following the passing of a European Directive, the United Kingdom has until 2003 to set the ethics committee structure on a statutory basis, with an anticipated improvement in regulation of research projects.

WHAT HAPPENS IF HARM RESULTS FROM RESEARCH?

There is always the possibility that someone will be harmed by involvement even in the best designed and controlled trial. The injury may be trivial or catastrophic but, irrespective of the degree of harm, the person concerned may well attempt to seek compensation for the harm allegedly resulting from his or her involvement in the specific trial.

More than 20 years ago, the Royal Commission on Civil Liability and Compensation for Personal Injury (the Pearson Commission) explored the routes available for compensation in such circumstances as part of its comprehensive review of compensation for personal injury. The Pearson Commission discovered that, in some – but not all – cases, *ex gratia* payments would be made to anyone who could establish that the trial had caused the harm complained of. The Association of British Pharmaceutical Industries also indemnifies against harm where, on balance, it appears that the damage was the result of involvement in the trial of new pharmaceutical products.

However, for some, the only way of obtaining compensation for harm suffered will be to raise an action in negligence in the civil courts. As we have already seen, success in such an action will not come easily although, arguably, the more stringent disclosure requirements might make success more likely where the grievance relates to an alleged shortfall of information. In other situations, even a well designed trial, approved by an ethics committee and properly carried out, can result in harm. Given, however, that the form of action available to the aggrieved participant remains that of negligence, it will be extremely difficult to win, particularly in the light of the scrutiny which the trial will have undergone.

For these reasons, the Pearson Commission recommended that compensation for injury sustained in the context of research should be available on the basis of strict liability. That is, it would not be necessary to show that the researchers had been negligent – merely, it would be sufficient to establish on the balance of probabilities that the harm resulted from involvement in the clinical trial. This recommendation has not been adopted in UK law although, depending on their final recommendations, the reviews of medical negligence currently being undertaken throughout the United Kingdom may yet have some impact in this area.

MEDICAL EXPERIMENTATION

At the beginning of this chapter we specifically distinguished between experimentation and research. The distinction is not only practical – that is related to the act itself – but also has legal significance. For those involved in experimental treatment, considerable interest will be found in the decision in the case of *Hunter v Hanley*. In this case, it was held that a doctor could be guilty of negligence if he or she deviated from usual practice – for example, by experimenting with treatments. This was, however, qualified as follows:

> ... but only if it could be established that there was a usual practice which was not followed, and that no doctor acting with due skill and care would have acted as the doctor in question did.

Thus, although directly in point, this case seems to equate the test for the permissibility of deviation from standard practice with a test that is not significantly different from the *Bolam* test which we have already discussed. If this is so, then this case does not necessarily hold out a significantly higher expectation of success for the patient who is involved in experimentation than exists for other patients alleging negligence.

It can be seen, then, that a very high standard of proof is required from persons alleging that they were harmed. There are two other aspects to be noted. First, the experimenting doctor is likely to have discussed the matter very extensively with the patient and will, as a result, have obtained a truly valid consent. Secondly, the courts may well take the view that medicine must advance and that, therefore, experimentation should not be discouraged when extreme circumstances demand its use. The criteria have, in fact been laid down recently in the case of *Simms v Simms* in which a highly contentious treatment was authorised in two cases of suspected vCJD; the risks of using an untried procedure were to be balanced against the certainty of death in its absence.

THE FUTURE

Medicine is not a stagnant discipline – partly because of the amount of research undertaken, and partly also because of new discoveries. Contemporary medicine is becoming increasingly preoccupied with the genetic basis of ill health and, inevitably, this will result in a drive to research in this area. Once again, the anticipated outcome is easy to describe as desirable – namely the hope of cure for illness – but the use of people for genetic research is, if anything, more troubling than their use in non-genetic research. This, of course, is because of the peculiar nature of genes.[2]

GENETIC SCREENING AND TESTING

Genetic research may be based on the population or be focussed on the individual. The former may take the form of population screening – for example to identify the incidence of a particular gene in the community – or may be by way of the genetic testing of individuals thought to be at high risk of inheriting particular conditions.

---

[2] The nature of genetic disorders will be considered in more depth in Chapter 9.

In October 1998, the Advisory Committee on Genetic Testing issued guidelines to Research Ethics Committees, the aim being 'to help committees identify the questions that they might raise with researchers.' The Committee described four kinds of genetic testing:

- Diagnostic genetic testing, which involves the use of testing in someone who is showing signs of a particular condition. The aim of this testing would be to help in managing the condition;
- Presymptomatic genetic testing, which would be carried out on people who have no symptoms or are otherwise healthy in order to find out information about their future health;
- Susceptibility testing, which would give information about the genetic aspects of conditions which might be partly genetic and partly not (so-called multi-factorial disorders);
- Carrier testing, which seeks to identify those at risk of passing on a genetic condition to others, even although they will never themselves suffer from the condition.

The Committee addressed a number of issues in respect of which ethics committees should be vigilant. One concern related to the question of confidentiality. Because genetic information is so sensitive, the ACGT advised that there must be an adequate system in place to ensure that there is no way that the individuals tested and the test results can be associated. A clear distinction must also be drawn between diagnostic testing and testing which is part of medical research. This is, in part, to protect people from being given information that they may not wish to receive.

Research Ethics Committees should also satisfy themselves as to whether or not it is intended that the information gained from tests is to be given to the individual or included in medical records, and the individual must be given full opportunity to agree to this or not. Truly valid consent is absolutely vital here. Additional questions may arise as to the disposal of samples taken for testing purposes. The ACGT's advice is that individual consents should be obtained for each specific use of any stored samples – that is, a general agreement in non-specific terms should not be taken as authority to re-use samples for different purposes. This issue has recently re-emerged following the disclosure of the unauthorised removal and retention of organs and tissue at post-mortem examination, and is being addressed in the review of the law in this area which is currently under way throughout Great Britain and Northern Ireland.

Special concern was expressed by ACGT about testing those who belong to families in which there is a risk of suffering from genetic disorders. In particular, ethics committees should look carefully at any research proposals which seek access to those members of a family who are apparently well. They should also have a clear plan about what they would do should it appear that the person does in fact have the gene which will predictably result in their developing a particular condition.

Children were singled out for special attention. The ACGT was concerned that the interests of the child should be adequately protected and it made the point that children's best interests were not confined to their *medical* best interests. The Committee's view was that testing would be unjustifiable when a child was presymptomatic and no therapy was available for the condition under review. Particular care must be exercised when the testing is intended to identify diseases or disorders which may affect children during childhood; those who have the authority to decide on the child's involvement must be given very full information and discussions on the matter must be sensitive. The best interests of the child must be paramount.

GENE THERAPY

Gene therapy has been much hyped; it is often said to hold out the best hope of alleviating suffering and of reducing the incidence of ill health in the future. Some believe that it will become the treatment of choice for genetically related disorders, particularly in those involving a single gene – that is, those conditions which can be attributed to a specific gene that is isolated from the influence of others. The procedure is, however, currently very much at the research stage. The recent death in the United States of a participant in gene therapy has done much to add to the intensity of ethical and clinical debate surrounding this kind of therapy and has re-emphasised the fact that, although commonly referred to as 'therapy', it remains research for the moment and, as such, it should be subject to rigorous scrutiny.

More than 2,000 people are said to be involved in gene therapy research worldwide, yet, as we have noted, only limited therapeutic benefit has so far been identified. Nonetheless, big business is enthusiastic about its future and biotechnology companies attract significant investment. And, of course, the idea of gene therapy has great appeal. However, few outside of the scientific community will be aware of the extent to which the technique has failed to live up to expectations. As *Scientific American* put it in 1999:

> Gene therapy took a standing eight-count last winter, after drug contenders sponsored by a host of biotechnology and drug companies failed to cure a single patient of disease. Yet, despite its current shortcomings, in laboratories and on Wall Street, there are signs that gene therapy is starting to stage a comeback.

One further issue remains to be discussed briefly. Although the potential value of gene therapy is clear, not *all* of its manifestations have been endorsed. Gene therapy can be split into two types – somatic and germline – and only the former is currently deemed acceptable. Somatic therapy affects the individual and his or her specific condition; by contrast, germline therapy, which is applied to the sex cells, results in genetic modifications which will be transmitted through future generations. In a sense, therefore, somatic therapy is very like any other form of medical treatment and, once available, will be subject to the same legal and professional controls. However, there are concerns that deliberately modifying the genetic make-up of future generations is a step too far. Additionally, it has been suggested that it would be unethical to do this, as it would mean treating tomorrow's children within the limitations of today's knowledge. For the moment, therefore, as we have said, it is to be presumed that germline therapy is unacceptable. It should be noted, however, that doubts have been expressed by some commentators as to the extent to which it is actually possible to make a clear distinction between somatic and germline therapy. Others see nothing unethical about germline therapy, suggesting that it is surely better to modify a harmful gene for all time than risk its emergence in future generations who would then be forced to undergo treatment which could have been avoided. One thing is clear – the ethical and scientific debate on this issue is far from over.

CONCLUSIONS

No matter the controversies, and despite the potential pitfalls, there is little doubt that human beings will continue to be used in research in ever increasing numbers. Problems there may be, but the alleged benefits of medical progress will seldom be challenged. With the advent of the age of the 'new' genetics, the possibilities of cure seem to come closer but, at the same time, the research needed to find such cures becomes increasingly intrusive. Although the potential of stem cell therapy may ultimately lead to a reduction in the scale of, and risks from, clinical research, this potential is as yet unproved and – if established – lies some way in the future.

No-one knows why people agree to participate in research, although it seems likely to be due to a mixture of altruism tempered by varying degrees of self-interest. Indeed, as we have already suggested, patients may hope for benefit even from trials which are expressly said to be non-therapeutic. Doubts must exist as to the actual quality of consent given in any research trial yet, on the other hand, we must beware of adopting an attitude that is too paternalistic. People already take risks – for example, in sports – and it would be widely regarded as unacceptable to stop them doing so. By analogy, it would be wrong to prevent people from agreeing to participate in clinical research which may benefit them and future patients.

For this reason, it is imperative that adequate safeguards are in place to ensure that such participation holds out minimal risk. Although, at present, the only human research which is given a statutory regulatory framework is that undertaken on human embryos, controlled by the Human Fertilisation and Embryology Act 1990, and research on incompetent adults in terms of the Adults with Incapacity (Scotland) Act 2000, the landscape of regulation is set for early change. It remains to be seen whether the new regulatory framework will be able to enhance standards and reinforce best practice in this important area of medicine.

CASES REFERRED TO IN THE TEXT

Halushka v University of Saskatchewan (1965) 53 DLR (2d) 436.

Hunter v Hanley 1955 SC 200.

Laskey, Jaggard and Brown v UK (1997) 24 EHRR 39.

Simms v Simms [2003] 1 All ER 669.

FURTHER READING

Association of British Pharmaceutical Industries. *Clinical Trial Compensation Guidelines*, 1991.

Beecher HK. 'Ethics and Clinical Research', *New England Journal of Medicine* 1966; 274: 274.

Garnett RW. 'Why informed consent? Human experimentation and the ethics of autonomy', *Catholic Lawyer* 1995; 36: 455.

Kinderlerer J, Longley D. 'Human genetics: The new panacea?', *Modern Law Review* 1998; 61: 603.

Learning from Bristol, CM 5207, 2001.

National Bioethics Advisory Commission *Research Involving Persons with Mental Disorders that may Affect Their Decision-making Capacity* (1998), Volume 1.1.

Paul C. 'The New Zealand cancer study: Could it happen again?', *British Medical Journal* 1988; 297: 533.

Pettit P. 'Instituting a research ethic: Chilling and cautionary tales', *Bioethics* 1992; 6: 89.

Report of the Royal Commission on Civil Liability and Compensation for Personal Injury (1978) (the Pearson Report).

Report of the Independent Review Group on Retention of Organs at Post-Mortem, Edinburgh, HMSO, 2002.

Royal College of Physicians of London. *Research Involving Patients*, 1990.

The Royal Liverpool Children's Inquiry Report, HC 12-II 2001.

'Gene Therapy', Scientific American, May–June 1999 (available at http://www.sciam. com.explorations.10149explorations.html)

8

ASSISTED REPRODUCTION

It is widely accepted practice to describe couples who are unable to have a family as being 'infertile' but this is not always correct. Infertility is an inability to produce *gametes* and this accounts for only about half the cases in which couples are unable to have children. In the remainder, the individuals produce gametes normally but, for one reason or another, fertilisation and implantation of an embryo in the woman's womb is prevented or is contraindicated. It is, therefore, more correct to speak in terms of 'childlessness' to describe such a condition. The distinction is more than a matter of semantics and has practical consequences. It has been noted in Chapter 2 that assisted reproduction has a very low priority in the majority of National Health Service resource allocation programmes. One line of justification for this is to argue that, while the underlying cause – for example, disease of the Fallopian tubes – is certainly a matter of medical concern, the result, childlessness, is a social rather than a medical matter. Thus, although unblocking the tube would come within the ambit of the health authority, the provision of *in vitro* fertilisation (IVF) would not. This perspective may be arguable on both economic and ethical grounds, but it is mentioned in order to show that health authorities which do not provide IVF *may* have a tenable point of view. In any event, it is reasonable to take a more open view and to define infertility as 'the involuntary, significant reduction of reproductive capacity' – a definition that was accepted by the Canadian Law Reform Commission and which conforms to popular usage. While the distinction we make should be borne in mind, the terms infertility and childlessness can be regarded as basically interchangeable for the remainder of this chapter.

It is generally said that some 10 per cent of couples who want to parent experience difficulty in doing so and that the underlying causes are distributed about equally between men and women. Thus, infertility is a significant disability in modern society in both numerical and emotional terms. At the same time, most people have an innate fear of interference with the natural order of reproduction. Fictional horror stories involving cloning or genetic manipulation of future generations are now too close to reality to be ignored and it is relatively recently in history that eugenic selection of the 'race' was regarded as an acceptable practice. As a result, many techniques associated with help in reproduction are banned in some countries – particularly in those with an unhappy record of attempted population control. Elsewhere, concern for the moral status of human embryos has led to, at the very least, an unsympathetic attitude to techniques that involve their wastage. It must also be said that the introduction of reproductive technologies has led to a revolution in feminist philosophy. The United Kingdom was one of the first jurisdictions to appreciate the extent of the legal and ethical problems associated with the so-called 'reproductive revolution' and, having set up a major inquiry into the practical and moral implications of human fertilisation and embryology in the early 1980s (the Warnock Committee), Parliament passed the Human Fertilisation and Embryology Act in 1990; the effect of this is to establish in the United Kingdom one of the most closely regulated systems for assisted reproductive medicine in the Western world. Nevertheless, it should be noted that the regulatory framework can be broadly described as liberal rather than prohibitive. Before discussing its influence on the treatment of those in need, it will be helpful, first, to look briefly at some of the causes of childlessness, even though they may be well known to the medical reader.

CAUSES OF CHILDLESSNESS

Causes in the man

The man may, of course, be unable to impregnate the woman because of impotence or psychological inhibition. Obstructive disease of the vas deferens is relatively rare, although the man may have had a previous vasectomy, which is now regretted. The commonest cause of childlessness in the male is true infertility due to azoospermia, which may be primary or the result of inflammation following disease in the genital system. Azoospermia may be relative, resulting in oligospermia, which it may be possible to circumvent. Indeed, nature itself may do so given time. Alternatively, the individual sperm may be physiologically or anatomically abnormal. Abnormalities in the man's seminal analysis are found in about 30 per cent of couples seeking treatment for childlessness.

An intermediate situation may arise which is attributable to the man and the woman together. In this, the woman develops antibodies to the man's semen and, as a result, the sperm are destroyed in the vagina and cervical canal. Immune disease of all types is on the increase and it is possible that this mechanism is a more common cause of childlessness than might be supposed; the hostile, reaction may be very specific to the sperm of one man.

Causes of infertility in the woman

Failure of ovulation is found in some 17 per cent of infertile couples. Again, this may be a primary condition in the ovaries or it may be secondary to hormonal deficiencies which can be remedied – physiological treatments of this type are not considered further in this chapter. In a further 20 per cent of cases, the woman's Fallopian tubes are blocked either as a result of anatomic disease or following pelvic inflammation. Whatever the cause, the end result is tubal insufficiency. Again, we do not address the option of surgical treatment of the condition as it has no particular legal connotations. Nonetheless, this may serve to remind us that the specific technologies that *are* discussed are unlikely to be used as a primary therapeutic resource in the treatment of childlessness.

The remaining relevant female preconditions comprise a varied group of conditions, most of which are significant in respect of assisted reproduction techniques. Thus, some women are subject to repeated miscarriages; others have no uterus or one that is anatomically inadequate; finally, there is a group of women who can conceive but who should not carry a child to term on general medical grounds. It is within this group that surrogate motherhood would provide an acceptable *medical* response to reluctance, rather than inability, to reproduce naturally.

For the sake of completeness, it is to be noted that no cause for infertility can be found in about 20 per cent of couples wishing to parent and there is, on the other hand, no reason why abnormalities should not be present in both the man and the woman – indeed, the mathematical chances of this being so are quite high.

TREATMENTS FOR CHILDLESSNESS

Rather as we have outlined the causes of childlessness, so we must consider the treatments available before we assess the legal regulation of assisted reproduction. Indeed, we might well ask: 'what *is* assisted reproduction'?

For present purposes, we can look on assisted reproduction as the provision of such services as are controlled, either directly or indirectly, by the Human Fertilisation and Embryology Act of 1990. This Act defines 'treatment services' as: 'medical, surgical or obstetric services provided to the public or a section of the public for the purpose of assisting women to carry children'. This is a very wide definition, which could include treatments such as hormonal replacement or secondary surgery on diseased Fallopian tubes and which will almost certainly be tried before entering the field of embryology. Clearly these are attempts to assist women to carry children but, equally clearly, there is no need for their specific regulation – indeed, they are not considered in the Act. Assisted reproduction in a legal and/or ethical context means treatment that involves the manipulation of gametes, the use in any way of the gametes or reproductive organs of third parties and the creation of embryos *in vitro*. This includes rather more techniques than are actually covered by the 1990 Act, and the Act itself has, in fact, been overtaken by more recent advances in technology. The treatments specified below include the basic techniques used in assisted reproduction as we define it; but we must emphasise that, for reasons of space, the list is incomplete – modifications of the old and the introduction of new methods are now almost daily occurrences.

Treatments for abnormalities in the male

These would include artificial insemination with the husband's (AIH) or partner's (AIP) sperm where the male is fertile but unable to consummate sexual intercourse and insemination by donor (DI)[1] in the event of male infertility or incompatibility. AIH, accompanied by concentration of samples of semen, can also be attempted in cases of oligospermia. For reasons which are not at all clear, a pregnancy is created by AIH or DI in only about 12 per cent of treatment 'cycles' even in the best of circumstances. Advanced treatments such as intracytoplasmic sperm injection (ICSI) or sub-zonal insemination (SUZI), which also seek to overcome oligospermia and abnormalities of the sperm, are, of course, now available under licence. Such techniques, however, involve the use of IVF (see below).

Treatments for abnormalities in the female

The basic treatment here is IVF where the woman's egg is removed from the ovary and fertilised in the Petri dish; the resultant embryo is then inserted in the woman's uterus. The process was originally developed for the management of childlessness due to blocked Fallopian tubes – in which case, the gametes come from the couple seeking treatment – but, effectively, IVF is involved in any treatment that requires embryo transfer – that is, transfer of an embryo from the laboratory bench to a receptive uterus. The live birth rate following IVF is of the order of 22 per cent per treatment cycle. IVF might also be considered for the treatment of childlessness resulting from the development of anti-sperm antibodies although, probably, AIH using modified semen would be attempted first.

The management of ovarian inadequacy will be by way of ovum donation from another woman. In the event that neither the man nor the woman can produce gametes, the treatment of choice will be embryo donation, where the embryo is formed from donated sperm and eggs. Again, both of these techniques involve IVF followed by embryo transfer.

Conditions within the remaining group involving the faulty carriage of a foetus are obvious candidates for management by surrogate motherhood, whereby another woman carries the baby with the intention of returning it to the childless woman after its birth. Surrogate motherhood is of two types. The more common, sometimes known as partial surrogacy, involves the impregnation of a surrogate by DI[2] using the sperm of the male from the couple seeking parenthood. By contrast, full surrogacy, sometimes referred to as 'womb leasing', results from the impregnation of the surrogate with an embryo derived from the childless couple. The distinction between the two procedures has both practical and genetic significance and we will see later that their legal regulation is also distinct. For the present, we need only note that there are far more conditions that provide a medical justification for full surrogacy than there are for partial surrogacy. In effect, the only condition for which the latter is the optimal treatment is where an infertile woman has neither ovaries nor a functional uterus – a specific and fairly rare condition.[3]

---

[1] Insofar as insemination by donor will, one imagines, always be artificial, the use of this abbreviation is to be preferred to the traditional AID. It also avoids any possible confusion with the condition of AIDS.

[2] There is, of course, no *technical* reason why donation should not be natural – as was, indeed, so in one of the first English cases to come to court. The Act, however, refers repeatedly to artificial insemination; the legal consequences could, therefore, be very different.

[3] Most such cases are, in fact, examples of the testicular feminisation syndrome.

THE HUMAN FERTILISATION AND EMBRYOLOGY ACT 1990

We can now look to how the law sets out to regulate these treatments which, in a way, break new ground in that, while they aim to improve reproductive capacity, at the same time they distort the physiology of the natural reproductive process to a variable, and sometimes extreme, degree.

The fundamental purpose of the 1990 Act is to establish the Human Fertilisation and Embryology Authority, the main functions of which can be summarised as reviewing information about embryos and any subsequent development of embryos and about the provision of treatment services governed by the Act; advising the Secretary of State; and providing advice and information for those offering, receiving and contributing to the provision of treatment services. Specifically, the Authority must establish a licensing committee which can grant distinct licences authorising three activities – the provision of treatment services, the storage of gametes and embryos and research in the field of reproductive medicine. The last of these has been briefly referred to in Chapter 7, but is largely outside the scope of this book; the second has major significance in relation to the first. But, by and large, treatment is our main concern and it is on that aspect that we concentrate.

Before going further, however, it is important to appreciate that the Act defines 'treatment services' for which a licence is required (see below) as treatment provided for 'the public or a section of the public'. While it is not easy to see why an individual is not 'a section of the public', it is widely assumed that this means that services that are provided on a purely individual basis and which are not otherwise proscribed are lawful in the absence of a license and, as a result, are, currently, unregulated. In effect, this means that isolated procedures involving donor insemination without storage of the semen can be legally undertaken on what may be described as a 'do-it-yourself' basis.

As to the requirement for a license, the Act first sets out a number of techniques for which the Authority may not grant a licence and which are, as a consequence, absolutely prohibited. Some of these are irrelevant to the individual seeking or providing treatment for childlessness, but others are of widespread importance. Fundamentally, it is currently unlawful for anyone to keep or use an embryo after the appearance of the primitive streak. This is taken to equate with a period of time not later than 14 days after the gametes forming that embryo were mixed; this period, of course, excludes any time during which the embryo was stored. In addition, the Authority cannot issue a licence which condones the cloning of human cells for reproductive purposes using embryos that have resulted from fertilisation. This part of the legislation caused considerable controversy when Mr Quintavalle, in an action brought in 2001, claimed that embryos derived from somatic cell nuclear replacement (CNR) did not result from fertilisation and, accordingly, were not covered by the terms of the 1990 Act. Mr Quintavalle was, in fact, successful at first instance. Both the Court of Appeal and the House of Lords, however, took a purposive approach – in short, that the *purpose* of the legislation was to prohibit cloning; CNR was unknown when the Act was passed but, now that it was here, it plainly fell within Parliament's *intentions* at the time. Simultaneously, Parliament passed the Human

Reproductive Cloning Act in 2001, which defined the offence of placing in a woman an embryo that had been created other than by fertilisation. Thus, human cloning for reproductive purposes remains unlawful, although it is now permissible to use the technique under license for research that is devoted to the replacement of defective organs – so-called 'therapeutic cloning'.

Beyond these absolute prohibitions, there are certain things that it is unlawful to do unless the actor has a licence for the purpose. The most wide-ranging of these is covered in the creation, storage and use of an embryo. Similarly, no-one can store gametes without a licence to do so. More particularly, a licence is required before one can use the sperm of any man in the course of providing treatment services for any woman 'unless,' as the Act says, 'the services are being provided for the man and the woman together'. This rather obscure wording has caused some confusion largely because it is used again in respect of parentage – a point to which we return later on. For the present, this particular section can be taken as excluding AIH and AIP, together with DI on an individual basis, from the restrictions imposed by licensing. By contrast, the use of the eggs of one woman in the course of providing treatment services for another woman is *always* subject to licensing.

Storage of gametes and embryos under licence depends heavily on the concurrent consent of the providers. In summary, an 'effective consent' must be in writing and can apply to the use, storage and/or disposal of the gametes and of any embryo created from them. The consent must include a decision as to how long the gametes or embryos may be stored and the person giving consent must state what is to be done in the event of his or her death or incapacitation. The person concerned must also have been given the opportunity to receive advice and counselling before giving his or her consent. In point of fact, the gametes cannot be preserved for longer than 10 years – or, in the case of eggs, beyond the 55th birthday of the woman donor – nor the embryos for longer than 5 years, although the latter period may be extended to 10 years or even longer if the embryos are to be used for treatment or if the providers are likely to become permanently sterile.

Thus, it will be seen that, if we exclude the research element – which probably provokes the greatest moral argument associated with assisted reproduction – the regulatory function of the 1990 Act is confined to 'treatment services' which involve the use of donated gametes or embryos and those which involve the creation of an embryo outside the body. This leads to some apparent anomalies. We need a licence, for example, to form an embryo in the Petri dish. If, however, we introduce the same gametes directly into the Fallopian tube – GIFT – we have created an embryo *within* the body. Therefore, provided it is done using the gametes of 'a woman and a man together', this more difficult and, in some ways, more unsafe technique can be performed in an unlicensed clinic; this situation is, however, currently under consideration. More generally, we have seen that an unlicensed sperm donation is not unlawful provided it is not a service offered to the public – and, indeed, since private insemination cannot be supervised, it would be hard to argue that it should be otherwise. By the same token, partial surrogacy lies outside the 1990 Act when it is a purely private matter – although, at the time of writing, there are strong moves towards the introduction of special regulatory powers. Full surrogacy, however, involves the creation of an embryo *in vitro* and is, therefore, already controlled – albeit by control of embryo production rather than by control of surrogacy *per se*.

The day to day regulation of assisted reproduction, and the introduction of new techniques, are governed by a Code of Practice issued by the Authority. It is, therefore, clear that, since the Code represents 'good medical practice' in the field, a clinic that persistently disregards its terms is liable to lose its licence. Yet, the Code itself, while being restrictive in tone, is, at the same time, and perhaps purposefully, very open in its language. Thus, in deciding whether to provide treatment, clinics are advised to bear in mind such variables as the patients' abilities to provide a stable environment for a resulting child, their medical histories, their health and age as indicators of their ability to provide for the child's needs and the effect of a new baby on existing children. Indeed, the Act itself emphasises that account is to be taken of the welfare of any resulting child including the need of that child for a father. All of which indicates admirable intentions. But such factors would not have to be considered before, say, issuing a marriage licence – and no-one would think of imposing such conditions on natural parenthood. Moreover, the Code is not directive – it does not say whether certain people will or will not be given treatment. It is, in effect, advisory only – clinics will 'bear in mind' or 'take account' of the various circumstances. This may be inevitable if the doctors' clinical freedom is to be respected but, at the same time, it does little to ease the position of either the patients or the clinics. In 2000, major publicity surrounded a couple who were seeking IVF treatment for the sole purpose of ensuring the sex of their fifth child. The Code of Practice says that centres should not select the sex of embryos for social reasons; what is the centre to do? Effectively, it can only refuse to provide the service[4] or refer the case to the Authority for adjudication – leaving everyone in an unsatisfactory state of doubt. Mr and Mrs Hashmi, for example, obtained permission, surrounded by strict conditions, to combine genetic tests with IVF in order to have a child who could provide stem cells for the treatment of an existing sibling only to have the High Court rule that the Authority had exceeded its powers. This judgement has, in turn, been reversed on appeal; the reasons for this have not been reported as we go to press.

Having considered the general aspects of the main Act, we can now go on to look at some of the specific legal results of the various treatment schedules available.

SOME SPECIFIC MEDICO-LEGAL ASPECTS OF ASSISTED REPRODUCTION

Artificial insemination by husband or partner

We have seen that the act of AIH is not legally controlled and it carries with it no significant ethical problems. Should the *reason* for AIH be impotence, that condition could form the basis for voiding a marriage in both England and Wales and in Scotland. However, the fact that AIH had been used might, in such circumstances, be regarded as approbation of the situation and, as a result, constitute a bar to a decree of nullity. The precise conditions would be important in individual cases, which must, at any rate, be very rare.

---

[4] Irrespective of the Code of Practice, members of the centre could refuse on the grounds of conscientious objection to the proposed 'treatment service' under the terms of the Act.

One would have thought, then, that AIH could be dismissed very rapidly in the present context. However, there is a growing tendency for married men to preserve specimens of semen against the possibility of disease or sudden death and this has two immediate legal implications. In the first place, retention, even if only for use within the family, is still subject to storage in a centre licensed to do so and to the stringent regulations as to consent that we have already outlined. In particular, the provider must state what is to be done with his sperm after his death. Secondly, in the event of it being used for insemination posthumously, he cannot, as the law presently stands, be regarded as the father of the resulting child who will, as a result, be legally 'fatherless'. For this reason, many clinics would consider posthumous insemination to be incompatible with the 1990 Act and with the Code of Practice – but they would certainly not be bound to refuse such treatment and the relevant 'consent' forms allow for such an eventuality.[5] The harvesting of sperm from a dead man is an extension of this process and is even more controversial.

Many will remember the publicity surrounding the case of *R v Human Fertilisation and Embryology Authority, ex parte Blood* (1997). Mrs Blood arranged for semen to be taken from her husband who was dying in an intensive care unit. A main issue arose from the fact that Mr Blood was not in a position to provide consent of any sort to removal; whether or not he was actually brain dead at the time (see Chapter 13) therefore assumed considerable importance. However, the Court of Appeal avoided this question, and concerned itself, instead, with whether or not the sperm could be used by Mrs Blood in view of the fact that the donor had given no effective consent to the *storage* of his sperm. Strictly speaking, both the storage and the use of his sperm were unlawful. Mrs Blood's case was eventually solved by recourse to European law which provides a right for European citizens to seek medical treatment in other European countries without hindrance. The case is, therefore, a poor precedent to tell us what the precise law is in these circumstances. Whether such a specimen could be used *immediately* and thereby constitute AIH would, we fancy, depend on whether a woman and a comatose man could be said to be receiving treatment together. On the face of things, it seems improbable – but stranger decisions have been made.

Medical ethics and the law may also be faced with the extension of this practice – that is, the removal and use of sperm from a man *after* he has died, a procedure that is becoming increasingly common in the United States. Current legislation in the United Kingdom does not cover such an eventuality but the case of Mrs U (*Centre for Reproductive Medicine v U*) indicates that it is not unlawful provided the consent procedures are satisfied. What Mrs U's case makes increasingly clear, however, is that the courts will uphold these provisions even though they may do so reluctantly; the fact that an argument between the staff and the widow actually arose demonstrates the depth of the objection to posthumous procedures that is felt by some clinics. The case also has considerable additional interest to healthcarers, in that it considers the question of when does counselling become undue influence.

---

[5] An attempt to change this situation was talked out in Parliament. It remains to be seen whether or not a similar Bill will be introduced in the future, since the Government has accepted the recommendations of an independent inquiry into this situation including its recommendation that the man should be able to be registered as the father of the child.

Insemination by donor

A number of persons are affected by the practice of DI and the law controlling it will become clearer if we look at them in turn.

The donor

Donors of sperm are, normally, only accepted when aged between 18 and 55. The treatment centre has a wide mandate to screen donors – especially in respect of genetic and sexually transmitted disease, but also including such imponderables as the donor's 'attitude towards the donation' – and to reject those considered unsuitable. In normal circumstances, a donor who has fathered 10 live children will not be used again. Currently, a donor can be paid £15 together with reasonable expenses for his donation. Very great importance attaches to written consent by the donor as to the specific uses to which his sperm is to be put – it will be seen later that, amongst other things, this governs the paternity of any child that is born as a result of donation.

Non-paternity of the donor is, in fact, ensured twice in the 1990 Act which says that where a donor has given 'effective' consent – that is, consent according to the Act – to the use of his sperm, he is not to be treated as the father of a resulting child. Consent to her insemination by a woman's husband, together with the ethical practice of a licensed clinic, also protects the donor's position.

The donor is guaranteed anonymity, both at the time and in the future, but the Authority is legally bound to keep a record of donors and this will include information as to their identities. The Authority can only release its confidential information as to a donor's identity when a supposed donor is defending an action brought by the child under the Congenital Disabilities (Civil Liability) Act of 1976 which is mentioned again below. The release of non-identifying information is discussed under the heading of 'the resultant child'.

The clinic

It will have been noted that those in charge of the clinic have a duty to select suitable donors, both in a general sense and in respect of the recipients. In choosing a donor, the clinic cannot guarantee a family resemblance but the recipient can express preferences as to the donor's characteristics. The search for a child of 'super intelligence' is not forbidden but it might well cause the clinic to question the motives of those seeking treatment – the possibility of it happening provides one good reason for disallowing competitive payments to donors.

Other associated duties rest on the clinic. In the words of the Code of Practice, it is for centres to ensure that the most up-to-date guidance is followed in testing for infections and that 'all reasonable steps to prevent transmission of a serious genetic disorder are taken'. Against this, the donor's rights to be given or not to be given genetic information about himself must not be forgotten (see Chapter 9). A duty of care extends beyond that which is owed to those under treatment and includes the potential child. Under a new section of the Congenital Disabilities (Civil Liability) Act of 1976, the clinic undertaking the treatment is answerable to the child if the child is born disabled as a result of an act or omission during the selection, storage or use of donated gametes or of an embryo created outside the body. The general rules governing proof of medical negligence, which have been discussed in Chapter 6, would apply – though what would be expected or what would happen if the abnormality was discovered during gestation is currently unclear.

The would-be parents

The couple seeking treatment is clearly hoping to found a family as near to the conventional as can be achieved and, here, the question of paternity of the child is of major importance. It is solved in two ways. Given that the woman is married, her husband will be regarded as the father of the child resulting from any artificial insemination unless it can be shown that he did not consent to the procedure. If she is not married, but she and a man are receiving treatment together, then that man will be regarded as the father of the child provided that the insemination was performed by a person licensed to do so. One or two points as to the meaning of 'receiving treatment together' need clarification here – the difficulty being highlighted by a judge of the High Court, Mr Justice Johnson, who asked, in *Re Q (parental order)* (1996), how can a man be receiving *any* treatment when the cause of the condition being treated lies in the woman? Any confusion has, however, now been cleared up and the phrase is taken to describe the circumstances in which the man and the woman who is inseminated intend to bring up the resulting child as their own or, in the words of Ms Justice Bracewell in *Re B (parentage)* (1996), are engaged in a 'joint enterprise' – in popular terminology, are 'partners'. The word 'partner' is not, however, used in the legislation and it is uncertain how 'permanent' the relationship has to be before the man qualifies for legal paternity – presumably this is something the clinic can consider as part of its concern for the child's need for a father. It is also to be noted that the consent of the 'partner' to the insemination is not specifically required but must, in the circumstances, be at least implied. In either the married or the unmarried state, the paternity conferred is 'for all purposes' – and this would include the completion of the child's birth certificate. For the sake of completeness, it should be mentioned that the Act makes no specific provisions as to paternity in the case of single, unattached women; the general exclusion of the donor as a legal father would, however, apply. Similarly, the Act is silent in respect of homosexual parentage.

Mrs Blood was not the only person to highlight some of the difficulties that can arise in the midst of apparent clarity. Consider the case of another Ms U – reported as *U v W (Attorney-General intervening)* (1997) – whose partner's sperm was of doubtful quality and who, herself, had great difficulty in implanting and retaining embryos that were inserted in her uterus. Hearing of a new treatment, they consulted an Italian clinic where Ms U's eggs were fertilised with sperm from both her partner, Mr W, and an unknown donor. Six embryos were inserted in Ms U and, as a result, she gave birth to twins, neither of which was genetically related to Mr W. Meantime, however, Ms U and Mr W had separated. Was Mr W the legal father of the twins? The judge concluded that Ms U and Mr W were being 'treated together' and that it was this, rather than the form of his consent, which dictated the issue of his paternity. So far, so good – *but* the insemination did not take place in a licensed clinic. It followed from this that Mr W was *not* the legal father – and, in passing, this particular requirement did not transgress European Union law which mandates that professional services should be provided unfettered throughout the Union – an interesting comparison with the judgement in Mrs Blood's case.

Fewer complications are likely when the couple are married and the husband consents to insemination. But what of the husband who does not consent? It has to be said that his position is not easy. We have already seen that the donor will not be held to be the father of the child and the legislation specifically protects him against the possibility of a husband's consent not being obtained. The husband is then in the position of any husband – he is regarded at common law as the father of any child born to his wife. He can rebut this by DNA or other testing for parentage but this also requires consent to testing the child which may not be forthcoming – and, bearing in mind the needs of a child for a father, the courts might be unwilling to enforce such a test. At the end of the day, he may be left with no more than a choice between accepting the position and recourse to the divorce court, though the latter would be by way of his wife's generally unacceptable behaviour, since insemination by donor does not, of itself, constitute adultery.

The resultant child

This is no place to discuss the moral basis for, or the psychological consequences of, DI as they affect the resultant child. We have seen above that his or her birth certificate is now 'normalised' – a fact which distinguishes the DI from the adopted child – and parents who have gone through the mental tensions of DI in search of a child are likely to be particularly devoted to that child. All in all, there is no absolute reason why a child should ever need to know that it was the product of DI. Yet there is a large body of opinion which holds that the child *ought* to know its true parentage. If this be so, we have still to balance such a 'right' against the interests of the donor – and, while the evidence from other countries is equivocal, it is at least possible that donors would be scarce, or more scarce, in the absence of anonymity.

The law is, as a result, a compromise. It has already been noted that the Authority must keep a register of treatment services provided insofar as they relate to identifiable patients, donors or resultant children. A person over the age of 18 can apply to the Authority for notice stating whether or not the information stored in the Register indicates that some person other than one or other of the applicant's apparent parents was his or her genetic parent. If it does do so, and if the applicant has been counselled as to the implications, the Authority must give such information as is required by regulation – but no more. As things stand, the information to be provided is of a very general nature only, and we have seen that disclosure of a gamete donor's name is strictly prohibited. The applicant can be a minor in the event of his or her prospective marriage; in these circumstances, the information given will include the possibility of a genetic relationship between the two parties. It is doubtful if this aspect of the legislation fully satisfies any of the interested parties and it has been decided recently that the provision of such non-identifying information about the applicant's parenthood as he or she requires is subject to Article 8 – the right to respect for private and family life – of the European Convention on Human Rights (R *(on the application of Rose) v Secretary of State for Health* (2002)). The Government has, at the time of writing, issued a consultation document on the subject and it may well be that the regulations will be changed in the near future.

Ovum donation

Ovum donation is, perhaps, the optimal treatment when the woman is sterile – that is, irreversibly unable to produce her own eggs. The theoretical basis for the treatment is, therefore, the same as that for DI with the sexes reversed. It might be supposed that we should be able to repeat the above discussion in explanation of ovum donation, simply substituting 'she' for 'he' and 'her' for 'him' as appropriate. In practice, however, there are some very considerable differences.

The donor

The most obvious of these is that, whereas male gametes are plentiful and easy to harvest, ova are produced sparingly and their recovery demands surgical expertise. Moreover, if this is to be an economical proposition, the ovaries usually must be stimulated to produce a relatively large number of eggs at one time; this is certainly an uncomfortable process which may, in fact, even entail some danger for the donor – although the evidence for this is, at best, incomplete.

Given these side-effects and given, equally, a strong demand for a scarce resource, it is not surprising that exploitation of donors is regarded as a very real danger and, for this reason, the Human Fertilisation and Embryology Authority is deeply concerned as to rewards for egg donation. Currently, a limit of £15, together with reasonable expenses, similar to that available to sperm donors, is placed on egg donation. The practice of 'egg-sharing' – or, effectively, payment for treatment services by way of simultaneous ovum donation – is, however, now allowed. As in every case of gamete donation, this is subject to serious pre-donation counselling. The egg donor cannot be regarded as the mother of any child born as a result of the treatment.

The recipient

This is because the woman who carries or has carried a child – whether this be as a result of natural or assisted means – and no other woman is to be regarded as the mother of that child for all purposes. It will be appreciated that this is particularly important in relation to surrogate motherhood, which is discussed below.

The technique

The second major distinction between sperm and egg donation is that the latter, to be effective, must involve the production of an embryo *in vitro*, and can, therefore, only be carried out by a person licensed to do so – and this despite the fact that the man and the infertile woman are clearly being 'treated together'.

Embryo donation

Embryo donation is to be distinguished from sperm and ovum donation in that both the gametes that constitute the embryo that is to be inserted in the woman's uterus are donated to the couple seeking treatment. The rules as to consent and the legal status of the donors are those that apply both to sperm and egg donation individually. Thus, the recipient woman will always be the mother of the resultant child; fatherhood will, at the same time, depend upon the giving of consent by her husband. Otherwise, egg donation and embryo donation do not need separate consideration.

IN VITRO FERTILISATION

The process of combining sperm and egg *in vitro* is common to several treatments for childlessness. The expression '*in vitro* fertilisation' (IVF) is, however, more often used specifically to imply treatment for blocked Fallopian tubes and it is in that sense that it is discussed here.

Normally, IVF involves the use of gametes from a husband and wife or from partners and, in that sense, the couple are being 'treated together'. However, it also involves the creation of embryos outside the human body and, as in the case of ovum donation, must always be performed by a person licensed to do so.

That having been said, there are no major legal hurdles associated with IVF – inserting an embryo derived from a man and a woman in the uterus of that woman is no more than a complex variation on a normal process. Nonetheless, it involves a number of ethical problems, some of which are associated with the Code of Practice imposed on licence holders and others, more fundamental, which depend on the status that is to be granted to the human embryo.

The Code of Practice

We have seen that the Code of Practice insists on what is, effectively, a screening process as to a woman's – or a couple's – suitability to receive treatment services. Since few of the recommendations are mandatory, the clinic has considerable discretionary powers – and these are more significant in the case of IVF than in, say, DI because the former can *only* be accomplished under licence. Thus, in one well-known case involving a woman who had formerly been a prostitute – *R v Ethical Committee of St Mary's Hospital (Manchester), ex parte H* – the clinic's refusal to provide services was not regarded by the courts as being unreasonable, although it was also clear that the clinic was under no legal *obligation* to refuse treatment. It is left to the individual reader to determine for him or her self whether the resulting temptation for infertile couples to 'shop-around' for treatment services is or is not acceptable.

The overall live birth rate for IVF is about 18 per cent of the treatments given and this stems from some 22 per cent of successful pregnancies. These, however, are very bald figures, which can be influenced by a number of factors. Firstly, the birth rate falls off steadily from a maternal age of 30 and does so fairly dramatically when the women are aged more than 36. The courts have, accordingly, held that discrimination of the grounds of age when selecting cases for treatment is not unreasonable – *R v Sheffield Health Authority, ex parte Seale* (1994). Secondly, both the pregnancy and the live birth rates are dictated by the number of embryos transferred to the womb. There is a major improvement when more than one embryo is used but, despite an increase in the pregnancy rate, the live birth rate is not significantly altered by the use of three rather than two embryos. On the other hand, the use of three embryos greatly increases the generally undesirable likelihood of triplet and quadruplet pregnancies which carry a risk of stillbirth and infant death that is some six times that of singleton pregnancies. The Authority's current guidance is that no more than three embryos should be inserted at one time but the clear preference, including that of the Royal College of Obstetricians and Gynaecologists, is that this should be reduced to two; figures indicate that this is being increasingly followed by clinics. It is, perhaps, worth noting that a woman, who was impregnated with three embryos when she had requested that no more than two should be implanted, received substantial damages following the birth of triplets (*Thompson v Sheffield Fertility Centre* (2000), unreported).

The status of the embryo

In general, IVF results in the creation of more embryos than are actually used. 'Spare embryos' are necessary side-effects of the process, firstly, because an uncertain number of eggs exposed may or may not become fertilised. Secondly, a surplus of embryos provides the opportunity for the pre-implantation diagnosis (PID) of genetic or chromosomal disease.

We should point out here, parenthetically, that some people will object to PID on the grounds that it debases the human embryo in general and discriminates against the disabled in particular. For our part, we suggest that, given the choice, PID is preferable to a late termination of pregnancy on genetic grounds – but that is not an argument that would be universally acceptable. Moreover, the argument is not yet over and has particular relevance in respect of X-linked disease. Assuming IVF is being undertaken within a family known to be at risk from such a condition and that we have no direct method of identifying the presence of the responsible gene, are we entitled to use PID as a method for rejecting all the male embryos that have been created? The legal answer is that we surely are; the moral answer is less certain. We have already drawn attention to a further complication; can a couple use PID to select the sex of their children purely as a matter of preference? The Code of Practice clearly says 'No'. But it has no binding legal force, and we must wait and see what answers are provided by the Authority and the courts. Neither has yet pronounced, simply because no clinic has been prepared to defy the Code of Practice when asked to do so. At the time of writing, however, a case is pending to be heard in the European Court of Human Rights.

But, to return to our main theme – and whatever the reason for the surplus – embryos are being used and discarded at will and the major ethical divide as to the propriety of IVF hinges on the status accorded to those embryos. They clearly have no *legal* right to life as IVF, itself, is perfectly legal given the licensing requirements and United Kingdom law allows for the production and destruction of *in vitro* embryos for research purposes. The argument is, therefore, a *moral* one. Put at its most simple and at its extremes, one side holds that, at the least, such embryos have all the makings of human beings; the other will say that they bear no resemblance to human beings, that they cannot exist independently and that their status is no more than that of human cells in general. Once again, in a book that is primarily concerned with medical *law*, we must leave the provision of what is, effectively, an answer to the unanswerable to the individual reader. We would, however, point out that the disposal of embryos is more than another facet of the abortion discussion (for which see Chapter 10). Whether or not to terminate a pregnancy will be seen to be a matter that is to be decided by the pregnant woman and her medical adviser. The law relating to embryology is, by contrast, directed to parentage and the 1990 Act makes it clear that the creation, use and destiny of pre-implantation embryos are subject to the effective consents of both the sperm and the egg providers.[6] This may, and often does, include their donation or their storage against the possibility of use in the future; as a result, there is no *need* for a 100 per cent wastage of apparently unwanted embryos. To this extent, the human embryo is given some legal protection and the Code of Practice exhorts clinics to take full account of its special status when considering how its development should be brought to an end.

This review of the possible legal consequences of IVF is still not quite complete. We have already noted that more than 5 per cent of live births will end up as triplets or quadruplets even if not more than three embryos are inserted in a given treatment cycle – and the proportion and the multiplicity, will be very much greater if the advice in the Code of Practice as to the number of insertions is disregarded. Is it lawful to reduce such multiple pregnancies to twin or single births by destruction of some within the womb? The answer is 'yes', provided the conditions of the Abortion Act of 1967 are observed – a matter we discuss again in Chapter 10.

SURROGATE MOTHERHOOD

There remain for consideration those 'treatments' that are available for the woman who is childless because of abnormality of the womb, who suffers from persistent miscarriage or who is unable to carry a child by reason of general ill-health. The size of the topic is such that we have isolated surrogate motherhood as a separate subject although it will be seen that it is illogical to do so. We have not the space to discuss the important social and moral arguments – including those relating to the status of women – that dominate our cultural attitudes to surrogacy and, as a result, we are adopting an essentially *medical* approach to this section. This has its advantages in that it emphasises the fact that surrogate motherhood is no more than an aspect of the management of childlessness in a somewhat different guise. Those who oppose surrogate motherhood yet accept IVF must explain why they will discriminate against the woman who is infertile because she has an abnormality of the womb in favour of one who has abnormal Fallopian tubes. Such a position is difficult to maintain – and is probably untenable.

As has already been described, surrogate motherhood can be divided into two major categories. The common version is partial surrogacy in which the surrogate is impregnated, usually by way of DI, by the male of the 'commissioning couple', to whom the resultant child is intended to be returned at birth. In this case, the surrogate is genetically related to the child she carries. The more uncommon variant is full surrogacy – or 'womb-leasing' – in which embryos formed from the gametes of the commissioning couple are inserted in the surrogate's uterus. The surrogate, then, has no genetic relationship to the child she surrenders, whereas the commissioning couple and the child constitute a normally genetically related family. Insofar as such a relationship is generally regarded as desirable, the results of full surrogacy are 'better' than are those of partial surrogacy. Moreover, we have noted above that full surrogacy

---

[6] Which may give rise to difficulty in the event of a change of heart in either following the creation of the embryo. But this aspect is, we believe, beyond the scope of this short book.

is the *medically* preferable treatment in far more conditions than is partial surrogacy – indeed, the latter can be regarded as the treatment of choice for childlessness only when adoption is the sole alternative. On the other hand, partial surrogacy is a simple process, which has probably always been practiced more widely than we imagine. Full surrogacy involves considerable expertise and, since it requires the creation of an embryo *in vitro*, it can only be carried out under licence. There is little wonder, therefore, that partial surrogacy has become the norm for this type of infertility treatment.

Partial surrogacy as a procedure is not controlled by the 1990 Act. True, it involves DI but, as we have seen, DI is subject to licensing only when it is a treatment offered to the public – and the great majority of surrogacies result from private arrangements. As a result, any need for control lies in the control of those *arrangements*, and it is here that we come to the main legal concern about surrogacy in general – that is, the possible commercialisation of the procedure. Seeking to address this particular issue, Parliament enacted the Surrogacy Arrangements Act in 1985 – notably, *before* the wide ranging Act of 1990 – for the specific purpose of making it a criminal offence to profit financially from surrogate motherhood whether it be through initiating or negotiating an arrangement. Advertising for the purpose is also expressly banned. However, while they may not be able to advertise their needs or their potential services lawfully, the principals – i.e. the commissioning couple and the surrogate – are expressly excluded from the criminal sanctions associated with participation. Otherwise, there is nothing unlawful about a private surrogacy arrangement. We will see later that any payments made to the surrogate may seriously jeopardise the future of the family and no arrangement made can be enforced. But the courts that have considered the matter have always been at pains to deny any criticism of those seeking to found a family in this way and, indeed, there is no objection to the use of an agency provided it is one that makes no profit. The Brazier Review Committee has recommended that all such agencies should be licensed, but no action has been taken as yet on this Report. Thus, the law surrounding the status of the principals is a complex mixture of statute and common law which lack of space prevents us from examining other than fairly superficially.

There is no doubt as to the status of the surrogate. She has carried the child and is, therefore, the legal mother of the child irrespective of whether or not it is genetically hers. But suppose she is married, as is often the case? What, then, of her husband? Clearly, he is the legal father of the child by both common and, so long as DI was used, statute law – unless he can show that he did not consent to the procedure. Equally, the commissioning male will not be the legal father, for he has consented to his sperm being used for DI.

However, if the surrogate is not married, then, provided it is a private arrangement, the commissioning male *will* be the child's father as a matter of common law, although, as in any case where an unmarried woman is made pregnant, this might be subject to proof by standard tests for paternity. But we are still not out of the woods – suppose the parties have decided to enlist professional help? They cannot go to their general practitioner for he or she can only act with impunity if the man (the donor) and the woman (the recipient) are being 'treated together' and, although it might look as though it does so, the phrase does not apply to a commissioning male and a potential surrogate because they are not going to bring up the child together. It follows that the only professional assistance available is through a licence holder and, in that case, statute law applies; the commissioning man is a consenting semen donor who cannot, by law, be the father of the child.[7]

The end result of this amalgam of law would be, in general, to the disadvantage of the child and this is anathema to legal policy in the United Kingdom. The situation could be rescued by adoption but this has technical difficulties and is not an entirely satisfactory solution from the child's point of view. Moreover, there is something slightly unreasonable about a couple being forced to adopt a child that is half theirs genetically and something quite absurd in the case of the child who is born as a result of full surrogacy. Parliament, accordingly, introduced the Parental Order.

Briefly, a married couple may apply for a parental order, which allows for a child, who has been carried by a woman other than the receiving woman, to be treated in law as the child of the 'commissioning couple', provided that the gametes of one or both of the commissioning couple were used to bring about the creation of that child. Fairly stringent conditions have to be satisfied:

- the application must be made within 6 months of the birth of the child;
- at the time of the application, the child's home must be with the couple, who, as stated, must be married and at least one of whom must be resident in the United Kingdom;
- each of the couple must be aged 18 or more;
- unless they cannot be found, both the 'legal' father of the child and the surrogate must have given free and unconditional consent to the making of the order;
- the child must be at least 6 weeks old before the surrogate's consent can be valid;
- the Court must be satisfied that no money or other benefit (other than for reasonable expenses incurred) has been given or received by the commissioning couple in respect of the making of the order unless it has been authorised by the court.

It will be seen that any financial transactions virtually inhibit the granting of a parental order save that reasonable expenses are allowed; the court decisions that have been taken indicate that 'reasonable' can be interpreted fairly liberally.[8] A further, and important, distinction from the adoption procedure lies in the fact that the court can adjudge a refusal to accept an adoption order as unreasonable and one which can, accordingly, be overridden; no such judicial power exists in the case of a parental order. It follows that applications for adoption and parental orders are not mutually exclusive; if one fails, the other can still be pursued.

It is, in many ways, surprising how smoothly the great majority of surrogacies are achieved. Nonetheless, it will be appreciated that the complexities are such that disagreements are bound to occur; we will end by considering how the courts will settle disputes. The answer is by no means clear cut for, as we have seen, the terms of any surrogacy contract are unenforceable. As a result, the courts have a relatively free hand. The overriding consideration is the welfare of the child and this will be assessed on a

---

[7] There is nothing to stop him claiming to be the father and proving this by DNA testing, though the court might not always allow the necessary testing of the child if it was not in the child's interests – see *Docherty v McGlynn* (1985).
[8] But the Brazier Committee was clearly concerned about this.

case to case basis – it would, for example, be perfectly legitimate for the court to take the financial status of the parties into consideration. Lying at the heart of the matter, however, is the weight to be placed, on the one hand, on the 'bonding' which takes place between a carrying mother and her child and, on the other, on the significance of a genetic association between a child and its rearers. No rule of thumb can be laid down. The impression is, however, that the courts will tend to support the carrying mother in a dispute involving partial surrogacy and the commissioning couple in a case of full surrogacy. But all considerations are subservient to the ultimate welfare of the child and, in the end, the decision may hinge on little more than the judge's intuition.

CONCLUSION

The conclusion to be drawn from this rather lengthy discussion of the treatment of childlessness is that, perhaps inevitably, the law has settled on a form of compromise – and a compromise between what can be extreme views. Thus, on the one hand, we have a body of opinion which holds that the manipulation of what are seen as human beings in the Petri dish is morally wrong and should be prohibited absolutely. Diametrically opposed are those who believe that reproduction is an intensely personal matter which should be free from bureaucratic interference and left to the discretion of the individuals concerned. Clearly, it is an area where, in the words of the late President Franklin Rooseveldt, you cannot please all the people all the time. The question is – does the current legislation please most of the people most of the time?

We believe that it probably does. Respect for the embryo, as, at least, a potential human being, is maintained by strict general rules which limit the uses to which it can be put, while the interests of those who have contributed to the genetic structure of the embryos are protected by a comprehensive system of consent to their destiny. Limitation of treatment to licensed clinics may appear restrictive of personal autonomy, but it can be seen as little more than ensuring that the childless are treated by the best clinicians available rather than by potential mavericks. Certainly, Parliament has been adamant in excluding commercial elements from the provision of the building blocks of infertility treatments; this is to be expected in the light of a long-standing national opposition to trading in body parts or tissues of any sort (see also Chapter 13).

Experience has shown that there are some aspects of the law which cause difficulty and which do not command majority support, but one of the advantages of the form of legislation adopted is that it is flexible and, as has been shown in the context of cloning, can be modified without great difficulty in the light of experience and in response to changing technical expertise and public attitudes.

CASES REFERRED TO IN THE TEXT

B (parentage), Re [1996] 2 FLR 15.

Centre for Reproductive Medicine v U [2002] Lloyd's Rep Med 259.

Docherty v McGlynn 1985 SLT 237.

Q (parental order), Re [1996] I FLR 369.

R v Ethical Committee of St Mary's Hospital (Manchester), ex parte Harriott [1988] 1 FLR 512.

R v Human Fertilisation and Embryology Authority, ex parte Blood [1997] 2 All ER 687.

R (on the application of Rose) v Secretary of State for Health (2002) 69 BMLR 83.

R (on the application of Quintavalle) v Human Fertilisation and Embryology Authority [2003] 2 ALL ER 105.

R (on the application of Quintavalle) v Secretary of Sate for Health [2002] 2 All ER 625.

R v Sheffield Health Authority, ex parte Seale (1994) 25 BMLR 1.

Thompson v Sheffield Fertility Centre (2000), unreported.

U v W (A-G intervening) [1997] 2 FLR 282.

FURTHER READING

Brazier M. *Surrogacy: Review for Health Ministers of Current Arrangements for Payment and Regulation* (Cm 4068, 1998).

Brazier M. 'Regulating the reproduction business?', *Medical Law Review* 1999; 7: 166.

Dunstan GR. 'The moral status of the human embryo: A tradition recalled', *Journal of Medical Ethics* 1984; 10: 38.

Freeman M. 'Is surrogacy exploitative? in McLean SAM (ed.), *Legal Issues in Human Reproduction*, Gower Publishing Co, 1989.

Hagger L. 'The role of the human fertilisation and embryology authority', *Medical Law International* 1997; 3: 1.

King MB, Pattison P. 'Homosexuality and parenthood', *British Medical Journal* 1991; 303: 295.

Lee RG, Morgan D. *Human Fertilisation and Embryology*, Blackstone Press Ltd, 2001.

McLean SAM. 'Creating postmortem pregnancies: A UK perspective', *Juridical Review* 1999; 323.

Wagner M, St Clair P. 'Are *in vitro* fertilisation and embryo transfer of benefit to all?' *Lancet* 1989; 2: 1027.

9

GENETICS AND PREGNANCY

Most intending parents hope that the foetus they will bring to term will be born healthy. There is nothing in this aspiration to cause concern. We simply want our children to have the best start in life, in the same way as we will try to maximise their opportunities throughout their lives. In the not too distant past, the capacity to influence the health of a future child was very much at the mercy of fate. Modern medicine, however, has been able to make a real contribution to the potential health of embryos and foetuses by warning women about risks during their pregnancy, encouraging healthy behaviour and discouraging dangerous practices.

Rapid advances have also been made in medicine's prenatal diagnostic skills. Testing the cells of the foetus is now a routine procedure in many pregnancies, and this allows prospective parents access to information as to whether or not their child suffers from a range of genetic and chromosomal disorders. Although treatment is seldom available following genetic diagnosis, the fact that a genetic problem has been established offers a woman the choice as to whether or not to continue with the pregnancy. Foetal monitoring can detect distress and mandate a change in the management of birth, and treatment within the womb – or even *in vitro* – designed to correct medical or surgical problems before the birth of the child may soon become commonplace. Despite criticism that pregnancy and childbirth are becoming overly medicalised, the fact is that the capacity to discover at least some aspects of the health status of future children has been a bonus for many people. Even so, the fact that such knowledge is available raises its own ethical concerns.

The rapidly growing mass of information linking physical and mental defects, disorders or ill-health to genetic inheritance has added a new layer to our capacity to uncover potential problems either before establishing a pregnancy or during its course. An increasing number of health problems, including, even, personality traits, are now seen as being genetically linked. This, of course, has the potential to affect reproductive decisions even before a pregnancy is established. Testing of intending parents could lead them, for example, to conclude that their genetic combination is such that parenting should be avoided, or to request that specific tests are carried out either before a pregnancy is established – by using *in vitro* techniques – or at the earliest possible stage in the pregnancy.

GENETICS AND REPRODUCTIVE CHOICES

The completion of the Human Genome Project, coupled with rapid progress in diagnostic capacities, seems set to change the face of reproductive options permanently and irrevocably. What was once left to chance may now become a matter of deliberate choice. Although it is not yet widely used, the ability to select genetic characteristics, or to avoid the transmission of certain inherited conditions, has already influenced our culture.

One fictionalised vision of this can be found in the movie 'Gattaca'. In this film, we were carried forward to a time in which genetic testing of parents, and of foetuses and children, was widespread. People who chose not to seek such testing had so-called 'faith children' and their behaviour was frowned upon. Moreover, the future of faith children was restricted, not simply by the possibility that they might inherit a disorder, but also because they were deemed to be inferior and suited only to certain tasks and employment opportunities. Meanwhile, genetically 'superior' children were given every opportunity to perform at the highest possible levels. Of course, the moral of the film lay in the triumph of the faith baby Eugene who, by dint of personal effort – and a certain amount of dishonesty – succeeded in penetrating the highest levels of his society, thus defeating the genetic pigeonholing which infested it.

Fantasy apart, while the genetics revolution will deliver ever increasing amounts of information to those hoping to reproduce, it has to be said that, for the moment, our diagnostic ability far exceeds our therapeutic capacity; essentially, our available choices are restricted to continuation or termination of pregnancy. This, may, of course, change with the development of gene therapy but, realistically, it is unlikely to do so soon.

Thus far, we have addressed what might be called the 'normal' pregnancy, in which children are conceived as the result of sexual intercourse between their parents. Now, however, assisted reproduction, or the creation of pregnancies by methods independent of sexual intercourse, which we have discussed in the preceding chapter, not only enables those who are sub-fertile or infertile to establish families but also offers new opportunities for genetic testing in the fertile.

The creation of embryos outside the uterus provides the opportunity to establish their sex and genetic make-up at an early stage. Thus, if a couple is at risk of passing on an X-linked disorder, it is possible to implant only female embryos and, thereby, avoid producing an affected child. This technique, known as pre-implantation genetic diagnosis (PID), is likely to be used increasingly often. However, many will see it as a controversial procedure. Although possibly only a minority would dispute the right of people to choose not to risk having a handicapped boy in the circumstances outlined, the inevitable discarding of the male embryos poses a major ethical dilemma.

Moreover, the technique can be used in a variety of situations in which the basis for, and the consequences of, the decision-making are less clear cut. For example, we now can pinpoint some of the genes which may cause cystic fibrosis. This seriously disabling condition will be evident from the time the baby is born and may result in considerable suffering and a shortened life-span. Nevertheless, the mere finding of the gene does not predict the likely severity of the disease nor does it tell us how it would respond to treatment. The question, therefore, is whether or not it is ethically acceptable to use genetic information to prevent the birth of such a child – a question which becomes even more cogent now as effective treatment becomes available, and children born with this condition are living increasingly long lives of better quality. On the other hand, we cannot ignore the interests parents have in making reproductive decisions which are right for them in the circumstances. For example, would it *ever* be reasonable to deny a woman (or couple) the right to decide against having a child suffering from a serious genetic condition, and would the answer be different if the woman (couple) already had one or more similarly affected children?

Such questions pit the 'interests' of future children against the interests of existing individuals whose right of reproductive choice is clearly, albeit often indirectly, recognised. Additional problems are posed by our ability to identify pre-implantation or pre-natally those who will suffer from late-onset conditions, such as Huntington's disease and some breast cancers. If anything, the identification of this group is even more ethically controversial than is the detection of a childhood onset condition. The questions confronting the intending parents in these cases are highly complex. Assuming that he or she lives long enough, a child born with the gene which will undoubtedly lead to its developing Huntington's faces a bleak distant future. On the other hand, that same child may have many years of happy and productive life ahead of it before succumbing to the condition – indeed, a cure may have been discovered before that situation arises. Similarly, detection of the gene linked to breast cancer does not mean that the cancer is bound to develop and, again, therapeutic options are likely to have improved before it appears.

Yet, it is clear that the primary objective of looking for and discovering an adverse genetic inheritance in the embryo is to avoid its implantation and subsequent birth. This is deeply distasteful for many, perhaps particularly for those whose religious or ethical principles lead to a wholehearted condemnation of abortion – for the arguments underlying the morality or immorality of both procedures are not dissimilar. However, despite the objections to such screening, it is not unreasonable to suggest that most people sympathise with, even if they do not wholly support, the right of intending parents to make such decisions on health-related grounds. As will be discussed below, such choices made on other non-health related grounds may be greeted in a less sanguine manner.

DESIGNER BABIES?

Fuelled in part by interest in the media, there is considerable contemporary concern as to the possibility that genetics will provide us with the opportunity to create children who have been positively selected to meet certain, particular, desirable characteristics. Leaving aside the question of negative selection on the basis of health status, parents may also want to give their children the best start in life in other, social, ways. For example, it may be that tall people are generally better regarded socially than small ones. We may have an in-built cultural preference for fair skin, blond hair and blue eyes. We may prefer boys to girls. We may want our child to be beautiful rather than plain, athletic rather than cerebral or in the highest band of intelligence.

Naturally, we probably want all of these, even in an uncontrolled and unregulated pregnancy. The question, however, is: what if it were possible to do this by designing the ideal child, in whatever terms that ideal was framed? Since time immemorial, the primary influence we have been able to bring to bear on the characteristics of our offspring has been through the selection of a mate – it may well be that we are mainly attracted to people because they have physical and intellectual characteristics that we regard as desirable to pass on to our children. To a certain extent, therefore, we already practice, albeit subliminally and somewhat haphazardly, what genetics could now possibly do for us scientifically, and we do not regard this as wrong or contentious.

Although in many cases the relationship between genes and environment is unclear, some characteristics, such as skin, hair and eye colour are more obviously linked to genetic inheritance than are others. The possibility for the future, therefore, is that selection of this sort will become a commonplace, or at least regularly demanded, technique. In a society which values, or claims to value, reproductive freedom, it might be asked what would be wrong with parents making such choices? Unfortunately for those seeking a simple solution to this question, there are – seemingly inevitably – vastly differing approaches to it which lead to diametrically opposed answers.

Arguments against the creation of 'designer babies' range from its potential for disvaluing those who do not meet our cultural ideal to the unfairness of giving these children such an advantage over their peers. Others, however, maintain that every parent strives to achieve this advantage by battling, say, for their children to go to the best schools. Deliberate manipulation to achieve the same result would not, in their view, be any different. In addition, they would argue, the individual child, tailored to its parents' ideal, need not shed a negative light on those others who do not share their characteristics.

It might also be suggested that designing babies in this way treats them as commodities rather than individuals. So, this argument would run, the child is not valued for who he or she is but, rather, for whatever characteristics it has that we think are attractive or desirable. To counter this, it could be said that this happens in nature in any event. Not all parents forge good relationships with their children whose personality, for example, they may find difficult, and many parents will bond best with those children whose attributes they particularly value.

The arguments could go on, but the initial question remains – does the fact that certain biological variations occur naturally make it right deliberately to mimic them artificially? Equally, it could be asked, if we regard it as being ethically right to screen out those embryos suffering from health-related problems, where is the difference if we screen out what can be seen as other 'undesirable' characteristics? Even if firm answers to such questions are not currently available, they must be sought in advance of such choices becoming routinely available, as they may well do in the not too distant future.

Indeed, selection for reasons other than the health of the future child has already been the subject of medical, ethical and now legal interest. Perhaps the first case to come to the attention of the general public was that of the Masterton family. Tragically, the Mastertons – who have four sons – lost their only daughter in an accident. They wish to have another daughter, by using IVF, in order to re-establish the gender balance in their family. In October 2000, the Human Fertilisation and Embryology Authority rejected their request for authorisation of the procedure on the grounds that sex selection for social reasons was not acceptable under the terms of its code of practice. The Mastertons continue their fight, probably boosted by developments elsewhere which suggest that the harm perceived by the HFEA (and, perhaps, the public) is ethereal. The American Society for Reproductive Medicine, for example, recently proposed that sex selection on social grounds was not unethical and should be permitted.

The focus of contemporary interest in this area has now moved beyond sex selection. Genetic testing has the capacity, as we have said, to identify embryos which might – if implanted – result in the birth of a child affected with a particular genetic condition. Genetic medicine can, however, also detect genetic compatibility, an expertise that has advanced to the stage at which it is possible to undertake tissue typing to detect whether or not, for example, one person could be a suitable donor of tissue, such as bone marrow, for transplantation. Thus, those suffering from particular genetic conditions may receive life-saving treatment. This is not a new technology – it lies, for example, at the heart of the transplantation programme. However, the combined resources of the assisted reproduction and the genetics revolutions now make it possible to select embryos for their compatibility with others. This has proved to be extremely controversial and has ultimately involved the HFEA and the courts of law. Two cases that arose recently highlight the grounds for this dispute very clearly.

Raj and Shahana Hashmi have a son, Zain, who suffers from thalassaemia. They sought, and ultimately gained, the authority of the HFEA to use IVF to establish another pregnancy, to tissue type the embryos and to select for implantation only those embryos which would be compatible donors for Zain. Shortly after this decision, the Whittaker family, whose son, Charlie, suffers from Diamond-Blackfan anaemia were refused permission to do what was effectively the same thing.

The HFEA, however, was able to identify differences, which explained the apparently conflicting decisions. In the case of the Hashmis, the use of PID was considered permissible in terms of their remit because the embryos were selected because they, themselves, would not suffer from thalassaemia. In other words, the decision about which embryo(s) to implant was taken on the basis of the health of the embryo(s), and the value to the existing child was arguably, although unrealistically, deemed to be secondary. In the case of the Whittaker family, however, there is no genetic test for Charlie's condition and therefore the decision as to which embryo(s) to implant would not be based on their future health, but would be taken virtually exclusively in Charlie's interests.

The distinction between the two cases might appear slender but, while the HFEA deemed the first to be permissible within their remit, the second was thought to be moving into uncharted territory. Interestingly, the HFEA was roundly criticised for the Hashmi decision by the House of Commons Select Committee on Science and Technology. What was criticised was not so much the decision itself, but the basis upon which it was made. The Select Committee felt that a step too far had been taken by a body which, in its view, had exceeded its mandate and authority.

The Select Committee were later proved to be technically right. In a case brought by Josephine Quintavalle, a 'pro-life' campaigner, the High Court decided in December 2002 that the HFEA had, in fact, exceeded its authority in authorising the Hashmis to proceed with embryo selection. This, however, was on the rather legalistic grounds that the remit of the HFEA restricted it to providing services for the purposes of assisting women to carry children. This did not include the provision of services designed only to provide a source of compatible tissues for the existing child of a fertile woman.

The High Court did not, therefore, condemn the procedure *per se*; the ethics of this remain as undecided as they were before the case was heard. It has, in fact, been announced while this book was at proof stage, that an appeal has been successful although the reasons have not yet been reported. Meantime, the Whittaker family travelled to the US for treatment, and happily announced a pregnancy by which they hope to obtain the treatment for their son that they sought in the UK.

There is no doubt that these are hard cases. The concerns which we have already highlighted about creating 'designer' babies are undoubtedly real and extend further than we have as yet discussed. On the one hand, for example, it is hard for many people to imagine that harm results from the creation of a child with the capacity to give life to a sibling. Others would, however, question the morality of creating a new person whose sole purpose in life, it might be held, is to provide a readily available therapeutic source. The issue is enormously complex, and the HFEA – as we write – is conducting a further consultation exercise: 'Sex Selection: Choice and Responsibility in Human Reproduction'.

INTERGENERATIONAL JUSTICE

One further matter has to be considered before addressing the legal consequences of the genetics revolution. This is ideally expressed in the following quotation from Fletcher and Wertz:

> The completion of the human genome project will provide a basis for acting on a moral obligation for *future* generations, a claim that has appeared weak in the past. A generation *with* such knowledge who neglected to use it to minimize the risks in reproduction could hardly be said to respect the requirements of intergenerational justice.

This concept seems likely to become increasingly credible as the possibility of *eradicating* genetic disease appears on the horizon. Essentially, what is being said is that we have an *obligation* to avoid producing genetically compromised children when methods to prevent this happening are available. What we have hitherto seen as a form of choice may become a matter of duty.

Although it was possibly intended to deal primarily with environmental risks, the attention of the international community has recently focussed on the kinds of responsibilities which we may have to those who come after us. For example, the UNESCO *Declaration of the Responsibilities of the Present Generations Towards Future Generations* states that: 'The present generations have the responsibility of ensuring that the needs and interests of future generations are fully safeguarded.' The Declaration continues: 'The present generations should strive to ensure, with due respect for the dignity of the human person, the maintenance and perpetuation of humanity (recognizing that the role of women is central to this process). Consequently, the nature and form of human life must not be undermined in any way whatsoever.'

This Declaration could be seen as imposing an obligation on present individuals to secure the best possible genetic inheritance for future generations. Thus, it could be argued, as in the film 'Gattaca', that we should not allow a biological lottery to determine the genetic health of our children and our children's children. If we have the capacity to identify rogue genes, and we have the means to eradicate them, we should not be allowed to make up our own minds as to whether or not we will do so. Rather, we have a duty to ensure that we only transmit the best genes. To do anything else might be seen as reproductively irresponsible.

This complicates our earlier discussion which was concerned with the question of choice; imposing an obligation of intergenerational justice could be taken to invalidate any choice we make which does not lead to the elimination of sub-standard genes in our children. Although this may seem somewhat far-fetched, it is all too easy to argue in support of it. The state, for example, will have an interest in maximising health and the more we correlate disability with genetics, the easier it is to claim that healthcare resources should not be stretched by people being given unfettered discretion to have affected children. Thus it could it be said that we not only have an obligation to the individual child to ensure his or her best genetic inheritance but that we, also, have an obligation to our community not to 'waste' healthcare resources when this can be avoided.

Clearly, then, genetics can have – now and in the future – a powerful impact both on the original decision to reproduce and on the course of any pregnancy. These consequences will be primarily personal and ethical, but they may also be legal, and it is to this aspect that we now turn.

GENETICS, PREGNANCY AND THE LAW

Although conditions are likely to change, the consequences of genetic technology for people's legal rights are rather limited at the present time. As things stand, the interface between genetics and the law is concentrated on genetic testing and on the treatment of the foetus before birth.

Wrongful birth and wrongful life

Whenever genetic testing and/or foetal treatment are offered, it is possible that either the test result will be misread or misreported or that something may go wrong with the treatment. In either circumstance, people may seek to recover damages for any harm resulting. As we have already seen, it is not easy to succeed in a negligence action but it may, nonetheless, provide a route to compensation. The question is; who would have a claim in these circumstances?

The child

Does a child have a right of action against a person committing an error if he or she is born suffering from a genetic condition which was tested for, either before or during pregnancy, but the test result was misinterpreted in some way or was negligently performed? This is a difficult question to answer.

It might seem self-evident that the child is entitled to compensation if it can be shown that the tester has been negligent. However, as will be remembered from our earlier discussion in Chapter 6, a link between the negligence and the harm caused must be shown before damages can be awarded. It is difficult to identify such a link where a condition is substantially or wholly genetic in origin. The negligent management may have prevented parents from choosing to terminate the pregnancy but it did not *cause* the child's condition. In other words, the only 'harm' that the child can show is that he or she was born suffering from a genetic condition. This is what is called an action for 'wrongful life' and it has been consistently held in the courts of the United Kingdom that no such right of action currently exists – and, in fact, only one very unusual French case has been accepted in the courts of the European Union.

The reasons for this are essentially based on public policy. As we will see later in our discussion of end of life decisions, the law starts from the position that life is sacrosanct, that it is a 'good' thing, even when it is painful or unpleasant. Thus, policy would make it very difficult to accept that it can ever be a recognisable legal wrong to have been born, even with a debilitating condition. An action can never be based on not having been aborted if it is held that life is always a blessing.

We believe, however, that there may well be reasons to believe that this situation might change in the future. The reason for an extension of genetic screening, as will probably occur, is, presumably, to eradicate more harmful genetic conditions. If this is accepted, it could be argued that we are in fact recognising that life with a genetic condition *might* amount to a harm. This at least seems logical, although whether or not the law will adopt this position remains to be seen. Even so, it is possible that the adoption of screening programmes would signify a change in policy – from one which claims to value all life, to one which seeks to reduce the pool of harmful genes in the population as a whole. It could, of course, be said that there is nothing new in this; the routine screening of pregnancies in the UK for congenital problems already does this. It is well accepted that the purpose of pre-natal screening is to provide the option of pregnancy termination. Indeed, in some cases, it is clear that this is not so much an option as an anticipated outcome of an adverse finding.

However, not even a change in policy could avert the legal problems surrounding the actual cause, which would need to be established before such an action could succeed. Things might be different if the child's condition were one which demonstrably owed much to its environment, with a genetic base contributing no more than a predisposition to the condition. Let us imagine that a child is born suffering from a genetic predisposition to a condition such as phenylketonuria which would not materialise if the child were to eat a certain diet or were to avoid certain chemical or other hazards. In this scenario, a failure to identify or impart the available information correctly could result in an avoidable condition actually occurring. The child might, then, be well able to trace a causal link between the negligent failure to warn and the onset of the condition. This case differs from the usual concept of wrongful life, and would stand more chance of success, because the child is not claiming that he or she should not have been born but, rather, that he or she would not have suffered a particular harm had his or her parents been told how to prevent it occurring.

The parents

What legal rights might parents have in these circumstances? If adverse genetic information is not disclosed, or is reported wrongly, the consequence for the parents will, of course, be that they are denied the chance to opt for termination of pregnancy; they will then have the added costs, both emotional and economic, of bringing up a handicapped child.

An action in negligence of this sort is one for 'wrongful birth' and it has been raised successfully in the United Kingdom on a number of occasions. In such cases, the parents are claiming recompense for the costs involved in bringing up a child whose birth they would have avoided had they known of its condition. Such an action is to be distinguished from the closely allied claim for 'wrongful pregnancy'.

The latter arises from a situation in which one parent has been sterilised in order to avoid subsequent pregnancies and the operation has been unsuccessful. Often, people have completed their family and have made a decision that they do not wish to have another child. An action in negligence can then arise if the sterilisation has been undertaken negligently or the risk of its not being permanent has been inadequately conveyed to the couple (see Chapter 4). It will be seen that the wrongful birth action differs from one for wrongful pregnancy in that the former must be associated with congenital abnormality – whether that be genetic, chromosomal or multifactorial; the latter, however, refers to the birth of *any* child, including one that is entirely healthy. Strictly speaking, therefore, the wrongful pregnancy case is misplaced in a chapter devoted to congenital disease. Nonetheless, as we have said, the two circumstances share many similarities. Moreover, of course, there is no reason why a child born following an unsuccessful sterilisation operation should not also be genetically compromised – thus, there are good reasons for discussing what is an important aspect of medical law at this point.

Several 'wrongful pregnancy' actions have been heard in our courts in the past and damages have been awarded. Importantly, also, the courts have firmly held that there is no obligation on people to minimise their loss by terminating the 'unwanted' pregnancy; equally significantly, damages have been awarded for the birth of both disabled and healthy children.

However, a recent case, which reached the House of Lords, has changed what had for a long time been accepted law. In this case, the parents, Mr and Mrs McFarlane, had completed their family and Mr McFarlane underwent a vasectomy. Having later been assured that his sperm count was negative, he and his wife resumed sexual relations without using contraception. Mrs McFarlane later became pregnant and gave birth to a healthy daughter.

The McFarlanes claimed compensation for the emotional and physical suffering which Mrs McFarlane had to endure as a result of the pregnancy, as well as for costs associated with bringing up the child. As we have said, a number of previous cases had considered this question and, in some, compensation had been awarded in recognition of the fact that – no matter how healthy, and no matter how much loved the child might be – the parents had actively sought to avoid having to bear these costs by means of sterilisation. The costs had been seen as a foreseeable result of negligence.

In the McFarlane case, however, the House of Lords concluded that, while damages could be awarded for the pain and suffering of pregnancy and childbirth, they could not be extended to cover the costs of bringing up a healthy child. Despite the diversity of the judges' given reasons, it is fairly obvious that this judgement was essentially based on policy considerations. It has been argued by many for some time that costs should not be recoverable in this sort of case because, amongst other things, to do so would suggest that a healthy child is seen as an expense rather than a blessing. It has also been suggested that the child would be horrified to discover in later life that its parents had tried to be compensated for its birth. Others, on the other hand, would point to the fact that the parents had tried to avoid the pregnancy and that they should be helped with the additional pecuniary consequences, even although they may very much love the child. This would not mean that the child is the subject of a financial transaction, but, rather, is a common sense approach to the practical problems facing the parents.

In the event, since the House of Lords is the senior civil court in the United Kingdom, it seems that it will be impossible in the future for parents to obtain compensation for costs associated with bringing up a healthy child. Although many would see this as doubtful justice, such costs will not be met by the person whose negligence caused the circumstances in which the pregnancy occurred. It is, however, noteworthy that the House of Lords would not exclude the possibility of such damages were the child to be born handicapped for any reason. This lacuna has now been filled by the case of Mrs Parkinson in which it was decided that, in that event, the parents can recover the *difference* between the costs of bringing up the handicapped child and those that would result from rearing a healthy child. Somewhat innovatively, it has also been held in the case of Mrs Rees that a disabled *parent* who sustains an unwanted pregnancy can be compensated to the extent that her own disability contributes to the extra expenses of bringing up a child. Mrs Rees' case is, however, due to be argued in the House of Lords.

INTERVENTIONS BEFORE BIRTH

The adjustment of compensation in respect of negligence is more simple when considering treatment or diagnostic invasion of the foetus before birth. A straightforward negligence action can arise if a child is born following such therapeutic or investigative procedures and has been harmed as a result. However, the child would not be able to sue if, say, the investigation was for a genetic – or any congenital – condition, the existence of which is the cause of the harm complained of as once again the negligent action did not *cause* the condition. He or she might, however, succeed in obtaining damages for any additional harm, such as disfigurement, that had been caused during the treatment.

Where this would differ from the normal negligence action (for which, see Chapter 6) is that the child would be suing for damage which occurred before it was born. It is a legal premise that the foetus and the embryo do not have any legal standing – they are not legal persons. It is also generally agreed that, if an action is to be brought, there must be a legal person who has been harmed. This apparent paradox was brought firmly into the public arena by the tragedy of thalidomide – which is a good example of congenital disease resulting from pure environmental factors.

An unusual increase in the number of cases of phocomelia – or incomplete development of the foetal limbs – became apparent throughout the world in the late 1960s. Suspicions as to the cause of this finally centred on the drug thalidomide. This drug was an effective anti-nauseant that was marketed as being safe for pregnant women to take. Evidence suggested, however, that women who had taken it in order to alleviate the 'morning sickness' of pregnancy were at significant risk of giving birth to deformed children. Although the company which marketed the drug never conceded that it did in fact cause the harm complained of, an *ex gratia* payment was eventually made to the affected families after an intense media campaign.

Quite apart from the personal tragedies which resulted, the incident also raised interesting and challenging legal issues. As we have already said, a *person* must be harmed before an action for personal injury can be raised. Thus, even if it was accepted that thalidomide had actually caused the deformities, it was not clear whether or not the children could sue for the harm, which had occurred before they became legal persons. In other words, had they taken the case to court, it might have been thrown out before the problems of negligence and causation could be considered.

In the aftermath of this tragedy, the Law Commissions in England and Wales and in Scotland were invited to consider whether or not a right of action did arise in the circumstances. As they reached slightly different, although analogous, conclusions, it is worth briefly considering them separately.

England and Wales

The nature of the legal system in England and Wales is such that it relies on precedent. Thus, the Law Commission was obliged to search for any previous cases which were in point. It was, at the time, able to identify only two Commonwealth cases which appeared to suggest that an action would be competent and it concluded that, for the avoidance of all doubt, it would be preferable to legislate so as to clarify the position once and for all. The result was the Congenital Disabilities (Civil Liability) Act 1976.

This Act gives a right to sue the negligent individual to children who are harmed as a result of injury before birth. The right, however, derives not from a foetal 'right' but, rather from the rights of the parents. Thus, a duty of care must have been owed to the parents before the action will arise. This means, also, that the child's claim may be reduced if the parent(s) agree to accept a risk. The English legislation also prohibits a child from suing its mother – unless the harm results from a motor vehicle offence, where the mother will be covered by insurance.

Scotland

Scots law is, in part, based on a tradition that allows the Scottish courts to utilise principle rather than precedent when addressing novel questions. The Scottish Law Commission concluded that, although there had been no previous cases in Scots Law, if it was in the interests of the child to be deemed to have been alive at the time the harm occurred, then Scots Law would place no barrier in the way of making that assumption. Thus, no legislation was needed. Simply put, the legal presumption should be in favour of recovery when harm can be shown. Interestingly, there is no reason to believe that a child, under Scots law, cannot sue its mother. In addition, the right given in Scotland is a right of the child him or herself. The vagaries of law-making are illustrated by the fact that it was later demonstrated in the case of *Burton v Islington Health Authority* (1992) that the Scottish provisions would have prevailed in England and Wales. The Law Commission thought, however, that it was better to be safe than sorry and the point is, now, of academic interest only.

CONCLUSION

It can be seen that, although the problems which might arise as a result of the increased focus on genetics in pregnancy are not entirely novel, the drive to increase genetic testing and gene therapy *in vitro* and *in utero* will pose additional questions for the law. As we have indicated, it may well be that the availability of testing, for example, will add some weight to calls for recognition of wrongful life actions. It may also require re-evaluation of current law on wrongful birth actions. And, of course, it seems set to expand the liability of doctors. A parallel and seemingly inescapable opportunity for accident and negligence arises with each new technique or other development in medicine. The impact of the genetics revolution will be no different.

CASES REFERRED TO IN THE TEXT

Burton v Islington Health Authority [1992] 3 All ER 833.

McFarlane v Tayside Health Board [1999] 4 All ER 961.

Parkinson v St James and Seacroft University Hospital NHS Trust [2001] 3 All ER 97.

R (Quintavalle) v Human Fertilisation and Embryology Authority [2003] 2 All ER 105.

Rees v Darlington Memorial Hospital NHS Trust [2002] 2 All ER 177.

FURTHER READING

Brownsword R, Cornish WR, Llewelyn M. (eds), *Law and Human Genetics: Regulating a Revolution*, Oxford, Hart Publishing, 1998.

Buchanan A. *et al. From Chance to Choice*, Cambridge University Press, 2000.

Callus T. ' "Wrongful life" a la Francaise', *Medical Law International* 2001; 3: 117.

Dickens BM. 'Can sex selection be ethically tolerated?', *Journal of Medical Ethics* 2002; 28: 335.

Fletcher JC, Wertz DC. 'An international code of ethics in medical genetics before the human genome is mapped', in Bankowski Z., Capron A. (eds), *Genetics, Ethics and Human Values: Human Genome Mapping, Genetic Screening and Therapy*, xxiv CIOMS Round Table Conference, 1991, p. 103.

House of Commons Science and Technology Committee, Fourth Report of Session 2001–2002, *Developments in Human Genetics and Embryology*, HC 791.

McLean SAM. 'A moral right to procreation? Assisted procreation and persons at risk of hereditary genetic disease', in Haker H, Beyleveld D. (eds), *The Ethics of Genetics in Human Procreation*, Aldershot, Ashgate, 2000, 13–27.

Mason JK. 'Wrongful pregnancy, wrongful birth and wrongful terminology', *Edinburgh Law Review* 2002; 6: 46.

Michael M, and Buckle S. 'Screening for genetic disorders: Therapeutic abortion and IVF', *Journal of Medical Ethics* 1990; 16: 43.

Nuffield Council on Bioethics. *Genetic Screening: Ethical Issues*, 1993.

10

TERMINATION OF PREGNANCY

We use the words 'termination of pregnancy' rather than 'abortion' for three main reasons. First, abortion can be confused with miscarriage or the unexpected and unintended loss of the foetus due to natural processes; what we are discussing here is the intended ending of a pregnancy which would otherwise be expected to progress normally. Secondly, abortion is identified in the minds of many people as criminal abortion – that is, abortion performed or attempted outside the medical arena. And, finally, and on much the same grounds, we believe that the word 'abortion' is highly emotive. Its use is probably responsible for the sometimes passionate approach that is adopted to legal termination of pregnancy – and it is the *legal* termination of pregnancy that is our main focus of attention.

On the other side of the coin, it might be questioned why we devote a whole chapter to the subject. 'Surely,' it will be said, 'we have had an Abortion Act[1] for over 30 years. Its working well, there is no problem' – and this is true, but only up to a point. We have been spared the violence associated with abortion that we have seen developing in the United States only because the British have, fortunately, been able to look at the problems in a reasoned way, recognising that, within a diverse public, we must find a middle way between extreme positions. We have made it clear throughout this book that nothing in ethics – nor in medical ethics as interpreted by the law – is beyond dispute; the structure of medical ethics is not that of rules but, rather, that of a discourse within which widely differing views can be held and can be justified. It is fair to say that this is more true of the subject matter of this chapter than of any other and we suspect that, despite the apparent absence of generalised open hostility to the present legal situation, this variability is to be found as much among healthcare professionals as it is among legal ethicists. It is because we see termination of pregnancy as such a prime example of the interrelationship of law, ethics and medical ethics that we look at the subject in special depth.

---

[1] It is not generally appreciated that the Act started as the Medical Termination of Pregnancy Bill and the name Abortion Act was adopted only at the last gasp of Parliamentary debate.

Essentially, attitudes to the deliberate termination of pregnancy depend, on the one hand, on an appreciation of foetal status and of the foetus' 'right to life' and, on the other, on how far one supports the overriding importance of personal autonomy – which has been discussed in Chapter 4 – and, particularly, a woman's autonomous right to use her own body as she wishes. Both these concepts need to be examined before the response of the law to a difficult situation can be considered.

FOETAL INTERESTS

Any defence of foetal interests – or of what are loosely called 'foetal rights' – depends on establishing what constitutes a human person. The important consideration here is that of 'personhood', for it is this which distinguishes a human being from human tissue. Unarguably, human tissue is 'human' in that it has the necessary content and format of human DNA but, while that tissue may well have sentimental value for some, few would hold that it deserves special treatment by virtue of its chemical make-up alone.

For many, the starting point of personhood will be the union of the sperm and the egg to form the zygote – the process of conception. This is generally regarded as the standpoint of the Roman Catholic Church – although it was adopted by the Church only during the 19th century. The argument behind this runs that a manifest adult human person cannot have become one without, first, being a zygote; personhood, therefore, is a continuum of which the zygotic stage is no more and no less than the first phase. Despite its religious basis, the proposal is not without general support; the Declaration of Geneva, which is the modern equivalent of the Hippocratic Oath, says: 'I will maintain the utmost respect for human life from its beginning'. Human life would certainly include the human embryo but, much as in the case of human tissue, it is clear that human life is not necessarily the same as human personhood; moreover, to show respect is not an absolute requirement but is one that allows for a balancing of attitudes. Stronger positive arguments against the personhood of the zygote can, however, be mounted. In the first place, an untold number of zygotes – or, if it is preferred, pre-embryos – are lost as part of the natural reproductive cycle; it would be absurd to see the normal menstrual period as potentially indicating the death of a human 'person'. Secondly, the zygote or pre-embryo has no potential future life until it is implanted within the womb. Finally, and on a more practical note, it has been seen in Chapter 8 that programmes for the relief of childlessness would virtually cease were the early embryo regarded as a 'creature in being' – or a human person. At the same time, however, it will be realised that this forms the basis for the Roman Catholic Church's opposition to IVF treatment as a whole.

What, then, of the implanted embryo? Many of the arguments outlined above will apply save that, now, it has the *potential* for human personhood. Given the freedom to do so, it will develop into a full-term foetus and will join the human community at birth – and the fact that it becomes a potential human being at this point is the main plank on which many found their opposition to termination of pregnancy at *any* stage of foetal development.

The importance once attributed to quickening as a measure of a significant change in the status of the foetus should be mentioned for historical reasons. Before the 19th century, the law protecting a woman who was 'quick with child' was markedly different from that relating to early pregnancy. Quickening, however, is a product of maternal sensation and foetal activity – it cannot be assessed by an outsider and is, therefore, useless as a *general* measure of development, although it may well provide a very significant moment for the individual pregnant woman. The modern equivalent to quickening is viability – or that point in development at which the foetus, given the need, would be capable of existing outside the womb.

Viability is essentially an American term which springs from what is probably the world's best known legal case related to abortion – *Roe v Wade*, which was heard in 1973. Put simplistically, the American Supreme Court divided pregnancy into three trimesters. In the first, the American Constitution was held to give a woman full control over her own body; in the second, the State could intervene in a pregnancy in the interests of the pregnant woman – it could, for example, control the places where terminations could be carried out; in the third, the foetus was considered to be viable and the State could, then, intervene on its behalf if necessary. The Supreme Court left the definition of viability to the medical profession – probably wisely as the concept of viability is innately difficult, depending, as it does, not only on the age of the foetus but also on the conditions under which it was born and on the medical facilities that are available to assist its survival. To an extent, therefore, the definition of 'foetal viability' will alter as medical expertise improves; nonetheless, it is of profound importance in America in respect of both the civil and the criminal law.

The United Kingdom legislators and judiciary, however, think in terms of the foetus which is capable of being born alive rather than of one which is viable. At first glance, these seem to be much the same thing. However, in the most significant of the relevant court cases – *C v S* (1987), in which a father sought to prevent the termination of a pregnancy on the grounds of foetal maturity – capability of being born alive was, effectively, defined as the ability of the newborn to exist by the use of its own lungs with or without the help of a ventilator. While it is difficult to establish this point when the child is in the womb, it has the conceptual advantage of setting a standard which depends entirely on the anatomic and physiological development of the foetus – a milestone that can be placed, in general, at about the 23rd week of gestation.

Thus, it is difficult, if not impossible, to isolate a specific point in time at which we can bestow 'personality' on the foetus which will, at the same time, satisfy everyone. What does appear, however, is the development of something of a continuum in which the foetus is given increasing recognition as it reaches maturity and this is also reflected in the legal protection it receives from the law in the United Kingdom, which is virtually non-existent in the early stages of foetal life. This was encapsulated in the words of the judge in the very important case of *Paton v British Pregnancy Advisory Service Trustees* (1978), in which a husband was attempting to prevent his wife terminating her pregnancy:

> 'There can be no doubt, in my view,' said the judge, 'that in England and Wales the foetus has no right of action, no right at all, until birth'.

This denial of status to the foetus, which applies in both the criminal and the civil law, is certainly accepted throughout the Commonwealth. However, as we will see later, the normal foetus of 24 weeks' gestation is protected in the United Kingdom against deliberate abortion of the pregnancy unless termination is needed for the avoidance of a risk of grave damage to the health or to the life of its mother. Moreover, anyone who intentionally kills a foetus that is capable of being born alive is, at least in England and Wales, guilty of the offence of child destruction – this being by virtue of the Infant Life (Preservation) Act 1929.[2]

Even so, none of this identifies the foetus as a *legal* person. That status is reserved for the living child that has been fully born – not even the child that is in the process of being born can successfully claim legal personhood. Yet, despite this, it must not be supposed that either the moralists or the lawyers adopt a wholly cavalier attitude to the status of the unborn child. The difficulty lies in defining any reservations in the face of the rigid legal position, and this is bound to lead to uncertainties. Thus, we have the Warnock Committee[3] holding that the human embryo is, of itself, deserving of a special status and entitled to some protection in law – a protection which, as we have seen in Chapter 8, is provided by limiting those who may manipulate the embryo. As to the foetus, the Polkinghorne Committee[4] considered that the living human foetus should be accorded a profound respect. Perhaps, however, it is the law itself which has come closest to undermining its own rule. A very senior Scottish judge said, in *Hamilton v Fife Health Board* (1993) which involved the death of a child following injury in the womb:

> It is perfectly common in ordinary speech to refer to a child in the womb as 'he', 'she', 'him' or 'her' ... it was this child who sustained injuries to his person

while, as to England, the House of Lords, in *A-G's Reference No. 3 of 1994*, refused to accept the Court of Appeal's description of a foetus as 'no more than an appendage of its mother' and acknowledged it to be a 'unique organism' – the precise status of which was, unfortunately, left unspecified.

Nonetheless, the law remains crystal clear that the foetus has no rights of itself – such rights as it has only come into operation when it is born. It is, however, equally clear that damage to a foetus becomes damage to a person – and, therefore, subject to litigation – once that foetus survives to infancy; this is a matter of common law in both the civil and criminal spheres and, in the former, is backed up in England and Wales by the Congenital Disabilities (Civil Liability) Act 1976. Thus, we are left with the rather strange anomaly that, legally speaking, it is safer to kill a foetus than to injure it – although its *parents* might have a right of action in either event.[5]

WOMEN'S RIGHTS

The ability to control reproduction is central to the advocacy of women's rights. It is an integral part of feminist philosophy that women should be free to be 'pro-choice'

[2] There is probably such an offence in Scotland but it is an innominate one covered by the common law.
[3] The Warnock *Committee of Inquiry into Human Fertilisation and Embryology* was responsible for considering the whole future of assisted reproduction as long ago as 1984.
[4] Which was set up to consider experimentation using foetuses: *Review of the Guidance on the Research Use of Fetuses and Fetal Material* (1989).
[5] However, this is subject, in England and Wales, to the Infant Life (Preservation) Act 1929 (see above) under which the fact that a foetus was of 28 or more weeks' gestation constitutes evidence that it was capable of being born alive and is, therefore, automatically protected against being killed.

in relation to pregnancy and its prevention, whether this be by any means from, say, abstinence from sexual intercourse to the termination of a pregnancy of any duration. This, however, is not a specific and limited right but, rather, it is to be seen as an essential component to the recognition of women as equal partners in society – legal control of pregnancy devalues pregnant women by comparison not only with men but also with non-pregnant women. Even so, very few of those arguing for the importance of women's rights would suggest that the foetus merits no respect at all. Rather, it is a question of how much respect is to be given and at what point it is to be applied when balanced against the woman's autonomy or basic interests – and the feminist position is, then, very clear. As one of the present authors has written elsewhere: 'Showing respect for the embryo/foetus at the expense of women's rights is a monumental misunderstanding of the concept of respect'.

It is central to this argument that women must be permitted to make decisions to terminate or continue with a pregnancy free from outside controls and it is of interest that, in contrast to what we have already seen as something of a swing of the pendulum towards conferring some form of personhood on the foetus, this 'woman's right' has now been openly recognised by the law – albeit not directly in association with abortion. We have already mentioned the case of *Re S* (1992) in which, for the first time in England, a senior judge ordered a caesarean section on a woman in obstructed labour who was refusing the operation on religious grounds. A small string of similar decisions followed until 1997, when the first of two such cases – *Re MB* – was referred to the Court of Appeal. The Court then declared very firmly, and reiterated in *St George's Healthcare NHS Trust* (1998), that a woman carrying a foetus is entitled to the same degree of respect for her wishes as is anyone else and that this applied even although it might result in the death or serious handicap of the foetus she was bearing – the autonomy of the woman was placed above any interests of the foetus, including that of being born alive (see Chapter 5 for further discussion).

It is, of course, possible to interpret these decisions in many ways. At one extreme, they can be seen as a major victory for women's rights; at the other, they represent an inexcusable waste of human life. But, whatever one's reaction, it is clear that they typify the close relationship between medical practice and women's reproductive choice and it is the 'medicalisation' of the latter which underlies persistent calls for changes in abortion law – a law which follows a remarkably common pattern throughout the Western world.

History indicates that there was very little demand for the legal control of pregnancy until it evolved as a prominent issue in the early 19th century. It is also true that, at much the same time, medicine was developing a scientific foundation and, as a result, doctors – who were entirely male – were acquiring ever increasing powers. Thus, a school of thought has developed which holds that it was this drive for medical power that was behind the movement in favour of legal control. There is, however, no need to invoke such a causative relationship. Medicine itself was emerging from a state of quackery and was developing a set of moral values of its own – a main feature of which was a strong feeling that a doctor's primary purpose was to preserve life. A growing religious belief in the humanity of the foetus is another part to be fitted into the social jig-saw of the time and there is little doubt that these two developments were mutually supportive. But, be that as it may, there is no compelling reason to suppose that the medical profession wished to dominate women. As we mention below, it is just as likely, or more likely, that it was concerned to protect women from the amateur abortionist and this was almost certainly the main motivation behind the first prohibitive legislation which was introduced in 1813. The pity of it was that, in the absence of any legal alternative, the result of the legislation was precisely opposite to that intended. Women wishing to end their pregnancies were forced to look to the criminal world – and it took Parliament another 150 years to appreciate the anomaly it had created. Inevitably, the result was a compromise and we can now look at how that compromise evolved.

THE LAW ON ABORTION IN THE UNITED KINGDOM

England and Wales

Although it is often forgotten, the basic law on abortion in England and Wales is contained in a very old statute – the Offences Against the Person Act 1861 Under this Act, it is an offence for a *pregnant* woman to attempt to procure her own miscarriage *unlawfully* and it is an offence for an outsider to cause a woman to take any poison or 'other noxious thing' or to use an instrument on her with the intention of *unlawfully* procuring her miscarriage 'whether or not she be with child'. The penalties for offending against the Act were – and still are – very severe. It is to be noted that the Act says nothing about the foetus; the offence is procuring a miscarriage, not foeticide. It is, therefore, arguable, that it was designed to protect women from the ravages of the 'back-street abortionist' rather than to protect the foetus – but it is difficult to assess the intentions of the legislators of that century.

What is, perhaps, more important is that no-one was excluded as a possible offender – not even the medical profession. On the face of things, therefore, no termination of pregnancy was possible until the passing of the Infant Life (Preservation) Act in 1929 and, then, the relaxation of the law was effective only if the foetus was capable of being born alive and the life of the mother was in jeopardy. That was until 1936, when a gynaecologist, Mr Alec Bourne, challenged the law by publicly terminating the pregnancy of a young victim of rape. On his being charged under the 1861 Act, the trial judge, in effect, directed the jury that the Infant Life (Preservation) Act should also be applied to the immature foetus and that a threat to a woman's life was to include possible severe damage to her health – be that mental or physical. Mr Bourne was acquitted and the result of his case could then be taken to represent the common law position. It was also noted at the time that, as the 1861 Act referred to procuring a miscarriage *unlawfully*, there must be a way of doing so *lawfully* – and this would, presumably, include a termination conducted by a medical practitioner for the benefit of his or her patient.

Scotland

We suspect that this would always have been accepted in Scotland where the 1861 Act does not apply and the basic law lies in the common law. Attitudes to abortion have always been more liberal in Scotland than in the rest of the United Kingdom, perhaps in part because the Scottish courts are traditionally reluctant to interfere in matters which they see as being in the province of the medical profession. As a result, therapeutic termination of pregnancy has virtually never been prosecuted there. Even so, the fundamental conditions are much the same save that, in Scotland, a woman commits no offence in procuring her own miscarriage and an 'abortionist' – or a person who terminates a pregnancy for no medical reason – is guilty of an offence only if the woman is actually pregnant.

Northern Ireland

The Abortion Act (for which, see below) does not extend to Northern Ireland; this may be because of its geographic relationship to the Irish Republic where termination of pregnancy is unlawful save in very closely defined circumstances or to additional cultural factors. Thus, the law in Northern Ireland remains much the same as it was in England following Mr Bourne's case. The same situation holds in, say, New South Wales where the practical approach to termination of pregnancy is as liberal as any in the world. The reader may, then, well ask why was any specific legislation required in the United Kingdom?

The answer is simply that common law based on the result of a criminal trial may well leave open windows of uncertainty – and there is no doubt that the medical profession as a whole remained in doubt as to how far it would be supported in any re-runs of Mr Bourne's prosecution; moreover, the profession, itself, was constrained by its unqualified Hippocratic Oath. Times and moods changed after the war and the public demanded some answer to the continued parasitism of the unqualified abortionist. The answer was the Abortion Act 1967 which, even then, resulted from a private member's Bill rather than from government policy.

THE ABORTION ACT 1967

From what has been said, it will be clear that the Abortion Act 1967, which has been substantially modified by the Human Fertilisation and Embryology Act 1990, is not the primary means of regulating the subject. It does not decriminalise abortion; rather it is an enabling Act in that it tells us when it is *not unlawful* to terminate a pregnancy. The base-line conditions are that two doctors must certify, in good faith, that the statutory grounds are met, unless the reason is that the life of the pregnant woman is at stake or there is a risk of grave permanent injury to her health – in which case, only one certificate is needed; that it is carried out by a registered medical practitioner in an approved hospital;[6] and that the regulations as to documentation and notification are observed.

There are four major statutory grounds which render the procedure lawful. It is worth repeating them here in full:

a. that the pregnancy has not exceeded the 24th week and that the continuance of the pregnancy would involve risk, greater than if the pregnancy were terminated,

---

[6] This regulation is modified in the case of terminations induced by antiprogestin analogues.

of injury to the physical or mental health of the pregnant woman or any existing member of the family; or

b. that the termination is necessary to prevent grave permanent injury to the physical or mental health of the pregnant woman; or

c. that the continuance of the pregnancy would involve risk to the life of the pregnant woman, greater than if the pregnancy were terminated; or

d. that there is a substantial risk that if the child were born it would suffer from such physical or mental abnormalities as to be seriously handicapped.

There must be very few who would cavil at ground (b) if properly applied. On the face of things, the same would apply to ground (c) save that it will be seen that this is a comparative condition – it does not say, as one might have expected, that a life threatening condition is *present*. Death from termination of early pregnancy must be virtually unknown whereas, even in these days, deaths do arise from disease in late pregnancy or during childbirth; it follows, therefore, that the termination of *any* early pregnancy could be justified by statistics. This, however, is blatant sophistry and ground (c) is, in practice, rarely used. Ground (d) is clearly of a distinct nature and we return to it later. For the present, we will concentrate on ground (a) – which is that cited as justification for some 97% of legal terminations in Great Britain.

The most obviously distinct feature is that ground (a) is, uniquely, time barred – the rationale being that the interests of the foetus are seen as gaining importance with age while women's interests in termination are at their least urgent as defined in ground (a). The figure of 24 weeks was something of a compromise reached during the debate on the 1990 Act; it also sits tidily with the Infant Life (Preservation) Act which, as has been seen, defines the offence of causing the death of a foetus capable of being born alive. Beyond this, however, it will be noted that the ground is extremely liberal. To begin with, it is, once again comparative. No risk has to be present and the majority of clinicians would accept that the risks arising from a full term pregnancy will always be greater than those associated with early termination. It is equally obvious that to force a pregnancy on a reluctant mother is likely to cause her more mental anguish than to accede to her request for termination. One can go further. A risk to the mental and physical health of any existing sibling posed by a new arrival in the family is probably always likely to be greater than continuing the status quo, even if only on economic grounds. Moreover, the Act specifically states that, in determining whether grounds (a) or (b) apply, 'account may be taken of the pregnant woman's actual or reasonably foreseeable environment'. It is not difficult to appreciate that, within some ethnic minority cultures, the birth of a girl could result in considerable family disharmony and the same, or the reverse, could affect other echelons of society; it follows that the termination of pregnancy by reason of the foetal sex, which has been roundly condemned by many commentators, may be abhorrent to many but is, at the same time, perfectly legal. A doctor who obeys the letter of the law with the consent of his or her patient can never be acting in *bad* faith and the conclusion is forced that, provided the regulations are observed, it is well-nigh impossible for a doctor to perform an unlawful termination of a pregnancy of less than 24 weeks in Great Britain – negligence is, of course, an entirely different matter.

We have suggested that ground (d) is of a different nature. It is commonly referred to as the 'foetal ground' but this is a misconception. The ground is there not in the foetal interest but, rather, in that of the pregnant woman who cannot, as a result, be coerced into relinquishing a child she wishes to bear irrespective of any potential 'abnormality'; equally, however, she cannot be forced to bring up a handicapped child against her wishes. It follows that termination of such a pregnancy could, in fact, be covered by ground (a) and, in practice, grounds (d) and (a) are often combined in the authorising certificate. A major reason for the isolation of ground (d) is that the decision is released from the time constrictions of ground (a). This is important because the sheer complexity of the technology involved means that it may be impossible to diagnose an abnormality with confidence before the foetus is capable of being born alive. A number of cases have been reported in the past in which the doctors were unwilling to abort a recognisably handicapped foetus for fear of transgressing the law in this respect. However, since the Human Fertilisation and Embryology Act of 1990 came into force, liability to prosecution under the Infant Life (Preservation) Act has been removed from doctors acting within the terms of the Abortion Act.

This is not to say that the doctor performing a late termination is quite free from risk. It may be that the foetus is not only capable of being born alive but actually *is* born alive following termination. The doctor is then on the horns of a dilemma which is all the more acute because, for reasons which will be evident from the above and for additional reasons, the 'living abortus' is likely to be either physically or mentally disabled. On the one hand, he has contracted with the pregnant woman to relieve her of her foetus – and arranging for the adoption of a disabled infant may not be easy; on the other, the surviving foetus is, now, a legally recognisable human person – a 'creature in being' – and anyone who connives at its death is at risk of, at least, a charge of manslaughter, or culpable homicide in Scotland. The moral solution of this impasse is not easy to reach and is further complicated by the fact that the resulting infant, should it survive to that status, may well be brain damaged simply by virtue of its extremely premature birth – and we will see in Chapter 12 that the quality of life for a handicapped newborn is a factor which will greatly influence the management of its disabilities. The legal solution, however, seems to have been based on pragmatism. A number of relevant cases have been investigated at the level of the Coroner's court but, so far as we know, no prosecutions have followed the death of a living abortus.

A legal duty to terminate pregnancy?

Modern ante-natal care clearly includes a duty – subject to the consent of the woman – to investigate the possibility of foetal abnormality and a correlative duty to inform her of the result. Negligence in this context may result in the birth of a disabled neonate, in which case the woman can justifiably say: 'but for your negligence, I would have had a termination. I now have a disabled child and you owe me compensation'. Such an action is termed an action for 'wrongful birth' and, because the error is frequently located in the laboratory – as, for instance, in the diagnosis of a Down's syndrome trisomy – or in the department of radiology – involving, say, the misdiagnosis of a neural tube defect – the defendant may well be someone other than the obstetrician.

The history of actions for wrongful birth in the United Kingdom has had something of a roller-coaster aura. The law has, however, now been largely clarified in a series of cases – of which *Hardman v Amin* (2001) is a good model. As a result, it can be said that the mere fact of the existence of the Abortion Act sets up the conditions for an action in the circumstances envisaged. The woman may yet have to overcome the hurdle of causation – that is, she must show that she *would* have opted for termination had she been given the chance – but otherwise, given that the resulting duty of care has been breached, such an action will succeed. Since, however, compensation for the upkeep of an unwanted *normal* child is now unavailable (for which see Chapter 9), the damages awarded will be limited to the difference in costs between caring for a normal child and those involved in the care of the disabled child.

An action for wrongful birth is brought by the parents. A comparable action by the neonate – who might, for example, claim a right to have been aborted and, thus, saved the stresses of a defective life – cannot be entertained in the United Kingdom since the important decision in *McKay v Essex AHA* (1982). In view of the above, it is somewhat ironic that one of the policy reasons given for this was that to hold otherwise would impose subconscious pressures on the doctors to advise termination in doubtful cases. The more acceptable reason, however, lies in causation – no-one has *caused* the abnormality in the child.

Reduction of multiple pregnancy

A further dilemma faces the doctor who is treating a severely multiple pregnancy – that is one involving quadruplets or more. These can be very poignant cases as the great majority result from hormonal treatment of infertile women who are particularly anxious for a successful live birth. Inevitably, the more foetuses that are present, the less likely is it that all – or even any – will survive to infancy; the option of deliberate reduction of the pregnancy must, therefore, be considered. To some, the process, which has been dubbed 'embryonicide', is anathema – akin to the culling of animal herds. On the other hand, a woman with, say, septuplets, is almost certain to lose them all; to reduce the number and, as a result, to achieve, say; a twin live birth is, then, to preserve life rather than to destroy it. There can, then, be little moral objection to doing so – although there may still be profound objections to the use of an original technique which achieves such an unfortunate result. At one time, there was doubt as to whether the procedure was lawful within the precise terms of the Abortion Act 1967 insofar as the pregnancy is not *terminated*; the 1990 Act, however, specified that it is legal so long as one of the grounds for termination under the 1967 Act applies – which, of course, will always be the case.

Reduction of multiple pregnancy is to be distinguished from *selective* reduction whereby a disabled foetus is killed *in utero* while leaving its normal siblings in place. There is no doubt that this is now, and probably always was, lawful within the terms of the Abortion Act, s.1(1)(d).

It is clear, however, that it is not easy to apply the same logic to, say, the reduction of a normal and naturally occurring twin pregnancy. Given that the same legal proviso is met, however, it is just as lawful to do so as it is to reduce the number of sextuplets. Nevertheless, some would place the two on different ethical planes – and might add that disrupting an identical twinship may have paranormal consequences of which we know little. Others may, of course, see the whole concept of pregnancy termination as an unacceptable interference with the natural order. In short, there is ample room for conscientious objection to the deliberate termination of pregnancy – an objection which may be based on professional grounds as well as those that originate from moral attitudes or religious conviction.

OTHER PEOPLE'S INTERESTS

The conscientiously objecting professional

The 1967 Act recognises that no-one is under any duty to participate in any treatment authorised by the Act – apart from any duty he or she may have in providing treatment that is necessary to prevent grave permanent injury to the health of or the death of a pregnant woman. This so-called 'conscience clause' is not, however, all-embracing. The doctor, for example, who objects to abortion cannot abandon his patient without referring her to an alternative medical practitioner; failure to do so would almost certainly be regarded as medical negligence. Moreover, the Act, as presently interpreted, recognises conscientious objection only to *participation* in the procedure. It has been held in the House of Lords in *Janaway v Salford AHA* (1988) that a secretary cannot refuse to type reports referring to terminations of pregnancy and still remain immune to dismissal as an unsatisfactory employee. The rather vague terms of the Act do, however, still leave room for doubt as to its extent. What, for example, is the position of the hospital porter who objects to transferring patients to the operating theatre? Or what rights of refusal to supply the 'pills' would the pharmacist's assistant have in the event that antiprogestin treatment became available 'over the counter'? We will have to wait and see.[7] It is of interest in relation to the last possibility that drugs designed for so-called emergency contraception – or, technically, contragestion – are now available to women over 16 without a doctor's prescription. Emergency contraception and medical abortion are distinct procedures; it is doubtful if the 'conscience clause' in the Abortion Act is intended to apply to the former, although some people might see the two as being of the same moral order.

Apart from doctors, nurses are, perhaps, the one group who can certainly be said to be covered by the conscience clause. In fact, their position *vis à vis* the Act was, at one time anomalous. It will be recalled that a termination of pregnancy is lawful only if it is carried out by a registered medical practitioner; yet one of the most common methods employed for the purpose – prostaglandin infusion – is carried out almost entirely by the nursing staff. The House of Lords has decided, in *Royal College of Nursing of the United Kingdom v DHSS* (1981) that a termination that is performed on the instructions of a registered medical practitioner is, for the purposes of the Act,

---

[7] Some doubt may have been introduced by reference to *procedures* as opposed to *treatments* in the Human Fertilisation and Embryology Act 1990 which also, as has been seen, deals with abortion. It is just possible that cases such as that of Mrs Janaway might be affected thereby, but the problem has not been addressed in the courts.

undertaken *by* that doctor. It is, however, an interesting illustration of the complex-ities of the law in this area that, on a simple head-count, the majority of the judges who heard the case through each of its stages took the opposing view.

The father

It can be said, briefly, that the father of the foetus to be aborted has no rights of veto nor of representation in any decision making as to whether or not a pregnancy is to be terminated – and this is irrespective of the reason for the termination.[8] This has been shown to be so both in England (*C v S* (1988)) and in Scotland (*Kelly v Kelly* (1997)); it has been confirmed by the European Court of Human Rights (*Paton v United Kingdom* (1980)) and it represents the position throughout the Commonwealth – includ-ing, importantly, Canada where legal systems co-exist that are markedly different from that of the United Kingdom. This may seem strange in view of the fact that, as we have seen in Chapter 8, the mother and father have equal responsibility for the disposal of their embryo *in vitro*. In fact, of course, it is no more than the logical expression of the accepted right of any competent woman to control what shall be done to her own body.

PREGNANCY IN CHILDREN AND THOSE WHO ARE INCOMPETENT

Which brings us to no more than a note on termination of pregnancy in those who are legally children, that is, those aged less than 18 years, and in those adults who are unable to take decisions as to treatment by reason of mental disability.

The Abortion Act 1967 says nothing about the age of the pregnant woman. We have seen (in Chapter 4) that consent to medical or surgical treatment by a young person aged over 16 is as effective in law as is consent by an adult and that the con-sent of the parents is not required in such circumstances. There is, therefore, no doubt that a woman aged 16 or more can always seek and consent to a termination of preg-nancy. The position of the girl below the age of 16 is slightly more difficult but, as has also been discussed, her management will be governed by the very important House of Lords decision in the case of *Gillick*. Arising from that case, it is now common law in England and Wales that the parental right to determine the medical treatment of a child terminates 'if and when the child achieves a significant understanding and intel-ligence to enable him or her to understand fully what is proposed' – such a mature minor is, in fact, nowadays described in medico-legal terms as being '*Gillick* compe-tent'.[9] Understanding, however, has to be measured alongside the severity of the proposed measure – the more serious the treatment proposed, the greater must be the child's powers of discrimination. Moreover, it was held that the decision in the *Gillick* case did not give doctors an open mandate to proceed without parental knowledge or consent; indeed a number of conditions for so doing were laid down – the most

---

[8] This goes some way to confirming that ground (d) – which refers to the handicapped foetus – is designed to protect the *pregnant woman's* health rather than the interests of the foetus.

[9] We have also noted in Chapters 4 and 5 that '*Gillick* competence' is acknowledged by way of statute in Scotland.

important being that persuasion to involve the child's parents had failed and that the treatment was in his or her best interests.

But so long as these criteria are satisfied, there is no reason why a young teen-age pregnancy should not be terminated under the 1967 Act without parental knowledge and there is little doubt that many terminations are carried out in this way. The majority, however, will be non-controversial within the family and the only time the circumstances will come to light is when there is disagreement between the child and her parents; such instances will then be taken to the Family Court or, in Scotland, the Court of Session, for arbitration where, given sufficient understanding on her part, the court will almost always respect the choice of the child. The word 'choice' is used advisedly because the minor pregnant woman may, and often does, *refuse* termination on the same terms. The court will not take the interests of the foetus into consideration as both the Children Act 1989 and the Children (Scotland) Act 1995 dictate that those of the child herself will be paramount when any decisions are taken over matters concerning her upbringing.

The general considerations as to the treatment of handicapped adults who are unable to consent for themselves have also been discussed in Chapter 4. The questions raised as to termination of pregnancy are, in some ways, easier to resolve than is the case in many other aspects of treatment as, here, the conditions are governed by statute. It follows that the doctor who terminates a pregnancy in an incompetent adult is acting within both the civil and criminal law so long as one of the grounds for so doing is present – and this despite the fact that no-one is in a position to consent to the operation. The more difficult aspect is that the 'grounds' may be seen as being twisted so as to reflect the interests of the woman's carers rather than those of the woman herself – and the right not to be prevented from procreating is as compelling when it comes to an actual pregnancy as it is when dealing with possible future pregnancies. Clearly it is a situation which demands a careful clinical judgement that is reached in a sympathetic social atmosphere.

THE FUTURE

Some 170,000 terminations are carried out annually in England and Wales which is a rate of just over 15 per 1000 women between the ages of 15–44. The question remains as to whether the law has or has not provided a satisfactory framework within which to deal with these unwanted pregnancies.

For many, the existing legal system is too restrictive, the fundamental fault lying in the 'medicalisation' of the legal procedure. In essence, the complaint is that medicine and science are permitted by law to play a key role in the interpretation of human rights and their implementation in law and that nowhere is this more obvious than in relation to the management of pregnancy. As one of the authors has written elsewhere:

> The result is that the law has been informed, defined and controlled by medical information about the foetus – and this has had profound consequences on what pregnancy termination means to women and their rights to make choices about their own bodies.

In short, the basic criticism of the 1967 Act is that it was set against a practical rather than a rights-based framework. To redress this imbalance, say the critics, the best modification would be to remove all the laws which govern abortion and to leave each decision to the free choice of the individual woman.

The counter-argument might well run that, since few would advocate the establishment of a trade of abortionist, there is no alternative but to look to the medical profession for the necessary expertise for safe terminations of pregnancy. The doctors will then say that they can only operate in an acceptable medical environment and that, as a result, 'medicalisation' of abortion is the logical outcome.

We have seen that, in practice, termination of an early pregnancy will *always* be lawful provided the doctors involved observe the regulations. Put another way, this means that the medical requirements of the 1967 Act are not, in fact, incompatible with the exercise of a woman's choice. Consensus in the sensitive area of termination of pregnancy may never be achieved but, meantime, the terms of the Act seem to have provided the compromise it set out to achieve and which is, apparently, acceptable to the British public. Radical revision of its terms might well disturb this balance and even lead to replication of the violence that is seen across the Atlantic. No matter which position one holds in the abortion discourse, there is, perhaps, much to be said for the old adage – 'if the engine's working, don't try to fix it'.

CASES REFERRED TO IN THE TEXT

A-G's Reference (No 3 of 1994) [1997] 3 All ER 936.

C v S [1987] 1 All ER 1230.

Gillick v West Norfolk and Wisbech Area Health Authority [1985] 3 All ER 402.

Hamilton v Fife Health Board [1993] 4 Med LR 201.

Hardman v Amin [2000] Lloyd's Rep Med 498.

Janaway v Salford Area Health Authority [1988] 3 All ER 1079.

M B (an adult: medical treatment), Re [1997] 8 Med LR 217.

McKay v Essex Area Health Authority [1982] 2 All ER 771.

Paton v British Pregnancy Advisory Service Trustees [1978] 2 All ER 987.

Paton v United Kingdom (1980) 3 EHRR 408.

R v Bourne [1938] 3 All ER 615.

Roe v Wade (1973) 410 US 113.

Royal College of Nursing of the U.K. v Department of Health and Social Security [1981] 1 All ER 545.

FURTHER READING

Berkowitz RL. 'From twin to singleton', *British Medical Journal* 1996; 313: 373.

McLachlan HV. 'Bodies, rights and abortion', *Journal of Medical Ethics* 1997; 23: 176.

McLean S. *Old Law, New Medicine*, Chapter 4, 1999.

Mason JK. *Medico-legal Aspects of Reproduction and Parenthood* 2nd ed., Chapter 5, 1998.

Munday D, Francome C, Savage W. 'Twenty-one years of legal abortion', *British Medical Journal* 1989; 298: 1231.

Peterfy A. 'Foetal viability as a threshold to personhood', *Journal of Legal Medicine* 1995; 16: 607.

Whitfield A. 'Common law duties to unborn children', *Medical Law Review* 1993; 1: 28.

Williams G. 'The foetus and the right to life', *Cambridge Law Journal* 1994; 53: 71.

11

GENETICS, INSURANCE AND EMPLOYMENT

Of all subjects in the medical arena, it is probably the so-called 'genetics revolution' that has captured the majority of media and public interest in recent years. Whether it be associated with the cloning of Dolly the sheep or the production of genetically modified plants, the world's imagination has been excited by the possibilities of genetics – for good or for bad. Recent claims to have cloned the first human babies have done little to still the voices of dissent over the potential use of genetic technology. Geneticists themselves are also all too well aware of the intense searchlight under which they are working, not least because the history of the use of genetic information is not pretty.

The eugenics movement was at its height in countries such as the United States in the early part of the last century. The science of eugenics seeks to apply genetic knowledge in such a way as to ensure the best possible gene pool. On the one hand, as we have seen in Chapter 9, this could be viewed as a positive strategy, sparing many people the discomfort and distress caused by inherited disadvantageous conditions and facilitating informed reproductive choice. On the other, it could be used as a vehicle for discrimination and abuse of those deemed to be genetically unfit or inferior. Many years before Nazi dogma sought to eliminate Jews, gypsies and homosexuals (who were thought to be genetically inferior or perverse), a political programme was developed in the United States which sought to eradicate 'adverse' genetic traits from the population. Programmes of compulsory sterilisation were carried out in order limit the reproductive capacity of those thought to be genetically defective and unfit to reproduce. Perhaps inevitably, given that genetic understanding was in its infancy, the net was extended to cover not just those who suffered from particular diseases but also to include those who showed undesirable social characteristics, such as recidivism. As a result, large numbers of people were sterilised without their consent.

The modern geneticist must operate against this backdrop, which also colours the picture that is painted by the media. The reactions to 'Frankenstein food' and the ban on human cloning in many western countries are derived very largely from such sources which, inevitably, are tainted with the temptation to emphasise the sensational. Undoubtedly there are dangers lurking behind genetic science. But, despite this, it has to be accepted that much good may come from its application and it may well be that geneticists will provide the answers to many of the major health threats to which we are currently susceptible.

For the moment, however, the good remains a matter of aspiration, and the negative seems more urgent. Not least, legitimate concerns are expressed as to the possibility of discrimination flowing from genetic knowledge. This potential cannot be denied and it is, perhaps, at its most acute in the areas of insurance and employment, both of which are central to our capacity to engage with our society. In what follows, we will highlight the current UK situation and, in particular, will evaluate the extent to which the law may or may not protect against the misuse of genetic information.

GENETICS AND INSURANCE

The Association of British Insurers (ABI) describes its members as being 'professional risk takers' – that is, the function of insurance is to calculate the likelihood of a risk eventuating and to place, by actuarial calculation, a monetary value on the potential of it actually arising. Even so, the vast majority of insured people are currently accepted on standard rates, with only a few people being expected to pay significantly higher premiums. This is so despite the fact that the decision whether or not to provide life or health insurance will be based substantially on factors, increasingly knowable, that determine the actual and potential health of the individual.

It is beyond dispute that the insurance industry provides not just a valued service but one that is increasingly essential. The ABI recognises, in its code of practice on genetic testing, both the importance of insurance to contemporary life and the need for the industry and to act in an ethical way.

The 'mutuality' based system of insurance based on assessment of individuals' risks, which is that provided by the insurance industry, steps in to provide an additional resource in situations where the impact of 'solidarity' based cover – such as we obtain through the National Health Service, and in which the risk is spread – is limited. Any threat to the provision of such insurance is, therefore, significant indeed. Equally, other forms of available insurance, many of which lie beyond the field of healthcare, will have a critical impact on the way in which individuals interact and shape their lives. For example, life insurance is increasingly linked to the provision of mortgage cover, while private policies can help to ensure a comfortable old age through pension funds; despite the recent crisis in this area, these provisions may still supplement the otherwise limited state pension. It is the very centrality of insurance to life in the contemporary western world that underpins concerns about the way in which insurers may use genetic information. On the one hand, those actually or potentially seeking insurance cover do not wish to be excluded from the pool of the insured. On the other, the insurance companies need profitability for survival – and their survival is important to the entire group of those covered, or potentially covered, by their policies. Put simply:

> The essence of an insurance contract, whether it be health, life or otherwise, is that, in return for the insured's premium, the insurer agrees to assume the risk of an uncertain event in which the insured has an interest and undertakes to pay a benefit, in cash or in kind, if the event occurs.

It is obvious, therefore, that there may well be tensions between the interests of the public and the interests of the insurance industry. Although in the long run both will wish the industry to survive, the public fears the creation of an uninsurable 'genetic underclass', whilst the industry fears being rendered economically non-viable if the fullest range of information is not available to provide the data for their actuarial calculations. Establishing the correct balance between these interests will not be easy.

In addition, our ability to detect ever increasing numbers of genetic markers of disease, or even of lifestyle, will also force a potentially radical revision of insurance cover as it is currently conceived. As we have noted, insurance is about risk taking – but the more that is known, the less will be the element of risk. People will no longer be seeking protection from unknown or unknowable events in their future but, rather, they will be looking for cover in an increasing number of situations that are – in theory at least – predictable, and this must pose a serious problem for the insurers. If their task is to calculate risk and insure against its eventuation, a question mark will clearly hang over the provision of insurance if that risk becomes routinely predictable – as might be the case with at least some genetic conditions. Certainly, it would require a radical re-evaluation of what the industry does. For this reason, if for no other, it seems likely that the industry will not necessarily wish to walk too far down the road to requiring either the availability or the disclosure of all genetic information – at least in respect of some forms of insurance.

Thus, the genetics revolution poses an unusually broad set of questions both for individuals and for the industry. The fact that the interests of both may correspond in some situations does not mean that they will be the same in all circumstances. And, although the industry and individuals may share similar goals, each may also value certain principles over others and, thus, seek different routes to pursue or attain them.

Health related information is, of course, already used extensively in the insurance business. Questions about smoking habits, for example, are designed to elicit statistical probabilities as to life expectancy. In fact, genetic information has always been used, even if only indirectly, by way of looking at the family history. However, whereas in the past the calculations were of necessity rough and ready, they will become increasingly sophisticated as genetic testing and screening techniques continue to evolve. The first question, therefore, must be: what value has health-related information in general, and genetic information in particular, in resolving the tensions that we have outlined?

How relevant is health-related information?

We are, as yet, a long way from being able to identify or foresee all risks that beset us – and this is also true of genetically controlled risk. Even as we become better at identifying the susceptibility of individuals to particular conditions, with few exceptions, such as single gene disorders like Huntington's disease, we do not – and may never – understand the extent to which a genetic predisposition interacts with environmental factors. Thus, we may not be able to say with any certainty that a person with a genetic abnormality will become ill. Even with single a gene disorder, there is no way by which we can predict the time of onset of the condition, nor its severity – nor, of course, can we predict whether or not the person concerned will die from some other cause.

People are naturally sensitive about disclosing health information. However, one feature of the insurance contract is that failure to disclose relevant information that is *known* will result in the contract being null and void. There is, therefore, little purpose to be served in failing to provide an insurer with such information – no benefit would accrue in the long term if it could be shown that it was deliberately withheld; and, if this is the case with 'ordinary' health factors, it must also be true of genetic information. Nonetheless, in a report entitled '*Inside Information: Balancing Interests in the Use of Personal Genetic Data*' (May 2002), the Human Genetics Commission[1] emphasises '...the importance of ensuring that insurance companies only request the minimum amount of specific information about the applicant's family history that is needed to make an insurance underwriting decision.'

At first sight, then, genetics appear to raise no issues which cannot be identified and addressed. However, as we have already seen in Chapter 3, genetic information differs in some ways from other health-related information. Traditionally, the spread of knowledge about an individual's state of present, past or future health is limited by the commitment of doctors to maintaining it in confidence. Health related information is, therefore, acknowledged to be sensitive, even private. By contrast, genetic information also tells us something about other people – the existence of a genetic condition in person A means that it may also exist in his or her parents, siblings and offspring.

Since the applicant's health status may be relevant to the insurers' decisions as to whether or not to assume certain risks, it would be unimaginable that the industry should be denied access to it. Nonetheless, its probative value must be taken into account. In its response to the Report from the House of Commons Science and Technology Committee, '*Genetics and Insurance*', the Government noted that '[i]t is apparent...that, with the exception of Huntington's Disease, few data have yet been published which support the use of genetic test results for insurance purposes.' Indeed, we have already suggested that even the test for Huntington's cannot be regarded as absolutely predicting that this condition will cause the death of the individual.

However, most health related data relate solely to the individual – a possible exception being sexually transmissible disease. The major fear of disclosing genetic data stems from the possibility that they may also be used to disadvantage other family members. Penalties might arise not just in relation to refusal of insurance, or loading of premiums, but might also include either one company using that information against relatives or result in the industry pooling knowledge for the benefit of other companies.

In addition to the risk to insurability, the possibility is also raised that family members may have information thrust upon them which they might prefer not to know. The nettle of genetic information will not be readily grasped in many cases. Those who do not seek this information could, nonetheless, have it forced upon them and the threat to the patient's 'right not to know' is arguably exacerbated by the nature of genetic information.

Of course, this may be less of a problem once the gap between the identification of a disease and its treatment is narrowed or even closed. For the moment, however,

---

[1] A body which was established in 1999, and took over the powers of a number of pre-existing committees, most notably the Human Genetics Advisory Committee which had been established in 1997.

there is little doubt that forcing unwanted, and potentially unwelcome, information on people is undesirable whether this be done subtly or openly – yet this is precisely what a demand for access to genetic information could lead to. In addition, the existence of a gap between our therapeutic and diagnostic capacities may fuel an initial reluctance to discover important genetic information. Studies have shown that people are afraid to take genetic tests because they are concerned that they may become uninsurable, or lose their jobs, as a result of what is disclosed. Indeed, many fear that, as reportedly happened in the case of HIV testing, the mere fact of having had a test will be sufficient to result in the person concerned becoming compromised. The Government has also expressed its concern about the possibility that this may occur, regarding it as 'essential' that people should not be deterred from taking a genetic test because of their fears about the availability of insurance.

One solution, of course, would be never to take a genetic test. But, although, in some cases, this would make no difference to the present or future health of the individual, it might well do so in others. Even although there is, as yet, no treatment of the established disease, prophylactic measures may be available in some conditions. In others, in which the genetic component merely interacts with other factors such as the environment, lifestyle changes could be initiated to minimise or avoid its consequences.

So, while we can conclude that genetic information differs from other health-related data, we can see that, nonetheless, it is sought and used for precisely the same reasons. It would, therefore, be manifest nonsense to suggest that genetic information should not, or does not, influence the insurance decision – and, as we have seen, it already does. It might also be argued that withholding available information from the insurer increases the risk of adverse selection – in other words, the risk is that individuals who knew themselves to be likely to meet an early death would take out massive insurance policies. The industry could, then, find itself bankrupt. As a consequence, many others would be denied the benefits of insurance in order to meet the claims of the few. But, although the possibility of such adverse selection should be taken seriously, the House of Commons Select Committee on Science and Technology, reporting in 1995, felt that it was a risk which the insurance industry could currently withstand. Nonetheless, in its 5th report, the Committee repeated its view that it would be inappropriate to legislate to deny insurers access to all genetic information.

The ABI's first response to the Committee's 3rd report appeared in a revised Code of Practice issued in 1997. In recognition of the fears generated by the possibility of compulsion, the Association agreed that insurers could not insist on such tests being taken. Even so, the Code stopped short of not requiring access to genetic information that was already in the applicant's possession. This is a relatively unsurprising conclusion given the nature of the insurance contract. However, in a further concession, the industry's code also stipulated that insurers should not require access to genetic information on life policies associated with mortgages of up to £100,000. This voluntary moratorium has subsequently been revised. The moratorium now extends to £500,000 for life insurance and £300,000 for other types of policies and is subject to review.

A mechanism is also now in place whereby an applicant who wishes to complain about the decision of an insurance company can appeal to the Genetic Testing Code of Practice Adjudication Tribunal. In addition, a revised Genetic Testing Code of Practice, which took effect in August 1999, restates the position that applicants 'must not be asked to undergo a Genetic Test in order to obtain insurance.' Data are to be handled sensitively – and in line with the provisions of the Data Protection Act of 1998. Explicit consent is now required from the applicant before genetic information is processed.

Some protections for the individual, albeit a trifle limited, are, therefore, now in place. It might be thought, however, that the complexities and uncertainties of genetic information are such that it should always be protected by health-related privacy and that the industry should not be permitted access to it in any circumstances. There is a very real fear that discrimination would flow from the release of this information.

Discrimination is defined here as the inappropriate use of relevant information, or the apparently appropriate use of irrelevant information. While the Human Genetics Commission was not able to confirm that such discrimination actually operates, it identified a 'strong and persistent sense of unease among those who had provided genetic test results to insurers about the way this had been interpreted.' The Commission felt that this was an issue which could not easily be dismissed, and which should be kept under scrutiny. In one recent study involving families with genetic disorders, 33.4% experienced difficulties when applying for life insurance, compared with 5% of applicants in the general population group. Perhaps more worryingly, 13% of carriers of genetic disorders also experienced difficulties even although such persons present no actuarial risk on genetic grounds. The investigators concluded that such genetic discrimination as does exist is due to failure to interpret information correctly – and is not part of a policy within the industry.

Despite this, however, the Science and Technology Committee's 5th Report criticised the insurance industry in that it had failed to give the public sufficiently clear information about its policy and called on the insurers 'to publish a clear statement detailing exactly which genetic test results they will consider (both positive and negative) for which conditions and under which circumstances...'

Nonetheless, given the definition of discrimination which we have used, and given that genetic information has limited predictive powers, it might be concluded that discrimination does – indeed, must – already exist. Discrimination does not require exclusion – merely unfair treatment. Thus, even if it remains the case that very few people are denied access to insurance outright, misreading what genetic information is actually available might, even so, result in premiums being weighted in an unfair and, therefore, discriminatory manner.

On the other side of the coin, even if we believe that genetic information *should* be excluded on the grounds of fairness, there is no obvious way of doing so logically without excluding *all* health related information. Once known, genetic information forms an integral part of healthcare records. It is not distinguished from non-genetic information, nor is it easy to see how it could be. Neither can it be presumed that to do so would be to benefit patient care. Thus, the critical question is not whether we should prevent genetic information that is already available coming into the hands of potential insurers – we know we cannot do so – but, rather can we be sure that it is properly used?

Predictive and actuarial value of genetic information

In April 1999, the Genetics and Insurance Committee (GAIC) was established as an independent review body charged with asssessing scientific and actuarial information presented in support of the use of genetic tests in insurance. GAIC is a non-statutory, advisory non-departmental public body covering the entire UK. Its terms of reference are as follows:

- To develop and publish criteria for the evaluation of specific genetic tests, their application to particular conditions and their reliability and relevance to particular types of insurance.
- To evaluate particular tests against those criteria and promulgate its findings.
- To report to Health, Treasury and Department of Trade and Industry Ministers on proposals received by GAIC from insurance providers and the subsequent level of compliance by the industry with the recommendations of GAIC.

Already, however, it has been recommended by the Science and Technology Committee that the role of GAIC should be strengthened and its membership reconsidered 'if it is to inspire public confidence in its decisions.' It also indicated that the ABI may not be the best body to regulate the use of genetic test results, and recommended that it should act urgently to reassure the public and the Government that its Code of Practice is being followed.

The ABI's code of practice states that the provision of insurance has to be based on commercial assessments, which must be fair – that is, related to the actual risk presented. To meet their own definition of fairness, then, the members of the ABI, who are responsible for about 96% of the business of UK insurance companies, must actually know, or must be able to calculate, the risks presented. In its report *The Implications of Genetic Testing for Insurance*, the Human Genetics Advisory Committee expressed concern that the insurance industry simply does not have access to the kind of information which would allow it to make sound actuarial calculations, especially when dealing with multifactorial genetic influences.

Thus, it appears that, for the foreseeable future, the widespread provision of genetic information is unlikely to offer the kind of certainty in risk calculation which the industry's own code, and its own definition of fairness, require. Most of the information gleaned from tests would be of no real value and it is, perhaps, mainly for this reason that the industry does not currently require testing before deciding whether or not to insure an individual. Indeed, in the Government's view, any requirement to undergo a genetic test or tests prior to obtaining insurance would breach the rights of individuals to privacy and respect, as well as being in direct contravention of both the Council of Europe's Convention on Biomedicine and the ABI's own Code of Practice.

Even were it otherwise, we would still have to ask whether the second criterion for ethical use of genetic information – namely its *appropriate* use – is attainable. Genetic information is only appropriately used when its implications are properly understood *and* it is relevant. Much research of a complex nature is needed before this ideal can be realised. That is not to say, however, that the necessary information will not be available in the future and, for this reason, neither the HGAC nor the HGC has recommended a permanent ban on the use of genetics as an actuarial tool. Nevertheless, the reader will have appreciated by now that the use of *any* genetic information for insurance purposes is fraught with difficulty and needs to be carefully monitored.

There is, as yet, no existing law that tackles this issue directly. The House of Commons Reports, which, of course, have no legal force, have emphasised the primacy of privacy as the underpinning principle to be used in handling genetic information. But, as we have seen, the consequence of absolute privacy might be the collapse of the industry itself which would be an unfortunate and damaging outcome. Thus, the current position is something of a compromise.

Although the UK approach has been to regulate genetics by way of a series of ad hoc committees, other jurisdictions have been less slow to introduce direct legislative intervention. A number of countries, including Austria, Belgium and Norway, prohibit the use or transfer of genetic information. By April 1997, at least 15 of the United States had enacted 'genetic privacy laws', and more than 30 other states were contemplating such legislation. It remains to be seen whether or not the United Kingdom will ultimately follow suit.

GENETICS AND EMPLOYMENT

If insurance plays an important role in the lives of many individuals, it can surely be argued that employment exerts an even greater significance. Genetic issues will arise in this context that are similar to those we have discussed above. However, there are relevant and important differences. As we have already seen, the insurance industry is susceptible of control; imposing conditions on the ABI will ensure that virtually all insurance companies will follow the same policies. No such direct control is possible in the case of employers and, that being the case, we must rely on the rules of law affecting employment contracts, data protection and health and safety at work if we wish to regulate the use of genetic information in that field. However, just as in the case of insurance, problems are likely to arise from the different agendas followed by employers and employees. The employee wants a job; the employer wants a work-force which is fit and able to do that job. In many cases, these two aims will be totally compatible, but in others there will be conflicts of interest.

In addition, the proliferation of chemical and other hazards in the workplace means that an employee's state of health, particularly in terms of susceptibility, has become increasingly relevant to employment decisions. Ill health gives rise to financial burdens on the community as a whole, meaning that health has become a major economic as well as social issue. Moreover, as employers carry the legal burden of ensuring safety at work, the temptation to narrow the risks by excluding certain workers from employment – rather than by raising safety standards – is likely to be real.

There are, therefore, plausible arguments in favour of employers having access to maximal information about would-be employees' liability to disease as well as about their current state of health. The UK Human Genetics Advisory Commission restated this in their 1999 Report *The Implications of Genetic Testing For Employment*, and noted that the increasing availability and cost-effectiveness of genetic tests might well encourage the use of genetic screening in the workplace. Even so, at the time of this Report, the HGAC identified only one employer – the Ministry of Defence – which was using genetic tests in employment decisions. By the time of the HGC's Report *'Inside Information'*, the Ministry of Defence reportedly had ceased to test aircrew recruits for sickle cell carrier status, 'although selective testing may be carried out where there is a clinical indication.'

The current position

Although there has been some legislative activity in the United States in this area, less attention has been paid to the possible impact of genetics on employment in the United Kingdom. At present, no legislation exists in the UK which directly regulates the use of genetic testing either before or during employment. Indeed, in its report, '*The Implications of Genetic Testing for Employment*', the HGAC indicated that there may be some situations in which genetic testing would be appropriate, and declined to recommend a complete ban on the use of such tests for employment purposes.

However, this does not mean that no protection at all is afforded to the would-be employee. Some is provided through those statutes that outlaw discrimination on the basis of gender or race. In addition, the Data Protection Act 1998, which seeks to control the uses to which personal data can be put, will have some impact. Additionally, in 1999 the Data Protection Registrar (now re-styled as the Information Commissioner) issued a consultation document entitled '*Concerning the use of personal data in employer/employee relationships*'. Amongst the recommendations of this draft code of practice was that:

> Employers should respect their employees' privacy and human dignity and no intrusive action should be taken unless it may be readily justified as wholly reasonable in the circumstances.

Health related information is deemed in terms of this Code of Practice to be 'sensitive personal data', which means that it may only be processed in limited circumstances. Specifically, the code indicates that sensitive health data 'includes any genetic susceptibility to physical or mental ill health.' The code also precludes employers from requiring employees to undergo genetic testing (or equivalent susceptibility tests) 'unless it can be objectively justified on either strong public, or employee, health and safety grounds.' Any such test can be carried out only with the consent of the individual concerned and must be interpreted by an appropriate expert.

Equally, international directives are not silent on this issue. Although not specifically relating to employment, Article 6 of the UNESCO Declaration on the Human Genome and Human Rights of 1997 provides that discrimination on the basis of genetic traits is not permissible where it 'has the effect of infringing human rights, fundamental freedoms or human dignity.' Genetic discrimination is similarly outlawed by the Council of Europe's Convention on Biomedicine.

Discrimination is possible both before and after employment. There are subtle differences between the two, however, which merit their being considered separately.

Pre-employment genetic screening

Discrimination

The most feared impact of easily available pre-employment genetic tests is the individual's consequent inability to obtain a job by reason of his or her genetic endowment. Although the practice is not widespread for the moment, there is real reason to imagine that, in the future, employers could make a strong case for testing potential employees, especially as the tests become cheaper and more accurate.

The UK House of Commons Committee on Science and Technology felt that, while, for the moment, there was no valid reason for insisting that genetic information be disclosed to an employer, this position might not last indefinitely. The Committee therefore recommended that genetic privacy should be ensured by legislation and that the availability of such information should be restricted. As to the last, it was considered that genetic screening for employment purposes should be permitted only where:

- there is strong evidence of a clear connection between the working environment and the development of the condition for which the screening is conducted;
- the condition in question is one which seriously endangers the health of the employee;
- the condition is one for which the dangers cannot be eliminated or significantly reduced by reasonable measures taken by the employer to modify or respond to the environmental risks.

The Committee also recommended that prospective employees should not be coerced into undergoing genetic screening but acknowledged that, where an employee refuses to undergo screening and this results in harm to him or her, the employer should be given a statutory defence to any consequent litigation.

Additionally, the HGC recently restated its view that 'generally' the principle of respect for persons should operate to prohibit employers from requiring a potential employee to undergo a genetic test as a condition of employment. Such recommendations have not, as yet, found a place in legislation and they remain, essentially, a statement of what is 'best practice.' They, therefore, provide very little protection for the aspiring employee. However, as has already been indicated, other legal devices might be available for the purpose. Thus, a successful legal challenge to an employment decision could be based on a form of indirect discrimination. Court cases have shown that the test for whether or not a decision is discriminatory will rest on the assessment of whether the reasons are 'acceptable to right-thinking people as sound and tolerable.'

Further legislation to outlaw discrimination comes in the shape of the Disability Discrimination Act 1995, which expressly precludes discrimination based on a person's state of health. Section 1 of the Act defines 'disability' as 'a physical or mental impairment which has a substantial and long term adverse effect on a person's ability to carry out normal day to day activities.' No protection is, therefore, provided under this legislation for the unusually susceptible person or for one who carries a genetic disorder because they clearly do not meet the criteria for 'disability'.

It has been suggested that Articles 11 and 12 of the Council of Europe Convention mean, amongst other things, that genetic testing in the workplace would only be permissible if it were used to benefit the health of the person being tested and would not be allowed for purposes of exclusion. However, the United Kingdom has not signed this Convention and, in any event, international statements of this sort have relatively limited impact on domestic law.

A right not to know?

One further consideration, already mentioned in the context of insurance, is the claim that people have a right not to know their genetic status. It is predictable that this 'right' would be ignored routinely if pre-employment screening were to become more common and that this would give rise to numerous emotional and psychological problems. Again, there is no national law in respect of a right not to know, although some protection may derive from the obligation of confidentiality.

As we have seen in Chapter 3, this obligation provides only limited protection. By contrast, international agreements address this situation directly. The UNESCO Declaration requires that people's right to decide whether they want genetic information should be respected, as does the Council of Europe Convention.

But, although these articles may be used in support of a refusal to receive information, they do not, of course, prevent an employer from seeking it. Thus, theoretically, an employer could require that a test be undertaken and, then, meet the terms of these Articles by agreeing not to pass the information on. More subtly, however, these Articles influence the decision whether or not to test. Suppose, for example, that a prospective employee agrees to undergo a test but requests that he or she is not informed of the outcome and is then refused employment. The subject will not have been given precise information, but will still know that something is wrong; the spirit of the Articles will have been broken, albeit indirectly.

Testing/screening in employment

People already in employment may also fear that their genetic status could either compromise their career prospects or result in their removal from employment altogether. In part, this concern might be thought to stem from the imposition on employers of the ultimate responsibility for ensuring health and safety at work.

Health, safety and employment

The Health and Safety at Work etc Act 1974 imposes a responsibility on the employer to provide a safe working environment by preventing the exposure of employees to risk. Thus, the employer is required to provide the safest possible working environment and should consider removing an employee on health grounds only as a last resort. The Trades Union Congress also holds the view that people should only be removed from employment on health grounds if this is the only way to prevent harm to themselves or others.

However, these criteria may not always be met. Women employees constitute a particularly vulnerable group. Since childbearing is unique to females, it might be thought that special protection in respect of pregnancy, or the likelihood of pregnancy, would be provided for women under the laws which preclude gender discrimination. However, at least one United Kingdom case suggests that this is not so. In the case involving Ms Page, a divorced woman was removed from her job on the basis that it exposed her to danger when she was of child bearing age. An industrial tribunal held that, although she had been discriminated against, the discrimination was not unlawful as the employer was able to show that his actions were in the interests of safety. The woman appealed, arguing that she did not intend to have children and that, in any event, she was prepared to accept the risk. The appeal tribunal, however, rejected her appeal holding that her willingness to accept risk was irrelevant. The responsibility for her safety rested with her employer and, in any event, her plans might change and it was unacceptable that she might put any future children at risk. Thus, not all decisions that are based on gender will inevitably prove to be unlawful.

What seems essential – in both the employment and the insurance arenas – is to appreciate that, whereas *relevant* health related information may well need to be disclosed, there must, nevertheless, be doubts as to the need for disclosure of *all* such information. In the US, some states have begun to address this question by placing restrictions on the kind of information which can be legitimately sought, and attempting to restrict it to employment relevant information only. This may look good in theory but its practicality is less clear – not only is it difficult to disentangle the genetic from the non-genetic information in health records but there may be additional problems in defining what is 'job-related' and what is not. Finally, it does not inevitably provide a balance between the interests of the employee and the economic burdens imposed on those who have to make extensive workplace changes in order to provide a safe environment for the occasional employee who might be susceptible to workplace hazards by virtue of their genetic constitution.

From what we have already seen, there may, on occasion, be good reasons to identify genetic susceptibility in the interests of health and safety at work. Even then, it is surely also important that any screening undertaken should be carried out voluntarily and after adequate counselling. Otherwise, the right of the potential or actual employee to remain in ignorance of his/her genetic makeup would be seriously infringed. Given the likelihood that genetics will play a future role in employment decisions and practices, the law has a responsibility now to pre-empt their abuse or misuse.

The Human Genetics Advisory Commission recommended that 'appropriate mechanisms' should be put in place as part of the Health and Safety Executive's strategy to ensure that the use of genetic testing in the workplace is adequately monitored. The following is a summary of the Commission's conclusions as to what principles should be considered if and when genetic testing becomes a 'real possibility'.

- an individual should not be required to take a genetic test for employment purposes – a person's 'right not to know' his or her genetic constitution should be upheld;
- an individual should not be required to disclose the results of a previous genetic test unless there is clear evidence that the information is needed to assess either his or her current ability to perform a job safely or his or her susceptibility to harm as a result of performing certain work;
- employers should offer an available genetic test if it is known that a specific working environment or practice might pose specific risks to individuals with particular genetic variations. An employer should be able to refuse to employ a person who refuses to take a relevant genetic test in certain jobs which give rise to issues of public safety;
- any genetic test used for employment purposes must be subject to assured levels of accuracy and reliability, reflecting best practice. The results of any test undertaken should always be communicated to the person tested and professional advice should be available. Furthermore, test results should be carefully interpreted, taking account of how they might be affected by working conditions; and
- if multiple genetic tests were to be performed simultaneously, then each test should meet the standards set out above.

The HGC has sought to reinforce compliance with these principles by recommending that employers and other relevant groups should enter into a voluntary agreement to notify the HGC of any proposals to use genetic tests for health and safety or recruitment purposes.

CONCLUSION

The ability to obtain insurance and/or employment is much valued. Involvement in each often dictates the extent to which an individual engages with his or her community, as well as providing the means to satisfy basic needs and desires. History has shown that, with the best will in the world, leaving eligibility decisions to insurers or employers alone may be insufficient to ensure that the competing interests of commerce and of individuals are properly balanced.

At present, little protection exists in the UK for the individual seeking insurance or employment or for the worker already in post. Whilst our reliance on existing law might have been sufficient in the past, the genetics revolution may require us radically to review the position. Clearly, there are competing interests and the decision as to which should prevail cannot be made easily. However, some decisions need to be made in the near future and we suggest that Parliament is the appropriate forum for debate, discussion and deliberation on how to balance interests which, with the best will in the world, will sometimes compete.

CASES REFERRED TO IN THE TEXT

Ojutiku v Manpower Services Commission [1982] IRLR 418.

Page v Freight Hire (Tank Haulage) Ltd [1981] IRLR 13.

FURTHER READING

Black J. 'Regulation as facilitation: negotiating the genetic revolution', *Modern Law Review* 1998; 61: 621.

British Medical Association. *Human Genetics: Choice and Responsibility*, Oxford Paperbacks, 1998.

British Medical Association and the Association of British Insurers. *Medical Information and Insurance*, 2002 available from www.bma.org.uk or www.abi.org.uk

Gannon P, Villiers C. 'Genetic testing and employee protection', *Medical Law International* 1999: 4: 39.

'*Government Response to the Report from the House of Commons Science and Technology Committee: Genetics and Insurance*', Cm 5286/2001.

House of Commons Science and Technology Committee. *Genetics and Insurance* (2001, HC 174).

Human Genetics Advisory Commission. *The implications of genetic testing for insurance*, available at http://www.hgc.gov.uk

Human Genetics Commission. *Inside Information: Balancing interests in the use of personal genetic data* May, 2002.

Low L, King S, Wilkie T. 'Genetic discrimination in life insurance', *British Medical Journal* 1998; 317: 1632.

Miller PS. 'Genetic discrimination in the workplace', *Journal of Law, Medicine and Ethics* 1998; 26: 189.

Nuffield Council on Bioethics. *Genetic Screening: Ethical Issues*, 1993.

O'Neill O. 'Insurance and genetics: the current state of play', *Modern Law Review* 1998; 61: 716.

Sorrell T. (ed), *Healthcare, Ethics and Insurance*, London, Routledge, 1998.

12

IS LIFE WORTH LIVING?

At first sight, this may seem a curious question to ask. Both instinct and reason, assisted by rising social standards, tend to drive us towards ever longer life and to search for the strength and courage to exploit the pleasure of each day. This is not the case, however, for some. Suicide rates are increasing in most developed countries with, apparently, young men in the highest band. It can be supposed that a kind of anomie, or disconnection from their environment, leads to these tragedies – but, whatever the reason, it is clear that, for some, life is not worth living.

This may also be true in the medical arena. Some evidence from the United States, for example, suggests that the suicide rate amongst the elderly is rising rapidly in parallel with their growing fear of being kept alive long after their quality of life has deteriorated to an unacceptable level. Doctors and other healthcare workers are confronted more and more often by patients who do not wish to survive, and hard decisions have to be taken when people who are incompetent, and who have no hope of recovery, lie in our hospital wards.

Clearly, then, this is a question that is worth asking. In the context of this book, however, it is unnecessary to consider suicide in any depth, save to make passing reference to its historical and legal position.

SELF-KILLING OR SUICIDE

Some readers may be unaware that suicide was thought of as an honourable act in the ancient civilisations of the Romans and Greeks – so much so that regulations existed as to the provision of the means to commit suicide and, in some cases, magistrates were charged with the responsibility of doing so. Gradually, a different tradition entered the debate and attitudes changed radically as Christianity became the predominant religion in Europe. The perspective that life was a gift from God, and that only God could choose to take it away, came to dominate thinking on this subject. Theories that questioned this view were widely canvassed in the 16th and 17th centuries but were increasingly rejected, with the result that suicide became effectively outlawed and was, in fact, declared a criminal act in England and Wales.

At first sight, there is something rather bizarre about criminalising behaviour when the individual concerned is dead. However, a rationale can probably be found in the relationship between death and property. In practical terms, there was little, if any, advantage to be derived from criminalising a dead person, but much could be gained by relating successful suicide to a loss of property rights. Thus, the real consequences of the criminalisation of suicide lay in the state's capacity to confiscate property and its refusal to permit burial in consecrated ground. In addition, until the 19th century, the body of the person committing suicide was subject to desecration which was inflicted, at least in part, so as to ensure that he or she found no comfortable resting place in the after-life.

The 20th century, however, saw a reactive swing of the pendulum and the British Medical Association, amongst others, called for a re-evaluation and revision of the law. This revision was completed in England and Wales in 1961 with the passing of the Suicide Act, which finally removed suicide from the list of crimes known to English and Welsh law. However, the Act specifically retained the offence of assisting in the suicide of another. Nowadays, those who complete a successful suicide will – subject to the authority of the religion in question – generally be able to have a religious burial and their property rights will be undisturbed, subject to any effect that a successful suicide may have on insurance policies. Many such policies may be rendered null and void in these circumstances. In addition, as suicide itself was decriminalised, it followed logically that it should no longer be a crime to attempt suicide.

There is some doubt about the history of suicide as a crime in Scotland. One eminent legal writer of the 17th century suggested that attempted suicide would be a crime, but it seems likely that suicide itself was never recognised as such in Scots law. Whatever the historical position, and despite the absence of Scottish legislation on the subject, it is probable that assisting a suicide would still be unlawful in Scotland – it might, perhaps, result in a charge of culpable homicide. An interesting sidelight, which demonstrates the sensitivity of the subject, is that the word 'suicide' must not appear on the Scottish certificate of the cause of death.

While, as we have said, we have no intention of attempting an analysis of suicide, the subject has some relevance to the way in which life and death decisions are treated in our contemporary society. Many see suicide and suicidal attempts as 'cries for help'. Rather than accepting that life is truly without value for some people, the issue has been seen as a medical matter with those having a suicidal tendency, or who actually attempt suicide, being regarded as being in need of psychiatric support. Doctors and nurses confronted with an unsuccessful suicide will attempt to treat the individual and to restore him or her to life on the assumption that most people rescued in this way will be grateful to those who have helped them live and will not go on to another attempt.

The health professionals are, in fact, then on the horns of a dilemma. It may well be that the patient would have changed his or her mind given the realisation that death was imminent and would welcome revival. On the other hand, we have seen that it is a well recognised feature of modern medical ethics that a patient is entitled to refuse treatment irrespective of the reasons for so doing and notwithstanding a likely fatal outcome (see Chapter 5). The act of suicide could be said, of itself, to imply such a refusal; at least, resuscitation treatment will, in most cases, be non-consensual with all that that implies. But the doctor cannot know which of these scenarios is correct. The patient *may* be thankful for his or her escape from death. But it is not inconceivable that he or she might see aggressive treatment as an actionable assault – and the relatives might be particularly so inclined should the patient have been restored to a brain damaged state (see below). The decision to treat or not to treat a so-called parasuicide can be very finely balanced and there is no generalised solution – each case must be judged on its own facts. However, there are other equally complex and sensitive situations in which life or death choices are made, and these will form the substance of this chapter.

DEATH IN THE MEDICAL CONTEXT

A number of factors – medical and non-medical – have conspired to ensure that decision-making in this context has become relatively commonplace in modern society. Improvements in nutrition and the social ambience have helped to create conditions in which people can live longer and more happily. Clinical advances in treatment, such as the development of antibiotics, and technology, such as is found in intensive care units, have enabled healthcare workers to rescue many who would otherwise have succumbed to the disease or trauma from which they were suffering. For most of the time, this is clearly a matter for rejoicing – lives that would otherwise have been lost can be regained, with the possibility of many more fruitful years to come. Sadly, however, medicine cannot avert the inevitable. In the end, we must all die and this means that, at some stage, it may be reasonable to argue that continued treatment is no more than a futile intervention in the process of dying.

The concept of futility in maintaining life is intimately bound up with that of 'brain stem death' which we discuss further in Chapter 13. There, we will see that a person is dead when his or her brain is dead but, for present purposes, it is suggested that we look at the proposition from the other side – that is, that the body is alive so long as the brain is alive. That may seem self-evident, but we can see quickly that it involves a dangerous simplification, for the brain is not a single organ. Certainly, the person is dead when the brain is dead but only when brain death includes brain-stem death – because it is the brain-stem that controls the function of the lungs and, hence, that of the heart. Brain damage short of this – whether it be sustained at birth, as part of an active life or is due to degeneration in old age – is compatible with life but can lead to an existence of such poor quality that it might well trigger the question 'Is Life Worth Living?'. The persistent vegetative state stands out as the prime example of such a condition.

The persistent (or permanent) vegetative state (PVS)

This syndrome occurs most commonly in people whose brains have suffered severe injury but it can, and does, follow any condition in which the brain is deprived of oxygen for an appreciable time – such as an after-effect of overdosing by drugs. A diagnosis of PVS means that the individual has lost all sense of awareness. This condition must, however, be distinguished from a state of coma; although this latter state may have been induced by the same means that may cause PVS, the insult to the brain may be reparable. For this reason, the comatose are not treated as being dead or near death but, rather, will be treated aggressively with the expectation of, at least, partial recovery. By contrast, it is essential to the diagnosis of PVS that there is no prospect of recovery – indeed, the syndrome is now more properly referred to as the 'permanent' rather than 'persistent' vegetative state so as to emphasise the need for the condition to be permanently irrecoverable.

Although persons in PVS show signs of life, in that they can breathe unaided and may simulate sleep/wake rhythms, they will never experience that life. They will have no awareness, no capacity for independent thought or action and no future as a functioning member of society. This may produce an unbearable situation for relatives and carers, especially when such an existence can be prolonged for many years with relatively minimal medical care – assisted provision of food and fluids, treatment of infections and careful management of personal hygiene may be all that is needed in a technical sense.[1] Such persons are clearly not legally dead yet, equally, they will never again be fully alive.

Thus, they present the law with a particularly difficult situation. Our legal system purports to uphold the sanctity of *all* life. Questions of quality are, at least theoretically, irrelevant, yet those are precisely the questions that these unfortunate individuals present. For them, the nature of the condition means that no life of quality is possible, although continued existence is. They have, it might be said, no interest in whether or not they survive, nor whether this be for a short or a long time. Others, however, have very real interests in their status. Some will seek to prolong the existence of the person in PVS while still others will believe that an early death is preferable. The division of opinion is such that management decisions in individual cases can properly be referred to the courts and, indeed, a decision to withdraw nutrition and hydration from a person in the PVS cannot, at present, be taken in England and Wales without the authority of the High Court.

Although, at the time of writing, more than 20 instances have been adjudicated in the courts, the situation is typified by two early cases that were especially well publicised. The first concerned the case of Anthony Bland, a young man crushed in the Hillsborough football stadium tragedy in 1989. His injuries deprived his brain of oxygen and this resulted in his lapsing into PVS. He survived in this condition for 3 years, by which time it was clear that no improvement in his condition was possible. His doctors, and parents, believed that he should be allowed to die, but this required the removal of the nasogastric tube which was supplying him with food and water. His doctors petitioned the courts to provide authority for the discontinuance of nutrition and hydration; they sought a declaration that this would not be unlawful, thus ensuring that, in doing so, they would not be guilty of a criminal act. The case finally reached the House of Lords.

The Law Lords ultimately confirmed the required declaration, although it must be said that the individual judges reached that conclusion by different routes. For some, it was deemed that it would effectively be an assault on Anthony Bland to continue to treat him without his consent. For others, the futility of continuing treatment was

---

[1] Some cases have survived for more than 30 years but this clearly involves particularly dedicated nursing care.

the paramount consideration. Yet others felt that it could not be in his best interests to continue to provide treatment which had no prospect of improving his condition. Whichever rationale was given, the conclusion was reached that the doctors were under no obligation to continue to provide medical treatment.

That, however, was not the whole matter. One further hurdle remained – namely, could assisted feeding be described as medical treatment? If it was, the doctors were exercising their professional judgement; if not, they, and the court, were paddling in the dangerous waters of euthanasia. Most members of the public would probably see food and water as essentials of life – not as medical treatment. Within the medical context nutrition and hydration are generally seen as part of basic care – that is, an aspect of medical management that will be supplied irrespective of the condition so long as the subject remains a patient. On either count, we should continue to provide food and water even when people are terminally ill. A distinction was, however, drawn in Anthony Bland's case in that he required *assisted* feeding. He could not feed himself, and it was necessary for nurses and doctors to provide nourishment by artificial means. This, it was held, *was* medical treatment which could, therefore, be withdrawn on the grounds of medical futility.

This conclusion has by no means been accepted everywhere as uncontroversial. Some commentators have pointed out, for example, that assisted nutrition and hydration is needed in other, non-PVS, cases in which there is no suggestion that it should be removed. Moreover, it could be argued that, even if it is medical treatment, it cannot be withdrawn on the basis of its medical futility, as it is not entirely futile – it is intended to prolong life and achieves precisely that end. Even so, the House of Lords had made its declaration, feeding was discontinued and Anthony Bland died some days later. It is worth noting, however, that this decision was specific to its facts. It is still required that any later cases should be heard by a court of law, thus taking the final decision out of the hands of relatives and doctors.

A similar case arose in Scotland in 1996. In this case, the Court of Session was asked to authorise the removal of assisted feeding and hydration from Janet Johnstone who was diagnosed as being in PVS following an unsuccessful suicide attempt. In this case, the Lord President of the Court of Session indicated that the decision should rest on what was deemed to be in Mrs Johnstone's best interests – a test that was also used by some of the judges in the case of Mr Bland. It is interesting to note that one of the judges in that case, Lord Mustill, thought that the very nature of the diagnosis meant that Mr Bland had no interests whatsoever, far less 'best' ones. However, the Scottish Court of Session related the patient's 'best interests', at least in part, to the notion of benefit. Thus, if continuing nutrition and hydration provided no benefit to Mrs Johnstone, then it could not be said to be in her interests to do so.

The Lord President felt that the decision as to whether or not to apply for court authorisation in future cases should rest with those who have the responsibility for reaching 'treatment' decisions – that is, the healthcare team. However, the Lord Advocate – who is Scotland's senior prosecuting official – later indicated that the doctors' immunity from prosecution for homicide could not be guaranteed unless the removal of nutrition and hydration had been authorised by the Court of Session. Like their English counterparts, therefore, it can be said that Scottish doctors would be well advised to seek court authority in these cases, if only to clarify their own legal position.

More recently, it has been suggested that the removal of nutrition and hydration from patients in PVS contravenes their human rights as codified in the Human Rights Act of 1998. This problem was specifically considered in a case involving Mrs M and Mrs H where it was held that neither the right to the protection of one's life nor the right not to be exposed to cruel or degrading treatment were breached when withdrawing treatment in the patients' best interests.

EASING THE PASSING

It is not inappropriate to pause here and consider one further aspect of medicine's occasional flirtation with the criminal law – that is, the concept of double effect.

As will be seen later, doctors are not legally empowered to assist their patients in dying, although, inwardly, both the doctor and the patient may appreciate that it is the right course to follow. One way in which the law can be satisfied is by appealing to the principle of double effect.[2] Essentially this indicates that a doctor will not be deemed to have committed a crime if he or she intends no harm but, nonetheless, the treatment that is given in the patient's best interests simultaneously hastens the death of that patient. The classic example is where a patient is in severe and intractable pain. The attending physician may either increase the dose of the pain-killing drugs – thus potentially shortening the patient's life – or leave him or her to suffer. The doctor will not be legally sanctioned when the former course of action is chosen, so long as his or her primary intention is to relieve pain – despite foreknowledge that the action may shorten the patient's life. Double effect is not, however, an open-ended dispensation. The good and ill effects must, for example, be proportionate to each other – the patient must be terminally diseased if death is to be an acceptable inevitable ill-effect. Similarly, the good effect must not be produced by means of the ill-effect; thus, the doctor cannot kill a patient on the grounds that it is a certain way of ending his or her pain.

Even then, the incorporation of the principle into law introduces several problems, not the least being the near impossibility of knowing what an individual doctor's intentions are in any given case. Others have criticised what they see as the sophistry of separating intention from foresight. Nonetheless, the application of the principle of double effect is widely accepted as being part of good medical practice and case after case has shown that judges will be very sympathetic to the plea. In practice, of course, any relevant case will be heard before a jury – and a jury will be likely to take a common-sense approach when lawyers are arguing the finer points of legal theory.

WITHHOLDING AND WITHDRAWING TREATMENT

The permanent vegetative state, which we have discussed in some detail, is the extreme example of an apparently valueless existence. Yet there are many who, often as a result of cerebrovascular disease, survive in a semi-comatose state and are unaware of their surroundings. Clearly, such persons do not come within the definition of

---

[2] Strictly speaking 'double effect' is a moral construct, the legal equivalent being based on 'necessity'. Popular usage has, however, given double effect a legal connotation.

PVS, yet their condition may be equally distressing. We have already noted that the House of Lords in *Bland* was determined to avoid an incremental shift in future cases to the realm of euthanasia and did, in fact, insist that the case was to be judged on its specific facts. How, then, are these less clear-cut cases to be managed?

The concept of futility

There are some situations in which it will appear to a doctor that treatment should not be started because to do so would be futile. This is a matter for clinical judgement and the law would be reluctant to criticise a doctor for failing to start treatment deemed to be useless, even if relatives and others wanted it to be given. However, the concept of futility is by no means clear. Many clarifications have been proposed for medical purposes in an effort to reassure both doctors and patients as to the situations in which it can be invoked. Some have suggested that a numerical assessment be used – for example, it could be seen as futile to start a given treatment if it had been found not to work in a certain percentage of cases. Others would tie the notion of futility to the quality of the outcome. The need for such definitions shows that it cannot be assumed that clinical judgement alone can always decide what is and what is not futile – in particular, interests other than those that are purely medical may have to be weighed in the balance.

The notion of futility can also be used in deciding that the time has come to withdraw treatment. Where no purpose is served by continuing therapy, the doctor's commitment to his or her patient may mandate that the time has come to cease invasive or distressing treatment and to rely on the provision of comfort and basic care. Of course, neither withholding nor withdrawing treatment will inevitably result in death, and it will be argued that there is no intention to cause death. Rather, the objective is to maximise comfort or to avoid imposing burdensome interventions when no good can come of them. However, the situation is not always uncomplicated. As was said at the beginning of this chapter, we generally strive to survive, even at an almost animalistic level. The fact that treatment is being withheld or withdrawn on grounds which make sense to the clinician may provide scant comfort for those who are hoping for cure or, at least an alleviation, of their condition.

In 1999, the British Medical Association (BMA) produced guidelines, which were revised in 2001, to assist doctors who are faced with making these difficult choices. Interestingly, in view of the earlier discussion, the BMA suggests that removal of assisted nutrition and hydration might also be acceptable in seriously brain damaged persons where they were being provided solely for the purpose of sustaining life. Briefly, the guidelines indicate that – in the absence of the patient's known wishes – the consultant in charge of the patient should make the ultimate decision, taking account of the patient's current and anticipated quality of life. In order to ensure that good medical practice is followed in the case of nutrition and hydration, the guidelines also recommend that the decision should be subject to independent review by a doctor not otherwise involved in the case, and that the reasons for the decision, and the findings of the review, should be carefully recorded in the patient's notes. Finally, the family and the healthcare team should agree that further treatment is inappropriate before nutrition and hydration are withdrawn.

Some guidance as to what would be the legal response can be found in the case of *Baby J*, which was heard in the Court of Appeal in 1990. J was a brain damaged child who suffered from repetitive epileptic fits and periods of apnoea that required ventilator treatment. Thus, his quality of life was very low but he was not dying. The hospital sought a declaration that it would not be unlawful to withhold further ventilation in the event of his having another attack. This was granted, the court holding, effectively, that the question was not about terminating life but solely about whether to withhold treatment designed to prevent death from natural causes. There is no certainty that one can extrapolate from the management of an infant to that of an adult; nevertheless, we anticipate that the courts would accept the withdrawal of *medical* treatment by doctors who considered it to be medically futile in the circumstances envisaged. It will be seen, however, that the problem of feeding was not addressed in the case of Baby J and we doubt if the recommendations relevant to this would be approved in any condition less than the permanent vegetative state.

Do not resuscitate orders (DNRs)

In some cases, the decision as to whether or not a life is worth living will be made in advance of a crisis developing. This situation will arise when it is felt that cardiopulmonary resuscitation (CPR) would be inappropriate. When this is so, the consultant in charge of the case and the healthcare team will decide, with or without the involvement of the patient, that no CPR should be initiated in the event of cardiac arrest and the patient will die.

Decisions like these can be taken on a number of bases. It may be that the patient's condition is such that CPR would have no clinical utility; or it may be decided that the patient's quality of life would be so poor as not to merit prolonging the process of dying. Guidelines drawn up jointly by the British Medical Association and the Royal College of Nursing in 1993, and revised in 2001, made it clear that, where possible, patients should be involved in these decisions but that, at the same time, information should not be forced on those who are unwilling to share it. The basic question is whether or not CPR would be of benefit to the patient; this is a medical decision, but it is recommended that the wishes of a person who wants to be resuscitated in any circumstances should be respected – subject, always, to the fact that a doctor cannot be compelled to provide treatment against his or her clinical judgement. Given that such orders are likely to be made only in the case of the most gravely ill, obtaining the patient's views will not always be possible. If it is not, then the opinions of the relatives should be sought, as well as those of the healthcare team. In England and Wales, it should be made clear the opinion of the relatives is no more than that; their role is not to take decisions on the part of the patient. The position in Scotland is not altogether clear in that, while, under the Adults with Incapacity (Scotland) Act of 2000, the incompetent patient's welfare attorney has considerable power in the provision of treatment, it is uncertain whether the same can be said of withdrawal of treatment. The courts are available in either jurisdiction in the event of disagreement. DNR decisions must always be taken on an individual basis – a 'blanket' policy would probably offend against the Human Rights Act of 1998. DNR orders should be regularly reviewed, as the circumstances may change, and their bases and extent must be carefully documented.

Although such orders are made most commonly in respect of older patients, this is not always so. One English case, *Re R*, concerning a young man of 23 recently found its way into court. His condition was such that he could not sit up, eat or communicate with others. It was also believed that he was both deaf and blind. In these circumstances, the hospital petitioned the court to authorise that he should not be resuscitated in the event of arrest – a policy that was supported by the young man's psychiatrist and mother. However, they also sought authority to withhold treatment, such as antibiotics, should he become victim to infection – strictly speaking, therefore, this case involved wider considerations than the mere consideration of a DNR order. In the event, it was agreed that CPR should not be undertaken should the appropriate circumstances arise; this was based on the supposition that it was unlikely to succeed. Perhaps more controversially, however, the court further opined that other treatments could be withheld because the patient's quality of life was so poor.

Withholding treatment and age

This case was something of an exception and, in recent times, the debate surrounding withholding or withdrawing treatment has been at its most acute in two distinct situations, broadly reflecting the whole human life span – that is, within the confines of geriatric and neonatal medicine. The major exception to this generalisation lies in the very specific circumstances of withdrawing ventilator support – a form of decision making which may arise at any time of life. We will address these dilemmas as separate entities.

The elderly

As we increasingly exceed our 'three score years and ten', we become more likely to succumb to the diseases and disorders that are typical of old age. No matter that social and clinical revolutions can keep us alive for longer, few will escape the degenerative conditions that are seemingly an inevitable part of ageing. These need not be life-threatening, but they are certainly not life-enhancing. This situation has already been explored in Chapter 2, but it merits brief repetition here. The gap between finite medical resources and apparently infinite demand for them has resulted – whether or not overtly – in choices being made between patients. It would be naïve indeed to imagine that age plays no part in these decisions – whether or not we agree that it should. What is significant for the purposes of this chapter, is that the concept of medical futility, however it is defined, is manifestly *not* the reason for deciding to withhold or withdraw treatment in cases where it is denied because of the patient's age alone. Rather, this is a political, not clinical, decision, based on – often unstated and generally untested – assumptions made about the quality of life for the elderly or its relative worth.

The severely ill neonate

Such decisions may also be made at the beginning of life. Here, however, the rationale generally equates more closely with the concept of futility – although a very early British case that was mainly responsible for alerting the public to the fact that some neonates were not being treated had little, if anything, to do with futility. In that case,

R v Arthur, heard in 1981, a paediatrician was accused of the murder of a neonate in his care. The child had been born with what seemed to be uncomplicated Down's syndrome and the parents expressed the wish that the child should not survive. Dr Arthur agreed with this, sedated the child and ordered 'nursing care only', meaning that the child should be kept warm but should not receive sustenance. The baby died aged 69 hours.

The charge against Dr Arthur was reduced in the course of his trial to attempted murder because pathologists gave evidence that the child, in fact, suffered from other disorders which might have caused death. In the event, Dr Arthur was acquitted. The judge directed the jury that the medical evidence indicated that Dr Arthur's behaviour was accepted as reasonable by a responsible body of medical opinion, and further said:

> I imagine that you will think long and hard before concluding that doctors, of the eminence we have heard…have evolved standards that amount to committing a crime.

Whatever the reasons for acquittal, they fly in the face of accepted law and legal tradition. A long line of later cases has, however, steadily and progressively exposed the tensions that often exist between our desire to protect the most vulnerable young babies and our judgements as to the quality of their lives.

In the same year as Dr Arthur's case was heard, a different decision was reached in the case of *Re B (a minor)*. In this case, a baby girl was born suffering from Down's syndrome complicated by an intestinal blockage. The parents refused to authorise surgery, knowing that the blockage would prove fatal if not dealt with. Their decision was challenged by a third party and the Court of Appeal decided that the life of the child would not be 'demonstrably so awful that she should be condemned to die'. The girl was eventually reunited with her parents following the life-saving surgery. The apparent lack of congruence between these two cases may be explained, in part, by the fact that, in the former, the death had already occurred whereas, in the latter, it remained to be averted. In a later case, the senior judge in the civil courts, the Master of the Rolls, has stated that the approach in *Re B* represents the law as it now stands.

In fact, there have been no further cases directly comparable to *Re B*. There have, however, been several in which the infant was suffering from serious physical disease with or without associated brain damage – *Re J*, discussed above, is a good example. In these, the courts have very firmly taken into account the quality of the child's life as at least one factor influencing their decisions. Further, they have inevitably taken accepted medical practice as being an important feature of the correct way to decide. Certainly, they have made it clear that courts will not impose an obligation on doctors to act against their clinical judgement.

In response to these cases, the Royal College of Paediatrics and Child Health issued guidelines in 1997, which sought to clarify the situations in which non-treatment decisions affecting infants might be appropriately made. Briefly, the guidelines provide five main situations in which doctors might consider withdrawing or withholding medical treatment from the very young. In line with the position already described for adults, treatment can be withheld or withdrawn – generally uncontroversially – when the child is diagnosed as brain stem dead. Secondly, doctors may decide that no further treatment should be given, or that existing treatment can be withdrawn, when a baby is in PVS. This may also be done when the child is so severely afflicted by disease that treatment only delays death. Fourthly, such decisions may be reached when, even though life can be saved, the child will be so physically impaired that it is not reasonable to expect him or her to suffer in this way. Finally, the situation may arise where it is felt that the imposition of further treatment is inappropriate because the child's condition will inevitably deteriorate and the family feels that it would be unreasonable to continue treatment.

These guidelines do no more than act as a template within which doctors can make decisions, generally with the involvement of the parents. Thus, they do not have the force of law, although it seems more likely than not that, if a doctor's decision was challenged, the courts would treat them seriously. Indeed, it is at least arguable that guidelines from such an authoritative source could be taken as the yardstick by which medical negligence is measured – and we see a similar situation arising at many points in this book. There can be no doubting, as already discussed in Chapter 6, that United Kingdom law pays considerable deference to what doctors regard as being the appropriate treatment. But a doctor who intends to withhold or to discontinue treatment of a child against the wishes of its parents would almost certainly be found to have been at fault if he or she had not taken a second opinion and, if appropriate, not have handed over the clinical care of the patient. Moreover, when it comes to proceedings in court, those who, by reason of age or disability, require expert assistance, will be represented in England and Wales by the Official Solicitor, who will, then, if necessary, muster his own medical opinions to present to the court. Whether or not the situation is satisfactory, it is the way the law works in this country.

Withdrawal of ventilator support

Maintaining a patient on ventilator support is, at best, a harrowing experience for the patient's relatives and the healthcaring staff. Very occasionally, it may also be so for the patient when he or she has some remaining cognitive function. At worst, it can be regarded as futile, for two main reasons – either the patient will never improve or physical improvement is likely to be accompanied by such residual brain damage as to make life intolerable. Most patients who are disconnected from ventilator support are so managed because they are, in fact, dead and disconnection before death is very rare. Nonetheless, it can and does occur and can be justified both morally and legally as being good medical practice.

Justification is commonly based on the patient's 'best interests'. Even so, as we have seen in the case of *Bland*, it is difficult to equiparate an action which will probably result in death with 'best interests' and, at least partly, for this reason an alternative process of decision making has been developed which depends on what is called a 'substituted judgement' test. Here, the decision-maker tries to put him or her self into the mind of the person who is now unable to express a view, and seeks to come up with the decision they would have reached if they had been able to. Commonly, this process will depend on evidence of what the person had said to relatives and friends before the onset of incapacity. One of the first cases in which this test was applied in these circumstances was that of Karen Quinlan in 1976 in the United States.

Karen Ann Quinlan was diagnosed as being in PVS at the age of 21, and her parents requested that life-support be discontinued and she be allowed to die.

Evidence was led from family and friends that she would not have wanted to survive in this condition, and although this was not, at the time, deemed sufficient *per se*, her father was appointed as her guardian and was given the authority to decide on withdrawing treatment, subject also to his obtaining the agreement of her doctor and the hospital ethics committee. Ms Quinlan was eventually removed from the ventilator. Her case was somewhat atypical in that, contrary to all expectation, she survived for several years. The *principle* of futility had, however, been accepted.

Despite its apparent simplicity, the American approach to proxy decision making by way of substituted judgement carries as many difficulties as does the British use of 'best interests'. The fear is always present that, when relatives and others are claiming that someone would have preferred to die, they are consciously or unconsciously doing so as a way of ending their own emotional trauma. Irrespective of this, they may, with the best will in the world, reach the wrong answer. However, the alternative test of best interests is equally open to allegations of subjective bias on the part of the decision makers. Perhaps we will never find a wholly satisfactory solution to taking treatment decisions on behalf of those unable to do so. Meantime, the authors feel that a rigidly controlled substituted judgement test is to be preferred insofar as it, at least, attempts to respect the autonomy of the unconscious patient. Such a test was approved in the case of *Cruzan v Director, Missouri Department of Health* (1990), where the court indicated that it was entitled to seek clear and convincing evidence of Ms Cruzan's purported wishes. But it must be said that, in practice, what others think is best generally comes to much the same thing as what others think the patient would have wanted.

We suspect that the dearth of relevant UK cases is due, in the main, to the fact that withdrawal of ventilator support is, now, an accepted and often an inevitable facet of modern intensive care. Meantime, it is perhaps worth restating the relatively obvious – that mechanical treatment is no different from any other form of therapy in respect of consent. Thus, in those rare cases where the patient is ventilator-dependent but is, at the same time, mentally competent – as, for example, in the event of localised brain stem haemorrhage – the patient retains the right to reject support. It is for this reason that we have already discussed the main English case of relevance – that of *Ms B* – under 'refusal of medical treatment'.

PATIENTS' RIGHTS

What has been said thus far has concentrated largely on situations where the patient is unable to express an opinion, or where his or her opinion may be superseded by other considerations, such as futility. However, there may be other situations in which the views of patients themselves as to what is in their interests can be, and are, strongly expressed. This may come about in three distinct situations. The first is where the patient has made what is often called a 'living will' or 'advance directive'. The second arises when patients refuse treatment which their healthcarers believe to be to their advantage and, in some cases, life-saving. The third, which bridges the gap between refusal of treatment and euthanasia, arises when patients request the doctor to assist them in dying.

We have already discussed the advance directive and refusal of life saving treatment in Chapter 5, where we have seen that the acceptance of both relies on the assumption that, if we are entitled to autonomous control of what is done to us in life, then we should, equally be allowed to control the manner of our dying. However, not everyone believes that such a view should be unqualified and, in certain circumstances, the law, which has a fundamental interest in the preservation of life, will intervene in order to prevent it being effected. What is, perhaps, the more controversial aspect of such control is to be found in the field of physician assisted suicide or PAS.

Assisting someone to die

Although we have, thus far, been looking in the main at situations in which the patients concerned will have little or no say in the management of their case, there will be many severely disabled persons who will be in a position to decide whether or not they wish to continue living. Suicide may be an option in these circumstances but, in some cases, this may be a psychological or physical impossibility. In particular, careful precautions by the hospital and the healthcare team will deny the hospitalised individual the opportunity of self-killing. Indeed, a hospital could expect severe censure for negligence if an individual were to succeed in committing suicide while under hospital care.

So we are confronted by the scenario in which a patient may assess his or her life as being not worth living but, at the same time, may need a doctor's help to bring it to a close. The doctor is, however, currently precluded from providing such assistance, first, by way of the common law of homicide and, second, by the Suicide Act of 1961, section 2 of which makes it a serious offence to counsel, procure, aid or abet a person's suicide.[3] Such difficult circumstances may arise in at least two main ways. First, patients may ask their doctors to advise and assist them to die in the least uncomfortable way. Evidence from home and abroad suggests that this is not uncommon and, indeed, it seems that a number of doctors will agree to do so even though they risk prosecution for so doing. It is important to appreciate that this form of PAS involves no more than the physician prescribing and advising the patient on his or her own use of a mode of suicide. However, the situation is transformed into that of active voluntary euthanasia should the doctor, say, actually inject a lethal substance at the patient's request.

Most opinion polls show that a majority of the public would like to see a change in the law so as to decriminalise both of these procedures, yet the law in most countries has remained obdurate, preferring to hold on to its traditional view that it should not appear to sanction the deliberate taking of life. Some, however, will see both a moral and a pragmatic difference between PAS and euthanasia and this has been recognised in the US State of Oregon where, as a result of a citizen's initiative,[4] the Death with Dignity Act was passed by a slender majority in 1994.

The Act was subject to court challenge but was later endorsed by the voters with a majority of 60–40%. It allows individuals to obtain assistance in their dying, by way of a legally prescribed dose of lethal drugs, when they apparently have less than

---

[3] The law in Scotland is uncertain. The 1961 Act does not apply there and there is no offence of abetting suicide. It is probable that such an action would be prosecuted as recklessly endangering life.

[4] A way by which US citizens can require the legislature to consider reformation of the law by gathering a sufficient percentage of voters together.

6 months to live and they have made repeated requests for assistance. Many feared that the statute would inevitably lead to, either, large numbers of people making use of its terms, or doctors taking matters into their own hands, rather as Dr Kevorkian famously did with his 'suicide machine' in Michigan. In fact, few people have asked for help in dying, and fewer still have received it. Most of those who succeeded were aged over 70 and all were suffering from terminal conditions. There is, therefore, no evidence from the Oregon experience of a logical progression from permission to abuse. It is, however, noteworthy that the doctors' participation is limited to the prescription of a lethal drug – it does not extend to its administration.

The second group of patients who may request assistance are those who foresee their physical inability to end their lives or who have already lost that ability. This group is exemplified by the victims of progressive neurological disorders such as motor neurone disease – a group which poses particularly acute ethical problems insofar as its members are experiencing well-nigh unendurable suffering, yet the doctrine of double effect cannot be employed in their management. These conditions merit particular consideration.

One example of the former subset was a 42 year old Canadian woman, Sue Rodriguez. Ms Rodriguez was suffering from motor neurone disease and was aware that, as the condition progressed, she would be increasingly unable to walk, talk, swallow or evacuate her own body wastes. She wanted to spend as much quality time with her family as possible and, therefore, did not wish to commit suicide while she was still physically able to do so. However, she also realised that, when her quality of life became too dreadful, she would probably be unable to take that final step without assistance. Accordingly, the only acceptable way out in her view was to obtain authority for a doctor to provide her with the means to end her own life at a time of her choosing. She petitioned the Supreme Court of Canada, claiming that the Canadian Charter of Rights and Freedoms should be interpreted so as to give her this right, which would also have had the effect of not criminalising any doctor who provided assistance. Her petition was refused by a very narrow margin (5:4) largely because of the competing interest of the State in protecting its vulnerable citizens. In the event, Ms Rodriguez found a doctor willing to assist her and she died as she had wished to. The doctor was neither traced nor prosecuted.

A similar issue also arose in New Zealand in the case of *Auckland Area Health Board v A-G*, although this case was complicated by the fact that the patient was unable to express his wishes at the advanced stage his disease had reached. Once again, the court authorised the removal of assisted respiration, in this case based on reasoning similar to that used in the Bland and Johnstone cases – there was no clinical justification for continuing to provide treatment when recovery was impossible and discontinuance was compatible with good medical practice.

There was, therefore, some conflicting precedental evidence to draw on when the interesting case involving Mrs Pretty progressed rapidly to the House of Lords and, thence, to the European Court of Human Rights. Moreover, the case demonstrated substantial differences from those discussed above. Mrs Pretty also suffered from motor neurone disease and the severity of her disease precluded her ending her own life. Rather than involve her doctor, however, she sought an assurance from the Director of Public Prosecutions (DPP) that he would take no action against her husband should he end her life by means that were unspecified. Thus, the case was, in fact, about euthanasia (see below) rather than about assisted suicide as we have defined it above. Nonetheless, it was consistently argued as a possible infringement of section 2 of the Suicide Act rather than as a potential murder or 'mercy killing'.

As a result, much of the argument was couched in terms of statute law and, predictably, the DPP found himself unable to prejudge a breach of the criminal law. Mrs Pretty contended, by way of judicial review, that this breached her human rights under the European Convention. In the event, neither the House of Lords nor the European Court of Human Rights found a breach of Article 2 (a right to life which did not translate into a right to death), Article 3 (Mrs Pretty's suffering was due to disease and was not 'inflicted' by the DPP's refusal) or Article 8 (there was no disrespect for private life by way of interference with her autonomy – an aspect of the judgement which is open to criticism). The method of pleading was unusual and the case tells us very little, save as to the current attitudes of the legislature and the senior judiciary. Lord Bingham quoted the House of Lords Select Committee on Medical Ethics with approval:

> The message which society sends to vulnerable and disadvantage people should not, however obliquely, encourage them to seek death, but should assure them of our support and care in life,

a message which, some would say, shows a lack of understanding not only of those who find themselves in an intolerable situation of the type described, but also of those who are afflicted with intractable pain or other forms of suffering and are seeking relief by way of death.

ACTIVE EUTHANASIA

Which brings us to active euthanasia, which many would see as the 'last chance' solution to an insufferable life.

For present purposes, euthanasia can be defined as 'the act of killing someone painlessly in order to relieve suffering'.[5] We have referred to it in the case of Mrs Pretty – wherein, then, lies the difference between euthanasia and assisted suicide? The difference lies in the fact that the final lethal act in the latter instance is undertaken by the patient; the former involves the active participation of an outsider. This intrusion may be voluntary – that is, requested by the patient – or involuntary, which implies either unrequested or, possibly, unwished for intervention. We will return to the latter below but, for the present, we must note that there is no legal distinction to be made. Consent is no defence to the infliction of severe harm and motive is irrelevant in respect of homicide. As Lord Mustill said in the case of *Bland*:

> It is intent to kill or cause grievous bodily harm which constitutes the mens rea of murder, and the reason why the intent was formed makes no difference at all.

This, then sets the stage for the remarkable case involving Dr Cox.

---

[5] An alternative is 'an easy death' but this is, in essence, a description of hospice treatment, which does not concern us here.

Dr Cox's elderly patient suffered from incurable rheumatoid arthritis which caused her intractable pain – so much so that she had on several occasions begged him to end her life. In the end, he injected her with a more than lethal dose of potassium chloride and she died rapidly. His motive was undoubtedly humane but, as we have noted, the law is indifferent to motive in these circumstances. Double effect could not be pleaded with any credibility as potassium chloride has no pain-killing effect, and Dr Cox was convicted of attempted murder.[6] The fact that a very light sentence was imposed not only by the judge but also by Dr Cox's peers in the General Medical Council is proof of the generally sympathetic – or, some might say, irresolute – legal attitude to such cases.

It is, in fact, very difficult to find any cases in which a healthcare professional has been convicted of the homicide of a patient in his or her care. The defence of double effect is accepted in the vast majority – the assumption being that, even if the carer has overstepped the limits of the principle, it has been done with the interests of the patient at heart. Many readers will remember, say, the case of Dr Moor in 1999 which the judge clearly thought should not have been brought. We must not, however, be too complacent. Dr Shipman's case illustrates what is, in a way, the other side of the coin.

Dr Shipman, it will be recalled, was convicted of the murder of at least 15 of his elderly patients. His method was to inject large quantities of opiates which are, perhaps, the drugs of choice for the treatment of severe pain. But none of his patients was in pain – or, at least, not pain of sufficient severity to warrant large doses of a dangerous drug. Double effect was not in issue. His intention to kill – if not his motive in killing – was clear and his conviction was uncontroversial. Dr Shipman has, of course, no place among those doctors who are striving, in all good faith, to do their best for their patients in areas of uncertain law. It is, however, important to recall his case, as some would see him as a grim warning of the 'slippery slope' leading to *involuntary* euthanasia once we officially approve of *voluntary* euthanasia and assisted suicide. This argument is, demonstrably, rather weak in this case as Dr Shipman's behaviour occurred when both are clearly outlawed; no link between relaxation of the law and Shipman's behaviour can therefore exist.

There are, of course, many other arguments both against and in favour of legalising physician assisted suicide and voluntary euthanasia; we need not analyse them here because our purpose is to demonstrate what the law is, not what it might be.

However, it is worth spending a little time considering attitudes and practices elsewhere to see what, if anything, can be learned from them.

The Netherlands

The Netherlands provides what is probably the best known example of relaxed laws related to voluntary euthanasia and assisted suicide. Both have been practiced for several years with the knowledge of the State and what was once a *de facto* situation has been legalised very recently. In essence, euthanasia remains a crime but doctors

---

[6] A charge of murder was not brought because the body had been cremated without reference to the Coroner and the cause of death could not be ascertained.

who assist their patients to die are provided with a statutory defence. They will not be penalised for so doing so long as they conform to rules laid down in statute. It is estimated that about 2–3% of all deaths in Holland are the result of (primarily) voluntary euthanasia or, more rarely, assisted suicide. However, the system has come under serious attack, as it appears that a number of deaths which could not be described as voluntary are included among those described as lawful euthanasia. Equally, it is widely recognised that some doctors do not follow the guidelines. Still others – some estimate as many as 50% – are reluctant to admit to having practised euthanasia because they still fear prosecution. It remains to be seen whether some of the confusion that has been generated will be dispelled by the existence of clear legal rules.

CONCLUSION

It is clear by now that individuals have only limited control over the consequences of a decision that life is not worth living. Doctors and courts, however, have considerable power which extends beyond the purely clinical assessment of medical futility and encompasses the taking of, and acting on, quality of life decisions. Whatever one's views on the deliberate termination of life may be, it might be thought paradoxical that those who have competently assessed their own life quality as being so low as to welcome release cannot choose the time and format of their own death. Equally, although decisions as to whether or not a life is worth living involve profound and emotional issues, they must, nevertheless, be taken on a daily basis in our hospitals by doctors and others on whom we, thereby, place an enormous responsibility. At the end of the day, it may be, again, one of those areas which are left to evolution rather than revolution.

CASES REFERRED TO IN THE TEXT

Airedale NHS Trust v Bland [1993] 1 All ER 821.

Auckland Area Health Board v Attorney-General [1993] 4 Med LR 239.

B (a minor), Re (1981) [1990] 3 All ER 927.

C (adult: refusal of treatment), Re [1994] 1 All ER 819.

Cruzan v Director, Missouri Department of Health 110 S Ct 2841 (1990).

J (a minor) (wardship: medical treatment), Re [1990] 3 All ER 930.

Law Hospital NHS Trust v Lord Advocate 1996 SLT 848 (Mrs Johnstone's case).

NHS Trust A v Mrs M, NHS Trust B v Mrs H [2001] 1 All ER 801.

Quinlan, Re 355 A 2d 647 (NJ, 1976).

R (adult: medical treatment), Re (1996) 31 BMLR 127.

R v Arthur (1981) 12 BMLR 1.

R v Cox (1992) 12 BMLR 38.

R (on the application of Pretty) v DPP [2002] 1 All ER 1; *Pretty v United Kingdom* (2002) 66 BMLR 147.

R v Shipman (2000) 68 Med Leg J 37 (unreported).

Rodriguez v Attorney-General of Canada (1993) 50 BMLR 1.

FURTHER READING

Biggs H. 'Decisions and responsibilities at the end of life: Euthanasia and clinically assisted death', *Medical Law International* 1996; 2: 229.

Blake M. 'Physician assisted suicide: A criminal offence or a patient's right?', *Medical Law Review* 1997; 5: 294.

British Medical Association. *Withdrawing and Withholding Life-prolonging Medical Treatment* 2nd ed., 2001.

Grubb A, Walsh P, Lambe N. 'Reporting on the persistent vegetative state in Europe', *Medical Law Review* 1998; 6: 161.

Jennett B, Plum F. 'Persistent vegetative state after brain damage', *Lancet* 1972; 1: 734.

Laurie GT, Mason JK. 'Negative treatment of vulnerable patients: Euthanasia by any other name?', *Juridical Review* 2000; 159.

Otlowski M. 'Active voluntary euthanasia: Options for reform', *Medical Law Review* 1994; 3: 161.

Resuscitation Council. *Decisions Relating to Cardiopulmonary Resuscitation – A Joint Statement from the BMA, Resuscitation Council and RCN*, 2001.

13

DISPOSAL OF THE BODY AND BODY PARTS

Surprising though it may seem, it is a general legal principle that a person does not own his or her body or its individual parts – in short, there are no property rights in one's body. This is broadly true so long as property is defined as something you can deal with as you wish – which would include selling it or using it for barter. The law as applied to the body is, however, extraordinarily vague and is sometimes contradictory. No-one, for example, would deny that you can cut off your hair, and even sell it, say, to a wig-maker. At the other end of the scale, the law would certainly step in – and most people would say rightly so – if you decided to cut off your hand for any reason other than for medical treatment. Much of the current law is based on a very old case – dating from 1603 – involving just such a scenario in which a beggar had his hand removed so that he might attract more sympathetic donations. He and his collaborator were found guilty of the offence of maim. Similarly, in recent times, a group of men who were indulging in sado-masochistic practices were found guilty of inflicting criminal harm on each other and the propriety of the charge was upheld in the European Court of Human Rights – this despite the fact that the men concerned had given their free consent and the activities took place in private (*R v Brown* (1996)). In this sense, therefore, the issue is about *control* rather than property as traditionally conceived. We will return later to the issue of property in the sense of rights to buy and sell.

LEGAL CONTROL OF THE BODY

A somewhat hazy pattern in the attitude of the law to our 'ownership' or rights of control over our bodies thus becomes discernible. We can dispose, non-commercially, of our body or its parts so long as it is in our best interests to do so or, at least, so long as it does us no harm. Thus, the common law holds that we can consent to surgical operations which would, otherwise, amount to a flagrant mutilation of the body (*Attorney-General's Reference (No. 6 of 1980)* (1981)). But this applies only if the operation is 'therapeutic' – that is, directed to the treatment of a recognisable disease – and, even here, we may be in difficulties. Readers may remember the case a few years ago in which a surgeon removed the legs of patients suffering from apotemnophilia, or hatred of one's limbs; there is no doubt that he believed that this was ethically acceptable therapy, yet the case provoked a public outcry. On the other hand, we will see that very considerable reconstruction of the sexual organs is widely accepted as the legitimate treatment for the gender dysphoria syndrome or transsexualism. The doctor is, however, forbidden by the Prohibition of Female Circumcision Act 1985 to undertake female circumcision for purely socio-religious or cultural reasons – and, interestingly, it is now doubtful whether male circumcision for non-therapeutic reasons is an acceptable part of ethical medical practice when the patient is too young to consent to the operation (*Re J (a minor)* (2000)).

This leads to a further reason why the law does not grant us exclusive control over our own bodies, that is, the public interest – in this case in not permitting the causing of personal harm. The rules were laid down over half a century ago when it was held that:

> As a general rule … it is an unlawful act to beat another person with such a degree of violence that the infliction of bodily harm is a probable consequence and, when such an act is proved, consent is immaterial (*R v Donovan* (1934)).

But that, it will be said, is as good a description of boxing as one is likely to find, yet boxing is a perfectly legitimate sport. The reason? The 'noble art' as it has been called has always been part of the British way of life and, until comparatively recently, its legitimacy has not been questioned nor has it been suggested that the spectacle of a boxing match is against the public interest. What, then, of 'total fighting' which is about as far from a 'noble art' as one can imagine and which has, even so, been licensed for public spectacle in England? Not only does this development reinforce the conclusion that the law in this area is ambiguous, but it demonstrates very effectively that the 'public interest' is, itself, an uncertain measure of lawfulness. 'Public interest' varies with the interests of the public which are, themselves, dictated by the changing nature of our whole social environment.

The difficulty in evaluating your rights of control over your own body is, then, twofold. Firstly, one has to ask who sets the benchmark that defines lawfulness? Put briefly, is it the State which undertakes to look after the welfare of its people or is it the people who influence the powers of the State by expressing their will? This is a question which has for a long time been encapsulated in what is known to legal philosophers as the Hart-Devlin debate. By and large, the Western world has decided that it prefers the freedom provided by social democracy to the controlled existence imposed by dictatorship, whether benevolent or otherwise. But even the most enthusiastic libertarian would concede that the State must look after its minorities and, particularly, its vulnerable minorities of whom the poor and the sick constitute important sections. If the force of law is needed for their protection, then laws there must be.

Secondly, once it is set, a legal benchmark becomes more deeply embedded with time and, as a consequence, more difficult to remove – and it is in this field that many of the seeds of medical jurisprudential conflict are sown.

Turning to the question of property rather than control, the greater part of the legal constraints on the ownership of our bodies stem from those that were applied to ownership of the *dead* body more than a century ago and, as we have already noted, it has since been a tenet of English law – recently confirmed in the case of *Dobson v North Tyneside Health Authority* (1996) – that 'there is no property in a dead body'. Yet, intuition tells us that this cannot be wholly true. There are, for example, large numbers of museum exhibits featuring dead human parts and dead bodies are to be found in the anatomy classrooms of most medical schools. Somebody must 'own' these whether or not they have any monetary value – and the law has, inventively, used them as a peg on which to hang its solution of the anomaly. Effectively, what has emerged is that, although a part of a dead body cannot, of itself, be 'property' – and, therefore, cannot, for example, be stolen – it can acquire a value of its own if it has been manipulated or worked on so as to alter its character. It follows from this that the person who has provided that extra gloss can be said to own the tissue. Thus, while it may be that no-one owns a part of a corpse, it becomes the property of the museum once the part has been embalmed and treated to enhance its value as an exhibit. This proposition was upheld in the unusual case concerning a Mr Kelly, a sculptor whose collaborator was convicted of theft, having 'stolen' a number of such specimens on his behalf (*R v Kelly* (1998)).

We suspect, however, that the majority of readers will think that this is not a satisfactory solution. Whatever may be the legal position, our moral intuition says that that part was not just part of a body, it was part of the body of a person that someone loved and it is for that someone to determine what is to be done with it. This leads to yet another aspect of 'property' – that is, the right to control the bodies of others, most commonly after death. This concern is probably at its most acute in the case of children, with whom parents have a special form of bonding. All will have been aware of the dissatisfaction expressed recently by the parents of a large number of children who had died following cardiac surgery at Bristol and whose hearts had been retained for further study in the hospital laboratory. Similar complaints surfaced at the children's hospital at Alder Hey in Liverpool and, later, in Scotland. All these incidents have been subjected to official inquiries whose reports are referred to at the end of the chapter.

Few aspects of medical ethics are entirely straightforward and, in most, there is a legitimate view to be taken from opposing sides. As we have already noted, many – and probably the majority – would feel that the disposal of a body is for the close relatives to decide upon and that any interference with that right should be subject to their authority. Moreover, they would say that the relatives must understand what they are authorising so that they can put specific limits on what is to be done. On the other hand, the utilitarian philosopher – that is, the person who believes that what is *right* is what provides the greatest *benefit* to society as a whole – would argue that further scientific study of dead parts is essential to improving our knowledge of disease and that the tissues should be available for the benefit of untold numbers of future patients. There is, of course, no reason why the two philosophies should not live together – the researcher can, for example, argue a case for retention which will be good enough to convince the relatives of its merit. They may, therefore, as a consequence, provide the necessary authority. It is a question of reaching the right balance. All would certainly agree that whatever is done should be done within the law and the law will attempt to steer a middle way in seeking to achieve that balance.

It can be seen, therefore, that claiming property rights is more complex than asserting a right to buy and sell. For example, the parents in the cases referred to above were not seeking to assert any such right in respect of their children but, rather, sought recognition of a disposal right; which is also a form of 'property'. The boxer, and arguably the man engaging in consensual sado-masochistic practices in private, is asserting a right to use his or her body as he or she wishes. Still others, of course, would argue that the rights that they should be allowed to claim include the right to buy and sell body parts or tissue – of which, more later. Given the wide range of concepts which fall within the notion of property, it is unsurprising that the law can, on occasion, seem confused and confusing. However, as much of the current concern in this area has centred on disposal of body parts, we will consider this issue in some depth in what follows.

DISPOSAL OF ORGANS AND TISSUES FROM THE BODIES OF THE DEAD

The legal response to the useful disposal of the dead body is by way of two main statutes. The Anatomy Act 1984 covers the very specific process of donation of bodies for an anatomic dissection that is directed solely to the study of human morphology; despite this limitation, the 1984 Act represents the common route by which a person bequeaths his or her *whole body* for medical use. By contrast, the Human Tissue Act 1961, which is of far greater concern to the practising doctor, deals with the removal and use of *organs* from the dead human body for, on the one hand, purposes of teaching and research and, on the other, for treatment in the form of organ transplantation. We will turn to transplantation later on in the chapter. For present purposes, we will confine discussion to post-mortem examination of the body and to the retention of tissues for non-therapeutic purposes following that procedure. In this respect, it is fair to quote the Interim Report of the Bristol Royal Infirmary Inquiry: 'The law regulating the removal, retention use and disposal of human material is obscure, uncertain and arcane'.

One of the reasons for this statement was that, as would be expected, the majority of post-mortem examinations of children and young persons are conducted on behalf of the coroner or the procurator fiscal (see Chapter 1) – an area in which the relevant law has been notoriously fragmented and indecisive. Disposal of a body in such circumstances is dictated in England and Wales by the Coroners Act 1988[1] which conflicts with the 1961 Act in several important ways – in particular, control of the body and its tissues is firmly in the hands of the coroner until the investigation of the death is complete. Once this is achieved, however, responsibility for the disposal of the remains reverts to the administrators of the deceased's estate.

This is, however, no place to recapitulate on the Coroners Act which is, as we write, under active consideration by the Government.[2] Rather, we will concentrate on the 1961 Act while acknowledging that that Act, also, will be subject to review and probable alteration.

---

[1] The procurator fiscal's authority in Scotland rests on the common law. A separate Coroners Act (Northern Ireland) 1959 governs the position in Northern Ireland.
[2] A similar revision is being carried out in Scotland.

Accepting that limitation, we can summarise the provisions of the 1961 Act as specifying that the body or parts of a body may be used for the purposes of medical education or research if a valid wish for such use was expressed by the deceased during his or her life. In the absence of such a request, the person in lawful possession of the body (for which, see below) may authorise a post-mortem examination and/or use of the tissues provided that, *having made reasonable enquiry*, he or she has no reason to believe that either the deceased, the surviving spouse or any surviving relative objects to him or her doing so.[3] Thus, the Human Tissue Act provides the deceased's relatives with no powers of possession or ownership. What it does do is to recognise the sensitivities of the next-of-kin and to provide them with a wide power of veto, a veto which, at least in theory, is subject only to the autonomous will of the living person to control the disposal of his own body after death – and, in general, only an adult or a competent minor can exercise that right. In addition, however, the Act makes separate provision for the performance of a diagnostic – or 'hospital' – post-mortem examination. In many ways, this is unfortunate. The motivation behind the life-saving provision of viable organs for transplantation and the inquiring nature of the post-mortem examination are quite different; yet the legal control of each is virtually identical.

Perhaps the most significant uncertainty in the Act for present purposes lies in the definition of the 'person in lawful possession of the body'. We suggest later, when we are discussing organ transplantation, that this is the hospital authority and it is generally agreed by authoritative writers that this is so – this interpretation was, in fact, written into the Transplant of Human Organs Bill 2001, a Bill which lapsed because of lack of Parliamentary time. However, the ultimate 'possessor' of the body is the executor or administrator of the dead person's estate who is responsible for its disposal; in the case of children, this will be the parents. There can be very few occasions when the parents of a dying child will not be close to the bedside. Their intention to accept their duty to bury or cremate the child will be evident and it follows that they will be legally, as well as in spirit, in possession of the child's body and can, therefore, agree to a post-mortem examination and removal of tissues. Again, however, this is subject to the Act and they must, therefore, establish that no other relatives object to their decision. Thus, strictly speaking, the parents cannot 'consent' to removal of their child's organs because another relative might veto that consent. Most would agree that this is an unsatisfactory conclusion, and this is one of the reasons why the issue of 'consent' to post-mortem examination is being thoroughly investigated following the recent disclosures.

As we discussed in Chapter 4, the most important aspect of consent in any form is that it should be 'real' – that is to say, persons must be fully aware of the nature and the extent of their consent or acquiescence, and this is particularly so in the case of the hospital post-mortem examination. The most common problem in this respect lies in the retention of material and we draw attention to one aspect of this that is often poorly understood by relatives of the deceased – that is, the difference between

---

[3] Very similar conditions are attached to the use of the dead body for anatomical dissection by the Anatomy Act 1984. As stated, we do not propose special consideration of the 1984 Act in this book.

organs, tissues and slides for microscopy. We define the first as whole functional organs such as the heart or liver and tissues as fragments of organs from which slides will be prepared. There is a world of difference between the effect on the sensitivities of the relatives in the two cases. Moreover, while the retention of whole organs in the long term is rarely necessary, pathologists will rightly maintain that the retention and, later, microscopic examination of tissue fragments is very nearly essential to a good autopsy. In addition, the availability of permanently retained microscopic material may be of enormous significance in any later legal proceedings. It is very important that relatives who are being asked to agree to a post-mortem examination are made aware of these differences. It is equally important that the possibility of short-term retention of organs for further study − including, most often, the brain and/or heart − is fully explained at the time when authority is being sought; how such organs are to be disposed of later may be a matter of profound significance to parents and other close relatives. There can be no doubt that the dead body is the legitimate subject of human emotion and this is particularly true in the case of children. This, however, is not to say that no similar respect is due to the adult cadaver − a wife may grieve for her husband as much as a mother does for her child. Clearly, a compassionate attitude to all post-mortem examinations is essential and there is much to be said for the introduction of bereavement counselling in which the involvement of the pathologist has been shown to be most effective.

At the same time, the public health importance of post mortem examinations must not be forgotten or obscured in the aftermath of death. The pathologist should not be constrained in his or her efforts to derive maximum benefit from an investigation − an investigation which, because of the moral significance attached to the dead body, should not be undertaken lightly. Once undertaken, however, it must be valuable. It is, therefore, essential that the pathologist be accorded temporary possession and custody empowering him or her to maintain good professional − and, indeed, ethical − standards. To this end, he or she may, as already mentioned, feel it essential to retain and further examine post-mortem tissues. The ultimate disposal of the body and its parts is, however, a matter for the executor or close relatives of the deceased; the use and retention of tissues are, therefore, subject to their authorisation. Obtaining this is a matter of good relationships, good ethics and, we believe, good law.

However, it has also to be appreciated that, once the death is the subject of an inquiry by either the coroner or the procurator fiscal, the medico-legal authority has overall control of the body *until his or her inquiries are completed*. The coroner or fiscal also has the power to retain tissues obtained at post-mortem examination but this is subject to it being directed to establishing the mode and cause of death. In the absence of an adequate and sympathetic explanation of the legal situation, the stage is set for misunderstanding between the relatives and the medico-legal authority. This is made more likely because the regulations do not say what is to be done with the organs and tissues once the inquiry is finished − an omission which is doubly unsatisfactory given that the medico-legal autopsy is a potential source of valuable research material. As with virtually every subject discussed in this chapter, there is no doubt that the relationship between the medico-legal authority and the relatives of the deceased will be closely examined in the comparatively near future.

DISPOSAL OF PARTS OF THE LIVING BODY

That, however, is not the end of the story. It has been noted already that the law as to the ownership of living body parts has derived in piecemeal fashion from that relating to the dead – and if there is dissatisfaction as to the latter, it is amplified time and again in respect of the former. The underlying reason for this is fairly obvious. Dead tissue cannot regenerate and its potential uses are circumscribed. Living tissue, on the other hand, can grow, it can replicate and it can be developed – and modern technology is such that there are decreasingly few limits to the uses to which it can be put. As a result, there is every possibility that questions as to the proprietorship of living tissue may escape the boundaries of the moral dilemma and become, in addition, problems to be hard fought in the economic arena. The Californian case involving Mr Moore provides the classic example.

Moore v Regents of the University of California (1990)

John Moore suffered from hairy cell leukaemia and his spleen was removed as part of his treatment. Unknown to him, his doctor and a research scientist had already discovered unusual properties of recognised commercial value in the organ's cells and, following the operation, they developed an immortal cell line. The doctor, the researcher and the hospital then obtained a patent with a predicted potential market in excess of $3 billion. Moore provided numerous blood specimens during this time, ostensibly still in pursuit of his health and well-being.

On discovering the true nature of the investigations, Moore felt, not unreasonably, that he should share in the profits and based his claim for recompense on the assumption that his property had been 'converted'; that is, that the hospital and the doctors had interfered with his interests in his personal property. To succeed, then, he had to convince the courts that his cells *were* his personal property. The Supreme Court of California was unwilling to accept this – and particularly resisted the view that ownership was of such a nature as to put a financial value on human tissue. Patent law, it was said, protects the inventive effort expended in scientific development, not the discovery of naturally occurring raw materials. They offered many reasons why Moore could not be said to own his cells. Several of these were of doubtful quality, but perhaps the most remarkable was that an extension of the law of property into this area 'would hinder research by restricting access to the necessary raw materials'. This is as clear an example as one is likely to find of the conflicting principles supporting, on the one hand, personal privacy and, on the other, the public or community interest.

In the end, Mr Moore did succeed in establishing a basis for his pleas but only on the grounds that he had not given truly informed consent to the use of his tissues and that his doctors had failed in the duties of loyalty and truthfulness that they owed to their patient. But whether the law on consent is sufficient to protect the undoubted interests of the *source* of a biological invention is debatable – and there are good reasons for supposing that it is not.

A rather similar situation arose in England when it was disclosed that thymus glands removed from children undergoing heart surgery were being passed to drug companies for use in the development of drugs affecting the immune system. It is important to bear in mind that, in these cases, the thymus glands *had* to be removed in order to perform the operations. The immediate legal question is, therefore, who *owns* redundant tissue that is removed at operation? The answer is that no-one really knows. We suspect that the hospital does for the purposes of its disposal but that the patient could demand that it be returned to him or her, subject to any public health considerations. Thus, again, this is a matter of control rather than an economic property right, even though, as we have already seen, the latter may ultimately be acquired by the application of skill to the tissue. It is worth noting that the very influential, albeit unofficial, Nuffield Council on Bioethics has recommended that tissue removed during the course of treatment should be regarded as abandoned material and, therefore, available to the first person who stakes a claim to it – which would normally be the hospital authority. But this would be acceptable without question only if the authority used the material in the way that most people would expect – that is, they would destroy it.

However, as we have seen from the case of Mr Moore, we are now faced with increasing commercial interest in discarded body parts and, indeed, the main concern with the use of human thymus tissue in England was that the hospitals were accepting a monetary award, albeit a very small one, from the drug companies concerned. There is little doubt that the majority opinion would be that specific consent is required from 'the source of the tissue' – i.e. the patient – if it is to be *used* rather than destroyed. But the rules of property as applied to human tissue are so complex that this would almost certainly require action by Parliament before it could be regarded as settled.

In conclusion, it is interesting to speculate on the underlying reason for the anxiety of the courts and the administration on both sides of the Atlantic to avoid placing a monetary value on human tissue – and the importance of *tissue* is to be noted insofar as, at least in the United States, the sale of, say, blood is regarded as unremarkable. Somewhat strangely, it seems that the antipathy stems from the notion of slavery and the buying and selling of human beings. We say 'strangely' in that there is a world of difference between, on the one hand, freely disposing of your tissues even for profit and, on the other, having them forcibly removed. Put another way, because you *may* sell your tissues does not mean that you *have* to do so. Equally, a right to sell your own tissue is not equivalent to someone else's right to buy and sell you. Even so, it is the 'slavery' concept that lies at the heart of the reaction, usually of horror, to the idea of selling one's organs for transplantation.

ORGAN REPLACEMENT THERAPY

It is well to stop for a moment and reflect on the unique morality attached to organ replacement therapy. The majority of treatments involve the use of devices, which can be manufactured at will, or of drugs, which are developed from chemicals that are widely available. The raw materials for transplantation therapy cannot, however, be constructed – at least for the foreseeable future. Their availability is limited absolutely by the size of the population. Treatment by transplantation is a trade in health rather than an absolute gain in health; or, put another way, any advantage to the population is to be measured in net terms rather than as a gross asset. Moreover, the advantage cannot be assessed on a purely numerical basis. A transplanted donor organ must be healthy and it will not be needed unless the recipient's organ is diseased; as a consequence, the process as is commonly visualised is trading a healthy life for one which is already compromised. Finally, it is to be noted that transplantation therapy does not *necessarily* increase the total of human happiness; the joy of the parent whose child has just received a transplant has to be balanced against the tragedy of the parent whose child was killed on the way to school. Perhaps the main moral dilemma thus raised lies in whether it is right that quality of life assessments should intrude on the decision-making process as to who should receive transplants. Such decisions are not the rela-tively simple matters of the allocation of expensive and scarce resources. Among many others, they impose the question of whether the donor has any right to control or influence the use of his donation; a whole range of human emotions is involved and, arguably, should be taken into consideration when the case is evaluated.

All this is, however, a largely philosophical argument which cannot, in practice, be applied directly to conditions of everyday life. The pure pragmatist will have no time for it. 'Healthy organs are available for use,' he or she will say, 'and we *must* use them for the general good'. Moreover, much depends on the nature of the transplant. Thus, in terms of kidney transplantation, two deaths will be postponed as the result of one life being ended prematurely. The ethical basis for transplantation therapy is, thereby, reinforced. On the other hand, cardiac transplantation provides no net gain in human terms – indeed, the result may well be less than neutral when assessed on the quality of the two lives involved; it is, therefore, far less easy to justify. At the other end of the scale, there is the concept of multi-organ transplantation whereby six or more lives could be rescued from one death. Relatively few would see this as anything other than an advantageous 'trade' and the person who conscientiously 'opts out' of such an arrangement stands on ground that is less than firm.

The short conclusion is that organ transplantation offers a valuable form of health service but that its advantages are not unmitigated. Its success depends almost entirely on the availability for use of those organs which become available for selection and, essentially, this can be achieved by way of any compromise between two extremes. At one, a government could introduce compulsory donation of organs in all suitable cases; at the other, individuals could be left free to dispose of their tissues as they wished on the basis that they were, thereby, disposing of their property. The heart of the problem lies in persuading the population that the treatment is both desirable and morally acceptable. We have seen that one avenue to this end is to increase the net gain in human happiness that can be derived from the programme – and this is largely a matter of its organisation in both technical and human terms. An alternative, and less widely discussed, approach is to reduce the dependence on death which figures so prominently in current popular thinking and to consider the advantages of living donation – a process which crystallises the argument as to the ownership of one's body parts within the context of transplantation as a whole.

LIVING DONATION OF ORGANS

The legal constraints

Donation of organs by the living is regulated by both the common and statute law. As has already been discussed, it is unlawful at common law to inflict serious injury on another person and the consent of the victim is, with well defined exceptions, no defence. It is, therefore, clear that one can only consent to donate a part of one's body if it causes one no appreciable harm or, at least, if the harm caused is greatly outweighed by the resultant benefits. The donation of bone marrow is a good example of the latter. The process, as is well known, is painful, it requires a general anaesthetic and, commonly, hospitalisation. All of which is 'harmful'; yet the advantages to a recipient can be so great that donation is regarded as both a laudable and a thoroughly legal practice. Indeed, the case of *Re Y (mental patient: bone marrow donation)* (1997), in which the advantages to the non-consensual donor were, at best, minimal, demonstrates how content the courts are to apply such a balance of benefit analysis. At the other end of the scale, it is clear that, no matter how selfless one felt, one could not legally consent to donate one's heart to a loved one and the surgeon who acceded to such a request would be guilty of, at least, manslaughter or culpable homicide.

Where, then, does that leave other organs?[4] Once again, it is a matter of a balancing exercise. An individual has two kidneys, yet he or she only needs one for a healthy existence. Moreover, the process of removal is, at most, a moderately severe operation to which a competent adult can quite legitimately consent. Moving on a bit, the loss of a lobe of a lung might result in, at most, slightly increased dyspnoea on exertion; but, on the other hand, the operation of lobectomy is rather more difficult than nephrectomy. Similarly, a person could manage quite well without a part of his or her liver;[5] but we are now in a field of technical difficulty where the risks of an operation are becoming less easy to justify – and, as has already been discussed, justification depends, in large part, on the procedure being to the patient's net advantage in relation to the donor's disadvantage.

Can we, then, say that this requirement is met – at least in the most common situation of live kidney donation? The person who has donated a kidney suffers the disadvantage that he or she risks damage to the remaining organ later in life. Against which, the psychological advantage of saving the life of someone one loves may be so great as to weight the scales in favour of donation. And this is where the ethical and legal difficulties begin. If we follow this argument to its logical end, we find that the *legality* of living donation depends on a psychological advantage and, hence, on a close relationship between donor and recipient. The greater the bond, the greater is the justification and, in the absence of a quite remarkable altruistic drive, it is quite possible to argue that it would be *unlawful* for a live person to donate a kidney for use to the first potential recipient on the waiting list. In short, not only can one refuse to donate – and no one can impose an *obligation* on another competent person to provide even bone marrow or blood – but one can also choose to whom one will offer this gift. Thus, a very good case has been made out for the organ being the property of the donor insofar as it is within his or her power to dispose of it as desired, subject only to the common law. But, if the organ is something that can be gifted, why is it

---

[4] An organ is legally defined as any part of the human body consisting of a structured arrangement of tissues which, if wholly removed, cannot be replicated by the body.

[5] While we do not want to complicate the picture unnecessarily, it has to be said that the liver can also regenerate by replicating itself; the problem then arises as to whether transplantation of a lobe of a liver is transplantation of an organ. Common sense suggests that it should be; we also believe it is to be so regarded insofar as the liver itself could not be replicated 'if it was wholly removed'.

not something that can be sold – and it is at this point in the argument that Parliament has felt itself bound to call upon statute law, which it has done by way of the Human Organ Transplants Act 1989.

The 1989 Act has two main functions. The first is to criminalise all aspects of financial trading in human organs – and this includes buying or selling organs from the dead as well as the living; the second is to regularise and control non-commercial organ replacement therapy using living donors.

As to the first, it is an offence for any person to make or receive payment for taking any active part in the transplantation programme and, somewhat unusually, this includes the principals – the donor and the recipient – as offenders. It is also an offence to advertise or to solicit organs for sale in any way. Payment does not include the reimbursement of any costs or reasonable expenses incurred by a person that are directly attributable to the supply of an organ. There are, however, no concessions beyond that and the ban on payment in money for organs is, effectively, absolute.

Ethical aspects

There is no doubt that the Act was triggered by the revelation that a number of Turkish immigrants to England had been involved in the sale of their organs through the medium of transplant surgeons. The combination of poverty and immigration smacked too much of exploitation and the restrictive Act was passed at exceptional speed – so much so that it has been cited as the classic example of Parliamentary 'knee-jerk reaction'. But, while the terms of the Act are intuitively attractive, the reasons behind it are less easy to justify when subjected to analysis. Those in favour of the ban would say that commercial donors are exposing themselves to unacceptable risk; but, as has been discussed already and will be considered further later, live donation is legally, morally and technically acceptable when it is conducted on a non-commercial basis. Secondly, the ethicist will say that free, unfettered consent is impossible when it is associated with financial pressure; but the financial pressure exerted by commercialism is no greater than the emotional pressure involved in free donation within the family. Thirdly, the process can be seen as exploitation of the poor by the rich; but monetary reward for any unpleasant form of employment is also a form of exploitation. Fourthly, many would hold that the commodification of the human body is intrinsically immoral; but there are many ways in which the human body can be used for profit which we do not condemn outright – we may rightly condemn those who profit from the exploitation of the body but we do not hold the principals to be criminally liable. Finally, it is said that allowing the sale of organs undermines the altruism which lies at the heart of the transplantation – and, say, the blood transfusion – service; but this is a particularly Western view which may well not be applicable universally. Moreover, one can ask if it is always true. Consider the person whose daughter suffers from a condition which can only be treated overseas and for a fee. If the daughter had been suffering from a renal disease, the parent would have been praised for altruistically donating a kidney to her. Why, then, is it *immoral*, or any less altruistic, for the parent to sell his or her organ in order to pay for the treatment of a non-renal disease? Such a scenario may be rare but it serves to illustrate that a rapidly imposed, blanket embargo may not be the best method of dealing with an exceptional situation.

It is also perfectly possible to look upon such an embargo as an interference with an individual's rights to behave him- or herself as he or she wishes, providing the action lies within the existing boundaries of public decency. This, however, implies that individuals have the power to dispose of their bodies as they wish – and the argument we have been pursuing has, now, come full circle. We do not for one moment suggest that there should be a free market in human organs. There is, however, a case to be made for payment – or other form of recompense – in special circumstances which could be overseen by an organisation such as ULTRA (see below). The International Forum for Transplant Ethics has recently said:

> Feelings of outrage and disgust that led to an outright ban on kidney sales typically have a force that seems to their possessors to need no further justification. Nevertheless, if we are to deny treatment to the suffering and dying we need better reasons than our own feelings of disgust.

Live donation not only eliminates the unsatisfactory concept of 'a life for a life', it also, of itself, offers scope for a significant increase in the number of organs available for transplantation. There are, therefore, good reasons why it should be encouraged. Yet, in fact, the proportion of live donations in the United Kingdom is only some 5% of all kidney transplants and is falling, whereas the proportion in the United States is nearly 25% – and the sale of organs is just as unlawful there as it is in the United Kingdom.

The 1989 Act in the United Kingdom divides donors into two categories – those who are genetically related to the recipient and those who are not. Donation by the former is not controlled save as to the provision of proof of relationship – and this, in itself, is sufficient to indicate that donation of a kidney is not so serious a 'maim' as to be unlawful at common law. The definition of genetic relationship is wide and goes as far as uncles and aunts of the half blood – at which point the genetic relationship must be at best tenuous but it still has to be proved by DNA or other testing in order to stay within the law. Whether or not it was intentional, the breadth of the permissible relationship reflects the ever-decreasing need for antigenic compatibility provided by the steady improvement in immunosuppressive drugs. It might be thought that Parliament was concerned to preserve the altruistic satisfaction of assisting a relative – and, thus, in preserving the net benefit test for undergoing a surgical operation – rather than to ensure some form of compatibility 'match' between donor and recipient, but this cannot be so as it will be seen that the law as it stands excludes the most intimate bond of all, that of husband and wife or partnership and, also, the not inconsiderable bond that often exists in a *de facto* or an 'in law' relationship. In point of fact, Parliament was probably most anxious to pre-empt the possibility of legal relationships being formed for the sole purpose of coercing donation.

Irrespective of the conditions laid down by statute, it is clear that lawful donation depends upon valid consent to what is, after all, a battery. There is no need to recapitulate what has already been said on this subject in Chapter 4, save to emphasise that the conditions are such as to dictate that consent must be of particularly well 'informed' type. Thus, we might usefully divert from the main discussion at this point to ask whether a child could ever give valid consent to be a donor and whether parental approval is significant in that connection. We have seen that an English minor aged 16–18 is empowered by statute to consent to medical and surgical *treatment* without simultaneous parental approval. This might be taken to exclude a *non-therapeutic* operation, although the same caveat may not apply to Scotland where the legislation is different in that, in general, reference is made to medical and surgical *procedures* – which clearly constitute a wider category than treatments. Even so, Lord Donaldson, when he was the senior judge in the English civil courts, said that, irrespective of statute, the common law right of children, who are able to understand fully what they are undertaking, to consent to treatment extended to the donation of blood or organs. However, he also said that:

> It is inconceivable the doctor should proceed in reliance solely upon the consent of an under-age patient, however competent he or she might be, in the absence of parental consent. (in *Re W* (1992))

Most doctors would be guided by that rule. Given that there *was* parental backing, American courts have supported the idea of 'altruistic benefit' in order to allow an incompetent child to donate to his brother and, surprisingly, the English courts have applied the same test to an incompetent – or non-understanding – adult (see *Re Y*, above). Nonetheless, such cases must be rare and, in practice, the authors' researches indicate that it would be exceptional for a British transplant unit to accept a child as a live organ donor.

Live exchange of tissues between persons who cannot pass the genetic test is unlawful unless it is authorised by the Unrelated Live Transplant Regulatory Authority (ULTRA). Thus, spouses, partners, 'in laws', good friends and even strangers *can* donate to each other – it is just that bit more difficult to do so, insofar as ULTRA must be satisfied that no payment has been made and that, in summary, the principals have been counselled and that consent was free from coercion. As an aside, it can be mentioned that these regulations do not apply in what is probably the most common form of unrelated live transplantation – that is, the use for donation of the *recipient's* heart when a person with lung disease is treated by means of a complete heart/lung transplant.

It is also clear that live donation is technically preferable to cadaveric donation for a number of reasons. Foremost amongst these are that the operation is of elective rather than emergency type, there is none of the urgency involved in keeping organs from a dead person 'alive' – or viable – and time is available for many investigations which cannot be undertaken during the limited period in which cadaveric organs remain useable. Live donation could provide significant relief for the chronic waiting lists for, especially, renal organ replacement therapy and it is surprising how little this avenue is exploited. As has been pointed out already, about 95% of organs for transplantation are taken from the dead and the most recent figures indicate that some 6000 residents in the United Kingdom are awaiting treatment. Public misunderstanding and mistrust are undoubtedly responsible for at least a proportion of this shortfall and an analysis of the basis for this is our main concern in the following section.

CADAVERIC DONATION

To say: 'There is a shortage of organs for transplantation' is to say so with regret. Yet we could make much the same observation by saying: 'There has been a marked fall in the number of accidental deaths' – which is a matter for congratulation.

The equation is not, however, as simple as that. No-one would want to see fit people killed accidentally, no matter what 'good' resulted from their deaths. Even so, beyond the borders of Utopia, some people are bound to die prematurely – and a significant proportion of these will, in fact, die from natural causes of, which subarachnoid haemorrhage is a major prime example. It is the shortfall between the baseline number of such deaths and the number of organ donations that is the cause for concern. The objective is to raise the Phoenix from the fire, not to start the fire itself. Reduction of the gap between the demand and the available is a matter for co-operation between the public, the medical profession and Parliament as the law-maker. We now look briefly at some of the areas where there may be room for improvement in that co-operative effort.

The rationale of brain-stem death

Until the later part of the 20th century, death of the person could best be defined as a permanent state of tissue anoxia. Thus, there is normally only a limited time – a matter of hours – in which to collect and use viable organs from the dead body once the heart and lungs have stopped. This time, as is well known, varies from organ to organ but, for present purposes, the important feature is that the brain cells are far and away the most sensitive to oxygen lack. It is, thus, possible for the major organs of the body to be 'viable' while, at the same time, the brain cells are dead. In normal circumstances, lethal cerebral injury will be followed by failure of respiration and, hence, of oxygenation of the tissues because breathing is under the control of the brain stem. The remaining bodily functions can, however, be maintained if the dead brain stem is substituted by a ventilator. The patient is, then, in the clinical and legal position of a 'beating heart cadaver'; respiration will not return if the ventilator is disconnected. The condition is that of 'brain stem death' which can be verified by the well-known series of standard and relatively simple tests which it is unnecessary to repeat here. It is, however, worth emphasising that, unlike the position in many developed countries, the diagnosis of death is not dictated by statute in the United Kingdom.

From the point of view of recovery of the organs, and *only* from that aspect, the condition of the ventilated cadaver is comparable to that of the living donor. Organ replacement treatment can proceed in nearly ideal conditions and the condition of any donated organs is greatly superior to those which have, themselves, been exposed to oxygen lack as a consequence of cardiorespiratory failure. Thus, the first hurdle the transplant surgeon has to surmount is that of convincing the public in general, and the casualty's near kin in particular, of the validity of 'brain stem death'. This may not be easy – it is hard to accept than a warm, pink body with a palpable heart beat is dead in the way that death is usually understood and, indeed, the concept has been widely criticised on just those grounds. Nevertheless, it has been considered and supported unequivocally by the foremost medical authorities in the United Kingdom and positive legal approval has been expressed, most notably in a case known simply as *Re A* (1992) in which a family attempted to force the hospital to continue to ventilate a child who had been diagnosed as dead. The House of Lords has also confirmed this from the opposite point of view in the well-known case of *Airedale NHS Trust v Bland* (1993) concerning the treatment of Anthony Bland who was in a permanent vegetative state – 'His brain stem is alive and so is he', it was said, the clear inference being that, had his brain stem been dead, he would also have been dead.

In a sense, the doubts and the argument are about nothing because, essentially, all death is brain stem death – the difference is that, whereas cardiorespiratory death normally precedes brain stem death, the reverse is true within the special conditions of the intensive care unit.

Cadaveric donation and the law

As we have seen, the law covering cadaveric donation is contained in the Human Tissue Act 1961 which is, in many ways, an unsatisfactory piece of legislation. Much could be written on the technicalities of the Act but, for present purposes, we will try to confine discussion to those aspects which influence the supply of organs for treatment.

In summary, the main effect of the Act is to divide donation into two categories:

a) *The deceased has expressed a wish during life that his/her organs be used for treatment, research or education after death.* In these circumstances, the person lawfully in possession of the body after death may authorise the removal of any part of the body in accordance with that request. Thus, the deceased has, in effect, 'contracted in' to the transplant programme. It is to be noted that no power of veto is granted in this section but, at the same time, the power of action is permissive – '*he or she may*' – rather than mandatory.

b) *The deceased has made no such request.* The person lawfully in possession of the body may then authorise removal of any part of that body if, having made such reasonable enquiry as may be practicable, he or she has no reason to believe that the deceased would have objected or that the surviving spouse or any surviving relative does object to the body being so used. Thus, anyone has the right to 'contract out' of the system during life and, in the absence of a previous direction by the deceased, the near kin can veto any positive action by the person in charge of the body.[6]

There are a number of difficulties attached to these conditions which have a bearing on the availability of organs. First, the legally valid wishes of the deceased can have been expressed either in writing at any time or orally in the presence of witnesses during his or her last illness. There is no logical reason to doubt that the completion of a 'donor card' satisfies the first requirement despite the fact that it is a printed document, and it follows that a donor card provides absolute authority for organ donation. It will be seen later that this fact is often either misunderstood or ignored.

Second, although there is now no doubt that the person 'lawfully in possession of the body' for the purposes of the Act is the hospital authority, it should be remembered that possession is not the same as ownership. The executors of the deceased undoubtedly have a right to possession of his or her body but such precedent as there is suggests that this is for the purpose of ultimate disposal – that is, where and

---

[6] It is to be noted that, absent the consent of the Coroner, no action can be taken if it seems that there may be an inquest or that the Coroner may wish to authorise an autopsy examination. Similarly, there can be no removal of organs in Scotland if the Procurator Fiscal has objected to such removal.

when the deceased should be buried or cremated. The hospital authorities must resign their possession if it is claimed by the executors but until that time – and the interval might include the window of opportunity for obtaining viable organs – they hold the possessory powers for the purposes of the 1961 Act. In practice, there are very few occasions when a suitable donor is not being maintained on a ventilator prior to death and there is ample opportunity for discussion between relatives, potential executors and, say, the hospital transplant co-ordinator. Argument as to possession would arise only in the event of violent disagreement – perhaps, for example, where the deceased was the *only* suitable match for an expectant recipient and the relatives were objecting.

Third, there is the very vexed problem of who is a surviving relative? The Act makes no effort to define such a person and there is little doubt that even a distant relation could veto cadaver donation. Equally, a person who might have been closest to the deceased – for example, a cohabiting partner – has no official voice. Perhaps more important is the question of the extent of the obligation on the person in possession to make enquiries of the relevant persons. This is governed by the words 'reasonable' and 'practicable' and it would certainly be unreasonable to expect so many enquiries to be made as to jeopardise the success of any later donations. Again, in practice, this is less of a concern than might be supposed. As has already been observed, the circumstances are almost always such that relatives are present at the bedside before death is certified; one close relation can then reasonably be taken to speak for the whole family. It might, however, be useful to have a list defining the term 'relative' if only to clarify who may *not* object to donation – and this may well form part of any revised legislation. It would not be illogical to adopt the list provided in the Human Organ Transplants Act 1989 as setting the limits but is unlikely that imposing such a restriction would make any measurable difference to the donation rate as a whole.

THE SHORTAGE OF ORGANS

Other potentially significant changes to the 1961 Act and its interpretation have been proposed with the main objective of improving the availability of organs. The first is to alter the permissive wording of the Act from 'may' to 'must' so as to make the search for donors an imperative. This could apply both when the wishes of the deceased had been expressed in life and when they had not. In the latter circumstance, the hospital authorities or the transplant team would be compelled to approach the relatives in order to establish the lack of objection to donation – a practice which is generally known as 'required request'. In the authors' view, this option would, however, place an undue burden on healthcarers and also restrict their clinical judgement. Healthcarers have at least a modified duty of care to the families of their patients. They must, therefore, have freedom to judge the extent to which the relatives are put under stress. The former situation is, however, rather different. It is almost universal practice for the transplant team to seek and to accept the views of the near kin even though the deceased has satisfied the 'living direction' requirements of the Act. To many, perhaps most, this would seem to be the caring and humane approach. It is, however, possible to look at the dilemma from the position of the patient's autonomy which, as we have seen throughout this book, is now a guiding principle underlying the doctor/patient relationship. The signing of a 'donor card' effectively provides the setting for the patient's last autonomous act; how, then, can we justify denying this jealously guarded privilege simply because he or she is no longer in a position to enforce it? This may seem a legalistic and unsympathetic approach. Nevertheless, objection by the relatives in the face of a valid donor card is a potent cause of lost donations.

The relatives' doubts might also be, to an extent, assuaged if it were a legal requirement that a certificate of the cause of death was presented to the deceased's representative before any donor operation was carried out. This has other important implications in that the Act requires that the responsible surgeon – who must, save in the case of removal of eyes or parts of eyes,[7] be a registered medical practitioner – should satisfy him- or herself *by personal examination of the body* that life is extinct. Given that the subject is a 'beating heart donor', this is a near impossibility unless the operation is postponed until a flat electrocardiogram is obtained following disconnection of the ventilator – a process which, of itself, goes some way to vitiating the advantages of beating heart donation. It would eliminate doubts if the surgeon were able to satisfy himself by way of inspection of a death certificate – but that is not how the law stands at present.

A more radical modification of the 1961 Act, designed specifically to improve the transplantation rate[8] would be to turn the existing law on its head and require people to 'contract out' of the system if they do not want to take part rather than, as at present, 'contract in' if they do wish to do so. In this way, any suitable cadaver would be immediately available as a donor unless he or she was known to have objected to being so used. While this approach has been advocated by responsible bodies such as the British Medical Association, and while it has been adopted in some European jurisdictions with apparent success, many would see it as a violation of the last respect due to an individual. Nor is it an administratively simple matter. Its efficient operation depends upon the availability of a centralised data base, which is neither a cheap infrastructure nor one that is immune to break-down. Moreover, it is difficult to believe that such a system could be introduced unless it included *some* deference to the wishes of the near kin, which would leave the situation much as it is at present. It is probable that the apparent, albeit limited, success of such schemes elsewhere is due not so much to the scheme itself as to the fact that public attitudes are modified once 'contracting out' is adopted as the norm.

And, there's the rub – improving the supply of cadaver organs is essentially a matter of convincing the public of its safety and of its grounding on good ethical principles. The question then is, can this be done without, at the same time, imposing elements of compulsion such as are evident in the alternatives discussed above? We believe that it can but, at the same time, that it will only be feasible when people appreciate that modern multi-organ replacement therapy represents far more than a life for a life; only then will individuals feel able to co-operate wholeheartedly in extracting what good they can from a personal tragedy.

---

[7] By virtue of the Corneal Tissue Act 1986, eyes or parts of eyes may be removed by a suitably qualified technician acting under the instructions of a doctor who has satisfied himself that life is extinct.

[8] We do not intend to discuss here the possibility of selling the organs of the dead which has none of the justifications applied to sale of organs from the living and which would involve such a change in attitude – both legal and social – as to be, currently, impracticable. As already mentioned the sale of organs from the dead is proscribed in the 1989 Act in the same way as is the sale of those from the living.

Even so, it is important than an enthusiasm for improving the number of donors does not reactivate the dormant fears of so-called 'body-snatching'. Elective ventilation is an example of such an, otherwise praiseworthy, initiative. In brief, this involves transfer of patients dying in the medical wards to the intensive care unit so that they can be immediately available as donors when death occurs. Although such a procedure may well capture a pool of organs which would, otherwise, be lost, it falls foul of the law in that the moribund incompetent cannot consent to an invasive procedure – and we have seen throughout this book how important is the concept of the inviolability of bodily integrity to modern medical practice. This conclusion might, however, be voided were the deceased to have left an advance directive or 'living will' requesting that such a procedure be followed.

THE USE OF ANIMAL ORGANS

We do not intend to discuss the use of animal organs – or xenotransplantation – in organ replacement therapy in any detail as the possibility lies many years ahead and, indeed, its potential may well be overtaken by developments in stem cell research. Nonetheless, techniques for suppressing the foreign antigen rejection mechanism are advancing rapidly and the subject is a matter of public, as well as scientific, interest.

Assuming that animal organs could ever be capable of sustaining human life – and there is, currently, no certainty of this – the problems of organ shortage could, in theory, be largely eliminated by their use. Not everyone would, however, welcome the innovation. Some would hold that the animal kingdom is a holistic entity and that we have no right to assume that we can use non-human species as reservoirs for the regeneration of humans. Closer to home, others would question the advisability of replacing human organs one by one as they failed; the end result might well be a vast increase in the number of those existing with senile brain damage. Yet others would point to the fact that the National Health Service could not possibly cope with the resulting financial load and xenotransplantation would become the prerogative of the rich.

For the moment, however, the practical difficulties are more important. The major hurdle of organ rejection could be minimised by the use of other primates and such replacements have been attempted outside the United Kingdom. There would, however, be particular antipathy to using our distant cousins in this way. The use of primates in transplantation is, in fact, banned in the United Kingdom save for research purposes. Effectively, we are left with the pig as the least unsatisfactory source of organs. Here, we encounter the really frightening possibility of transferring animal infection – and particularly viral infection – to man. As a consequence, animal donors would have to be kept in maximally sterile conditions with all of the associated suffering that entails. Which brings us back to our original, and what is probably the major, objection to xenotransplantation – that our right to enslave the animal kingdom in this way is, at least, questionable and may well be unsustainable.

On the other side of the coin, the recipients of a xenotransplant would be required to surrender fundamental liberties by being subject to a lifelong monitoring and surveillance regime, which might be seen as flying in the face of their human rights. Moreover, it is not clear that consent to this surrender is legally competent. As we have seen, there are limits to what individuals may consent to; this may well be one of them. In present circumstances, it would almost certainly be unlawful to transplant a pig's heart into a human – the chances of failure and death of the patient, even if delayed by a week or two, would be so high that no person could give valid consent and no surgeon could undertake the operation and still be certain of remaining within the law. This situation is likely to persist for several years to come. Meantime, the government has established a Xenotransplantation Interim Regulatory Authority (UKXIRA) which will oversee the development of the procedure pending the introduction of legislation. The authority of UKXIRA is required for clinical trials of xenotransplantation; only a few applications have been made and, to date, no such authority has been given. Xenotransplantation may well come in time but it is by no means certain that it will also usher in a braver new world.

CONCLUSION

The central pillar of this chapter has been the Human Tissue Act of 1961 and that, in itself, goes a long way to explaining why its tenor is generally one of dissatisfaction. Firstly, the Act is old – and it has remained unaltered during a half century that has witnessed a sea change in medico-social attitudes. Secondly, its drafting has always been the subject of criticism because of its uncertainty. And thirdly, and perhaps of greatest importance, it attempts to cover too much ground under a single umbrella. Medical research and teaching provoke responses that are greatly different from those appropriate to treatment by way of organ transplantation and the authors are strongly of the view that this should be recognised in the revised legislation that is bound to come. Meantime, the unsatisfactory state of affairs reminds us that a sympathetic doctor/patient alliance remains the ideal as much in death as it does in life.

Equally importantly, however, we have also questioned whether or not it is reasonable to continue to assert that there are, or should be, no property rights in the human body, or at least in its parts. Modern medical reality might provoke a re-evaluation of this mantra. At the same time, we have emphasised the complexity of the very concept of property itself, arguably requiring the law to take a more sophisticated approach to individual rights in respect of control, ownership and disposal.

CASES REFERRED TO IN THE TEXT

A, Re [1992] 3 Med LR 303.

Airedale NHS Trust v Bland [1993] 1 All ER 821.

Dobson v North Tyneside Health Authority [1996] 4 All ER 474.

J (a minor) (Prohibited steps order: Circumcision), Re [2000] 1 FLR 571.

Moore v Regents of the University of California 793 P 2d 479 (Cal, 1990).

R v Brown [1993] 2 All ER 75; *Laskey, Jaggard and Brown v United Kingdom* (1997) 24 EHRR 39.

R v Donovan [1934] All ER Rep 207.

R v Kelly [1998] 3 All ER 741.

Sidaway v Board of Governors of the Bethlem Royal Hospital and the Maudsley Hospital [1985] 1 All ER 653.

W (a minor) (medical treatment), Re [1992] 4 All ER 627.

Y (mental incapacity: bone marrow transplant), Re [1997] Fam 110.

FURTHER READING

Advisory Group on the Ethics of Transplantation. *Animal Tissue into Humans* 1996.

Downie R. 'Xenotransplantation', *Journal of Medical Ethics* 1997; 23: 205.

Dworkin G, Kennedy I. 'Human tissue: Rights in the body and its parts', *Medical Law Review* 1993; 1: 29.

Fox M, McHale J. 'Xenotransplantation: the ethical and legal implications', *Medical Law Review* 1998; 6: 42.

Harvey J. 'Paying organ donors', *Journal of Medical Ethics* 1990; 16: 24.

Interim Report of the Inquiry into the Management and Care of Children Receiving Complex Heart Surgery at the Bristol Royal Infirmary, 2000.

McLean SAM. 'Transplantation and the "nearly dead": The case of elective ventilation' in McLean SAM (ed.) *Contemporary Issues in Law, Medicine and Ethics*, Chapter 8, 1996.

Mason K, Laurie G. 'Consent or property? Dealing with the body and its parts in the shadow of Bristol and Alder Hey', *Modern Law Review* 2001; 64: 710.

New B, Solomon M, Dingwall R, McHale J. *A Question of Give and Take: Supply of Organs for Transplantation*, 1994.

Nuffield Council on Bioethics. *Human Tissue: Ethical and Legal Issues*, 1995.

Pallis C. *ABC of Brain Stem Death*, 2nd ed., 1998.

Report of the Royal Liverpool Children's Inquiry, 2001.

Report of the Independent Review Group on the Retention of Organs at Post Mortem, 2001.

White S. 'The law relating to dealing with dead bodies', *Medical Law International* 2000; 4: 145.

World Health Organisation. *Guiding Principles on Human Organ Transplantation*, 1994.

14

SEX, GENDER AND THE LAW

THE DIAGNOSIS OF SEX

In a very old but, nonetheless, influential article, Mr Justice Ormrod pointed out that 'the law is relatively indifferent to a person's sex' – and this is still true to-day. One can obtain employment, a driving licence or even a passport in whichever sex one wants to. Moreover, the criminal law is leaning the way of the civil law. Time was when rape could be committed only by a man on a woman; now, persons of either sex can rape those of the opposite or of the same sex – and the offence is no longer limited to penetration of the vulva.

Where, then, does any legal interest lie? An analysis of case law, together with the collateral statutory family law, leaves one in little doubt that, despite a relatively steady erosion of principle in accordance with changing moral attitudes, current public policy in the United Kingdom remains that of regarding the nuclear family as constituting a corner stone of our society. As a consequence, the law attaches very considerable importance to marriage which it defines as a union between 'one man and one woman'. Sex is, therefore, an integral part of marriage and we will see that United Kingdom law has been resolute that the sex of a person is settled at birth and remains unchanged throughout life. The birth certificate is, therefore, an important document. This is not so much because it is often used or needed – indeed, we have seen in our opening paragraph that it is not. Its significance in UK law lies in its status as a statement of historical fact. At present – and we will see that this state of affairs is unlikely to persist for long – the terms of the certificate can be altered only if it is discovered that a genuine mistake has been made. It follows that, although the medical details will be well known to the reader, we must, briefly consider how such mistakes can be made. Only then will we be able to analyse and understand the legal response to a 'change of sex'.

In ordinary circumstances, our sex is decided at birth by the doctor or midwife on the basis of our external genitalia and it is this that determines the sex that is entered on our birth certificate. Very occasionally, a mistake is made. Sometimes adrenal hyperplasia leads to overgrowth of the female pudenda and a false diagnosis of masculinity is made. More often the testes do not descend and the male external organs exhibit a degree of hypospadias; a male child may then be taken for a female. Hormonal deficiencies of many types may arise spontaneously or they may be transmitted genetically, in which case complex patterns of what is popularly known as 'inter-sex' may arise. One of these – the testicular feminisation syndrome – is particularly important in the modern medico-legal context. In this, the androgenic hormones are produced but cannot react with their target organs; the result is a genetic 'man' (for which, see below) with all the physical attributes of a woman save that 'she' has no ovaries or uterus and, generally, has, at most, a poorly developed vagina.

Many such 'errors' will either adjust themselves during adolescence or they will come to light at puberty when, say, there is some anomaly in the expected pattern of menstruation. A difficult medico-legal situation then arises – is the 'error' to be seen as such and the adolescent assisted into a change of lifestyle or is the adolescent's sexual adaptation to be preserved and, indeed, supported by hormonal and/or surgical treatment? The ethical arguments surrounding such cases are beyond the remit of this book – indeed, as is so often the position, generalisations can be dangerous and each case must be decided on its own particular conditions. It need only be said that decisions based on bona fide medical evidence and on the understanding of both the patient and his or her parents form part of good medical practice and are, therefore, both legally and ethically acceptable when undertaken in the patient's best interests.

It is worth noting at this point that decision-time may not rise until marriage. There is no doubt, for example, that many of the petitions for nullity of marriage on the grounds of non-consummation that were such a feature of medico-legal activity in the early 20th century resulted from misunderstanding the testicular feminisation syndrome. The case of Mrs W, whose gonads and genetic make-up were male but whose genitalia were ambiguous, is a good modern example which demonstrates the softening of attitudes that has evolved over the years. Every effort was made to bring up Mrs W as a boy but, by the time it came to marriage, it had clearly been an error of clinical judgement – and the court agreed that it was so.

If an error *has* been made and it is one that ought to be rectified, the Registrar can enter the matter in the Register of Corrections and the sex that was given on the certificate of birth can be altered; it is to be emphasised that, within the existing law, it is *only if* an error has been made that this can be done. We will see that this apparent rigidity has caused considerable difficulty in the courts of the United Kingdom and Europe but it is not an illogical position to adopt. The certificate of birth does no more than certify that 'John – or Jane – Smith was born on a given day'. It does not certify that 'I, the bearer, am John Smith' or 'I am Jane Smith' although, in the absence of other identification papers in the United Kingdom, it has to serve that purpose when identification and proof of age are required. It is fundamental to any discussion involving 'sex change' and the law that we consider how often, or how seldom, that requirement has to be met. In practice, we have already noted that United Kingdom law pays scant regard to the sex of its citizens. But we have also seen that this *laissez faire* attitude is discarded when statute law and, in particular, marriage law is involved.

In view of the fact that about 1 in 3 marriages ends in divorce, it is somewhat surprising that marriage in England and Wales is still referred to in the secular ceremony in the same way as it was in 1866: 'the union of one man and one woman, voluntarily entered into, for life, to the exclusion of all others'. For present purposes, we need to concentrate only on the words 'man' and 'woman'. We have recognised that mistakes can be made when a person's sex is decided on the grounds of the external genitalia and we have also seen that an error can be corrected. It follows, therefore, that additional diagnostic factors must be taken into consideration and, from the legal point of view, we can best consider these by way of the criteria laid down in 1970 by Mr Justice Ormrod – who was, himself, medically qualified – in the fundamental case of *Corbett v Corbett (otherwise Ashley)*.

The most obvious second diagnostic choice for determining sex lies in the gonads but they will also be seen to provide an unsatisfactory criterion. A woman's ovaries are concealed in the abdomen while testes are frequently undescended and, similarly, retained in the abdomen. Thus, the presence of, as well as the type of, gonads may be difficult to determine. Moreover, both testes and ovaries will be present in the very rare condition of true hermaphroditism.

It will be seen later that the law pays considerable attention to the chromosomal status of the individual. While the reader will be well aware of the facts, we must, because of the importance that has been attached to the matter in recent cases decided in the European courts, point out that to say that the chromosomal pairing XY represents a male and that of XX a female is an over-simplification. The general rule is to hold that the possession of a Y chromosome indicates a male rather than that the possession of two X's indicates a female. The distinction between the two statements is important as the sex chromosomes are notorious for the production of trisomies. According to the general rule above, the person carrying the common trisomy XXY is male whereas he/she would be female if we adopted the alternative rule. Similarly, the mirror image of the defective chromosomal 'split' – X(O) – is female because she has no Y chromosome but would not so qualify were the 'XX = female' rule to be adopted. Although this may seem to be unnecessary detail, it is, as we have indicated, of considerable practical importance because the presence of such anomalies, and their interpretation, have provided a main platform for those who seek to blur the traditional male/female distinction with which we are familiar.

These characteristics comprise what have been called the biological sex factors. We have not yet touched upon the sociological factors – the general appearance, how a person dresses and, above all, how a person *feels* about his or her sex. Taken together, such factors can be regarded as representing the person's *gender* and, occasionally, his or her biological sex and gender are at loggerheads. The extreme of such conflict results in the gender dysphoria syndrome or what is better known as transsexualism.

TRANSSEXUALISM

Transsexual symptoms may arise as a result of mistaken sexual identity at birth but these are a minority – the judge in *W v W*, which we have mentioned above, was at pains to emphasise that Mrs W was *not* a transsexual. The typical transsexual is a man or woman of undisputed biological sex who is convinced that he or she has been provided with the *wrong* physical sexual attributes. The conviction is more than an idle fancy and is, accordingly, to be distinguished from, say, transvestitism, in which a man gains pleasure from cross-dressing but will revert to 'normal' once his enjoyment has been fulfilled. The transsexual is not, or is only rarely, a homosexual in the true sense. The transsexual man may well be attracted to other men but this is because he sees himself as a woman – regular heterosexual associations will be established once his biological sex has been altered to fit with his gender. It can now be accepted that transsexualism is a genuine psychiatric condition – possibly congenital, in that our personal gender may well be pre-determined at birth – that merits treatment. The difficulty here is that 'treatment' in the form of psychotherapy that will reverse the condition is very rarely successful, largely because it is usually unwanted. In the end, the only *effective* 'treatment' – which is not necessarily the same as *successful* treatment – is to treat the mental turbulence by following the script and 'reassigning' the biological sex by way of extensive surgery and supportive hormonal treatment.[1] Needless to say, such extreme measures require careful pre-assessment and counselling. It goes without saying, for example, that the practical results of a female to male reassignment are likely to be less satisfactory than those in the reverse situation. Nevertheless, reassignment surgery is now well-supported by informed medical opinion – were it not so, such mutilation of the body might well be unlawful – and the operation is now available under the National Health Service subject to the restraints imposed by lack of funding which have been discussed in Chapter 2.

Thus, it will be seen that the 'converted', or treated, transsexual's place in society, which is controlled by his or her *gender*, poses no general problems other than those arising from a less than successful cosmetic result. He or she – and conversion from male to female is far more common than the reverse – will be accepted in his or her altered sex and life, including societally acceptable cohabitation, can go on undisturbed. That is until, as has been already intimated, we come up against any statute law in which sex is a determining factor – and marriage law is the most important example for present purposes.

Transsexual marriage

It has already been noted that lawful marriage is a union between man and woman. A supposed marriage between persons of the same sex is void – so far as the law is concerned, it never happened. Moreover, the official performing the marriage ceremony has a duty to ensure, so far as is practicable, that the conditions for a lawful marriage are satisfied and this was, of course, a main purpose behind the advance publication of the banns of marriage which gave the general public the opportunity to raise a question and inform the celebrant of any irregularities. Clearly, then, the transsexual seeking to be married has a major problem to overcome, a problem which will be decided, one way or another, on whether or not the acquisition of a new *gender* constitutes a change of *sex* for the purposes of marriage.

This was the fundamental question addressed in the case of *Corbett v Corbett* in 1971 which is one of those unusual cases, heard by a single judge, which never went

---

[1] The ethics of gender reassignment surgery can be applied to other conditions involving mutilation – for example, apotemnophilia or the body dysmorphic syndrome in which the patient develops a pathological hatred of part of his or her body.

to appeal yet which, even so, has remained as the expression of the law for many years. The Corbetts, of whom Mrs Corbett was a converted male to female transsexual, were married in Gibraltar. Later, the marriage broke down and Mr Corbett sought to have the marriage declared void on the grounds that the parties were of the same sex. Mr Justice Ormrod had a lot to say about sex and marriage, some of which can be regarded as a trifle irrelevant. But, in essence, he held that:

- marriage is a relationship that depends on sex and not on gender;
- biological sex depends on the original genital and gonadal configuration and the chromosomal pattern; and
- in the event of doubt, priority is to be given to the external genitalia.

Mr Justice Ormrod had no difficulty in the case at issue, as all the biological criteria were consistent – the marriage was void. But, in addition to saying that he would have opted for the pre-operative genital appearances had there been any doubt, he also said that the sexual constitution of an individual is fixed at birth and cannot be changed. These two statements are difficult to reconcile in the case of the converted transsexual whose genitalia and gonads *have* been changed. As a consequence, later courts have concentrated upon the one criterion that *is* immutable – that is, the chromosomal pattern, which has come to be the yardstick by which sex is measured in England and Wales.[2]

While this does lead to conformity in the law, it is unfortunate in that our X and Y chromosomes comprise the one biological sexual attribute we have which is of no practical consequence either to ourselves or to outsiders. The *Corbett* principle falls flat on its face, for example, when confronted by the testicular feminisation syndrome where we have a person recognised by herself and by all outsiders as a woman but who has male chromosomes. Moreover, the reasoning in *Corbett*, which was concerned only with family law, has also been extended and applied to the criminal law. In the case of *R v Tan*, a male to female converted transsexual was found guilty under section 30 of the Sexual Offences Act of 1956 which criminalises a man who lives off the earnings of prostitutes. Her conversion was excellent but she could not convert her chromosomes. This, again, is an unfortunate result as the basis of criminal activity lies in behaviour, not in anatomic niceties. This is well illustrated by the 1988 Australian case of *R v Harris, R v McGuinness* where two male to female transsexuals were accused of attempted indecency with a man – an offence which can only be committed by another man. One, who had not undergone reassignment surgery, was found guilty; the other, who had been converted surgically was found not guilty. Each had the same chromosomes but only one had male genitalia.

Thus, the Australian courts would certainly not extend the English interpretation of *Corbett* to the criminal field and there is evidence that Australia and other common law jurisdictions, which includes the great majority of the English-speaking world, would reject it even as to family law. In the United States, a male to female convert's marriage to a man has been declared valid on the grounds that she could act within marriage as a female (*M.T. v J.T.*). By contrast, marriages in the reverse situation have been declared void in the United States; they would, in any case, be voidable – that is, they could be extinguished – throughout the United Kingdom on the grounds of

---

[2] So far as we can discover, no comparable case has been decided in Scotland.

non-consummation. Thus, transsexual marriage is subject to a great deal of confusion and also involves an element of unfair discrimination between the sexes. This, it is said, would be dissipated in the United Kingdom if it were possible to alter the birth certificate; that done, it is widely assumed that the problems of same-sex marriage would no longer exist.

Transsexualism and Europe

It is clear that the control of peoples' sex lives is likely to involve their human rights as expressed in the European Convention on Human Rights which is now embodied in the Human Rights Act of 1998. As a result, the medico-legal history of transsexualism in the United Kingdom is closely bound with that in the European Union and we cannot consider the former while ignoring the latter. With this in mind, we must start from the premise that there are at least 20 member States of the Council of Europe in which the definition of sex is thought to be sufficiently wide as to validate transsexual marriage in the converted sex.[3] The European Parliament has also expressed its support for legislation along these lines. Small wonder, then, that transsexuals in the United Kingdom wishing to marry have turned to the European Court of Human Rights for relief, pleading, in the main, that the refusal of the United Kingdom to allow the birth certificate to be changed offends against Article 8 of the Convention, which provides for the right to respect for one's private and family life, and Article 12, which establishes a right to marry and to found a family.

The first challenge to existing United Kingdom law came in 1986 from a Mr Rees who was a female to male convert. Here, the Court of Human Rights noted the relaxed attitude to sex outside marriage that existed in the UK and the relatively small number of times that a birth certificate has to be produced. Accordingly, the application under Article 8 was dismissed by a majority of 12:3 judges. The application under Article 12 was dismissed unanimously since marriage was clearly a matter of union between two people of opposite biological sex; significantly, it was emphasised that the right to marry was 'subject to the national laws governing the exercise of that right'. Five years later, Ms Cossey, who was a very successful male to female reassignment, invited the court to reverse its opinion. It did not do so but the majority in respect of Article 8 was reduced to 10:8 and the unanimous finding as to Article 12 in Mr Rees' case now became a majority of 14:4. The very strong dissenting arguments stressed the rapidly changing attitudes to what are, essentially, private matters. It was pointed out that scientific understanding of the condition had evolved considerably and that the anomalies of the sex chromosome trisomies, discussed above, threw grave doubts on the validity of the chromosome test. Very tellingly, it was remarked that reassignment surgery was a treatment for a recognised psychiatric condition and that treatment was incomplete without full recognition of the new status. The whole court suggested that the United Kingdom should keep a careful watching brief on what was a changing and uncertain situation.

---

[3] These include Austria, Belgium, Denmark, Estonia, Finland, France, Germany, Greece, Iceland, Italy, Latvia, Luxembourg, the Netherlands, Norway, Slovakia, Spain, Sweden, Switzerland, Turkey and the Ukraine.

All the omens, then, pointed to the likelihood that the United Kingdom would lose the next case in which it was involved. Very surprisingly, it did not. In 1998, Ms Sheffield and Ms Horsham, both male to female converted transsexuals, fought a further case in the European Court of Human Rights, again, mainly under Articles 8 and 12 of the Convention. The first action was dismissed by a judicial majority of 11:9, first, because the unusual conditions in the United Kingdom meant that a birth certificate had to be produced so rarely that doing so was not an intrusion into personal privacy of such severity as to warrant interference with the State's administrative laws.[4] Second, the court considered that there had been no significant changes in the understanding of transsexualism since Ms Cossey's case and there was still no sufficiently common policy on the subject within Europe to justify a change of opinion. Again, however, the United Kingdom was rapped over the knuckles for its unenthusiastic approach to research on the topic. Interestingly, the applicants lost their case in respect of Article 12 by a majority of 18:2 which suggested that there was an attitude to social inconvenience which differed from that adopted on the specific issue of marriage. Indeed, the court rather bravely articulated their belief that the right to marry guaranteed by Article 12 referred to the traditional marriage between persons of opposite biological sex; Article 12 was seen as being mainly concerned to protect such marriage as the basis of the nuclear family.

On the face of things, therefore, recognition of transsexual marriage in the United Kingdom appeared to be by no means close at hand. Yet the pressures continued in the domestic courts as well. In 2000, Mrs Bellinger, who was a 'married' male to female transsexual, brought a case in which she asked that her marriage be declared valid. On the basis of previous experience, one would have thought that the action was hopeless. Nonetheless, she took it to the Court of Appeal where she lost by only a 2:1 majority. The President of the Family Court had some caustic comments to make on the dilatoriness of the Government's approach to the issue while the dissenting, and very senior, judge thought that there were now no compelling reasons why Mrs Bellinger should not be regarded as being legally married.

Almost inevitably, then, the walls were torn down and, in 2002, Ms Goodwin succeeded in convincing the European Court of Human Rights that the United Kingdom legislation violated not only Article 8 but also, and as a direct consequence, Article 12. Thus, the United Kingdom is now in breach of its European commitments. Parliament will have to find time to amend the law and the probability is that, within a year or so, transsexuals will be able to apply for revised birth certificates and to marry within their new sexual identity – irrespective of whether or not they have undergone reassignment surgery. The historian will be satisfied by the intention to preserve the original record but it is likely that the general public will be denied access to evidence of a change of sex.

It is unlikely that legislation that is consistent in every possible situation can be drafted but we have, in fact, been living with some anomalies for some time. Is it, for example, logical to forbid transsexual marriage yet to turn a blind eye to the marriage of a 'woman' who is the result of the testicular feminisation syndrome? The issue in

---

[4] Note that an applicant won a similar case against France because, there, the sex identified at birth has to be disclosed frequently.

both cases is that of *gender*. In similar vein, we could ask if it is logical to forbid 'marriage' between two lesbian women when marriages between women and male to female converted transsexuals are perfectly legal and have been celebrated in both secular and religious environments. Bridging the gap between the United Kingdom and the European Court of Human Rights may, in fact, be less painful than some have anticipated.

Transsexualism and the family

Such anomalies are not confined to marriage and, aided by the general inclination of the British public to respect their neighbours' privacy, they may spill over into the family circumstances. An apposite case was heard by the European Court of Human Rights in 1997.

Here, Mr X, a female to male converted transsexual, had lived with Ms Y in a stable relationship for some 10 years. Ms Y had a daughter, Z, by way of artificial insemination and an application was made to have X registered as the father of Z. An appeal under Article 8 – interference with family life – was launched when this was refused. Once again, this was turned down by the Court of Human Rights, the grounds being, first, that their lives as a family were scarcely affected by the lack of registration – Z had been given X's surname and X and Y together could, for example, apply for a residence order which would give X full parental rights. Second, it was by no means clear that it was in Z's best interests for X to be registered as her father. And, third, the Court considered that to allow such a change in the regulations might have unfortunate repercussions throughout family law – in short, it was a classic instance of the old maxim 'hard cases make bad law'.

Nevertheless, this 'birth certificate' case does not rest on the logic that lies beneath a refusal to alter the fact of a person's sex at birth. Reference to Chapter 8 will show that, under the Human Fertilisation and Embryology Act of 1990, X could have been legally registered as Z's father had he been 'a chromosomal man'. Thus, that part of the birth certificate relating to parentage is no longer sacrosanct as to fact and the refusal of the Court to make use of this avenue is yet another example of the remarkable staying power of the *Corbett* decision. This is all the more significant in that, while the 1990 Act speaks in terms of a 'man and a woman seeking treatment together', the Court of Human Rights translated this as 'male and female partners'. Such nuances are important in interpreting statute law. United Kingdom law cannot envisage Mr X as a 'man'; it would be far less difficult to accept a converted transsexual as a 'male or female partner' for it would be reasonable to regard the *adjectives* as being based on gender rather than biology. But the Court did not follow up this point and one wonders if, and if so how, forthcoming legislation will deal with such unusual scenarios.

Transsexualism and employment

The United Kingdom arguments that have, until Ms Goodwin's case, successfully sustained the status quo in respect of family law are, however, very much harder to accept in the field of employment. The aspect of employment law which is particularly relevant in the context of this chapter is largely that of discrimination between persons seeking employment and, particularly, discrimination on the ground of sex.

Until recently, and in ordinary circumstances, the fact that a person is a transsexual has not made a major impact on the employment market. It is, for example, perfectly feasible for a person to be regarded as a woman for employment purposes and as a man for the needs of national insurance. Much depends, however, on mutual co-operation and difficulty can arise if the employer and the employee cannot agree.

The transsexual is, then, in a difficult position. The basic test of discrimination under, say, the Sex Discrimination Act of 1975 is to compare the treatment given to a woman with that which would be given to a man in comparable circumstances and vice versa. But we have seen that the male to female convert remains a man in law. Thus, in the event of an accusation of discrimination by such a person on the ground of sex, the comparison is between a man with unusual characteristics and a man without those characteristics; there is, then, no discrimination *between* the sexes. As a result, the 'female's' only route to satisfaction is through the Council of Europe Directive of 1976, which describes the principles of equal treatment for men and women as regards access to employment and in relation to vocational training and working conditions in general. However, even here, it is clear that the transsexual is in an anomalous position.

The case of *P v S and Cornwall County Council*, which was heard in 1996, was, therefore, of considerable interest and importance. In brief, P, who was employed in an educational establishment, announced his intention of undergoing a sex reassignment operation. He was given 3 months' notice of dismissal but he insisted that he would do his remaining work dressed as a woman. The Board of Governors thought that the work could be done at home and, in fact, P did not return to work before his contract of employment ended. In the meantime, she had completed her surgical conversion. She then brought an action before the Industrial Tribunal alleging discrimination on the ground of sex. The Tribunal could not accept this but passed the case to the European Court of Justice in the belief that dismissal because of a change of sex could breach the Council of Europe's Directive on equal treatment.

The European Court of Justice does its work by referring a case to an Advocate General who investigates and submits his or her report to the full court for adjudication. In this case, the Advocate General, first, developed an ingenious argument which we will call the 'sex argument'. In summary, this went: to deny protection to those who are discriminated against by reason of sex, but who fall outside the traditional man/woman classification, is an obsolete approach. P would not have been dismissed if she had remained a man. Therefore the cause of the discrimination was sex, and, therefore, her dismissal offended against the Directive. In a second line of argument, the 'equality argument', the Advocate General emphasised that the objective of the Directive was equality between persons – a principle that requires no account to be taken of factors such as sex, race, language and religion. The court was invited to take a 'courageous decision' that rejected a 'quibbling, formalistic interpretation' of sex discrimination in favour of the general principles underlying the fundamental human right of equality between persons at the workplace. In other words, the fact that there were no specific provisions regulating the treatment of transsexuals in European law was irrelevant. Their right to protection could, however, be inferred from the

Council's intention to harmonise living and working conditions within the Union. The Court accepted the Advocate General's advice.

P v S was, as it had to be, rapidly absorbed into United Kingdom labour law. In one later case, a male to female convert was forced into sick leave due to harassment by her male colleagues and her employers dismissed her on grounds of incapability. The Employment Appeal Tribunal upheld the decision of the lower tribunal that she had been unfairly dismissed. In doing so, the EAT went a stage further in the development of the law and applied the 'sex argument' in *P v S* so as to bring the case directly within the Sex Discrimination Act of 1975.

In another, even more interesting, case, the Employment Tribunal considered that it was unable to do this but, nevertheless, followed *P v S* in applying the 'equality' terms of the Council of Europe's directive to their judgement. M was a male to female transsexual who wanted to become a policewoman. However, the West Midlands Police turned her down when her history was discovered, the reason being that candidates who would be restricted from carrying out the full duties of a police officer were unacceptable.

The tribunal did, indeed, find that the action of the police offended against the Directive as it had been interpreted in P's case, yet M never got to be a policewoman. Why not? The answer lies in Article 2(2) of the Directive which allows the State to exclude from the enforcement of the Directive those occupations in which the 'sex of the worker constitutes a determining factor' – or, in other words, those occupations that cannot be properly undertaken by persons of one or other sex. The activities of the police in England and Wales are governed by the Police and Criminal Evidence Act of 1984 ('PACE'). Amongst other things, PACE dictates that a person can be searched only by a police officer of the same sex, and the regulations surrounding intimate searches are even more stringent. Thus, because Ms M was legally a male she could not carry out a lawful search of a female. By virtue of her appearance, she could not search a male because that would cause embarrassment – something PACE was specifically designed to avoid. Once the criminal world had discovered her true state, they would be sure to exploit it – for example, by claiming a search had been illegal. In short, Ms M would never be able to carry out a substantial part of both routine and emergency police work and the Chief Constable was justified in discriminating against her – or, in Euro-speak, derogation from the directive was permissible. Opinion in this area is, however, developing rapidly and a Ms A has recently had a similar brush with the West Yorkshire Police. In this case, heard in 2002, the Court of Appeal rejected the arguments that had been successful in that of M and held that, even if a transsexual policewoman could not undertake some duties, the effect on police efficiency was minimal. The remedy of refusing her employment – and, thus, offending her rights to equality – was a disproportionate way of solving the problem.

There is now no doubt as to the basis for regarding discrimination against transsexuals as being unlawful. Special regulations introduced in 1999 hold that the dismissal of an employee proposing to undergo gender reassignment is contrary to European law. Discrimination in employment and vocational training based on grounds of gender reassignment is, therefore, prohibited. The importance of Ms A's case is that the discretion inherent in the let-out clause – which allows discrimination when the nature of employment so demands – is also strictly limited.

CONCLUSION

Thus, we have seen that the essential indifference of the British socio-legal system to sex and to sex change persists[5] – that is, so long as it remains a matter of private concern. The law will, however, take a second look when the interests of others are involved – including, in particular, those of children – and it has adopted a firm stance against altering the birth certificate in favour of defining sex in terms of gender rather than of biology. Considering that this is an attitude that is opposed by the majority of those countries forming the Council of Europe, it is surprising that it has subsisted for so long, although it must be said that the 'margin of appreciation' doctrine does, within limits, allow states to maintain a legal regime which conforms to the morals of its own state.

Refusal to alter the birth certificate of a transsexual runs hand in hand with a refusal to acknowledge a transsexual's right to marry in his or her gender sex. The United Kingdom's insistence that you cannot change an historic fact seems, prima facie, to be based on unassailable logic which leads one to suggest that, if there *is* to be a change of position, it might be best justified on medical grounds. The theory that is most often quoted in arguments that support full recognition of transsexual rights holds that gender is not an acquired attribute but, rather, is already present in the developing brain and is, therefore, to be included in those sexual factors that are settled at birth. We hold no position on the point but, if it *were* so, transsexualism could be seen as proof of an error made at birth – albeit an unavoidable error – which would justify an entry in the Register of Corrections. But how well that reasoning would stand up to a logical counter-attack is anyone's guess!

CASES REFERRED TO IN THE TEXT

Bellinger v Bellinger (2001) 64 BMLR 1. (Since declared incompatible with articles 8 and 12 of the ECHR: (2003) Times, April 11th, HL).

Chessington World of Adventures Ltd v Reed [1998] ICR 97.

Chief Constable of West Yorkshire Police v A [2002] IRLR 103.

Corbett v Corbett [1970] 2 All ER 33.

Cossey v United Kingdom [1991] 2 FLR 492.

Goodwin v United Kingdom (2002) 67 BMLR 199.

M v Chief Constable of West Midlands Police (1996) Unreported.

M T v J T 335 A 2d 204 (N J, 1976).

P v S [1996] All ER (EC) 397.

R v Harris, R v McGuinness (1988) 35 A Crim R 146.

---

[5] In a recent interesting twist to the scenario, a male to female transsexual was sent to prison in her gender sex. A decision in the case of a transsexual who had not undergone surgery would, however, be harder to make.

R v Tan [1983] 2 All ER 12.

Rees v United Kingdom [1987] 2 FLR 111.

Sheffield and Horsham v United Kingdom [1998] 2 FLR 928.

W v W (nullity: gender) [2001] 1 FLR 324.

X, Y and Z v United Kingdom [1997] 2 FLR 892.

FURTHER READING

Kennedy IM. 'Transsexualism and single sex marriage', *Anglo-American Law Review* 1973; 2: 112.

McAfferty C. 'Gays, transsexuals and the right to marry', *Family Law* 2002; 362.

Ormrod R. 'The medico-legal aspects of sex determination', *Medico-legal Journal* 1972; 40: 78.

Taitz J. 'Confronting transsexualism: Sexual identity and the criminal law', *Medico-legal Journal* 1992; 60: 60.

Thomson JM. 'Transsexualism: A legal perspective', *Journal of Medical Ethics* 1980; 6: 92.

Whittle S. 'An association for as noble a purpose as any', *New Law Journal* 1996; 146: 366.

15

MENTAL HEALTH AND MENTAL CAPACITY

There can be few areas in medicine where the conflict of ethical principles is exposed so starkly as it is in respect of the management of mental ill health. We have seen throughout this book that autonomy of the individual – that is, the right to make choices and to control what is done with one's body – has become the cornerstone of modern medical ethics. Yet, by definition, the person with mental disorder cannot make ordered decisions and, in the extreme position, someone must act on his or her behalf – this is, in short, paternalism, a concept which is now generally regarded as both outmoded and undesirable but which returns, in this context, as an acceptable, and in some cases an unavoidable, option.

The solution to the resulting problem is not, however, of the all or nothing variety. A person's mental disorder may be permanent, temporary or fluctuating; it may be severe or it may be minor; it may interfere with one form of mental activity but not with another. Put another way, mental disorder will interfere with the patient's capacity to make autonomous decisions to a variable extent and the degree of acceptable paternalistic intervention on his or her behalf varies directly with the degree of incapacity. This leads us to a succession of questions. How far can we respect the residual autonomy of someone with only partial capacity? Who is going to decide the patient's capacity in the prevailing circumstances? Who is going to establish what are the patient's best interests? And who is going to ensure that these best interests are catered for and how this is to be done?

An immediate answer may well be: 'the medical profession', but a moment's thought is sufficient to show that, while this is largely true, it is inadequate. Mental incapacity goes hand in hand with a relative inability to survive in the modern world. Thus, the mentally disordered form a vulnerable group and it is the duty of the State, not of the medical profession, to see to the safety and well-being of its vulnerable citizens. There are bound to be times when these requirements can be met only by isolation of the patient and, in the event that he or she cannot or does not consent, this will involve compulsory detention. How and in what circumstances this power is used is clearly a matter for the State and provides the basis for the Mental Health Acts[1] – which, it is worth pointing out, are there not only for the protection of the mentally disordered against a hostile environment but also as a means of regulating what might otherwise become an over-enthusiastic medical profession. We should also refer at this point to the new dimension that is developed from the concept of human rights within the European Union – as particularly exemplified by the Human Rights Act 1998 which reproduces the terms of the European Convention on Human Rights. For present purposes, the most important aspect of this lies in Article 5 which states:

> Everyone has the right to liberty and security of person. No one shall be deprived of his liberty save in the following cases and in accordance with a procedure proscribed by law

The relevant exception is to be found in: '(e) the lawful detention of persons for the prevention of the spreading of infectious diseases, of persons of unsound mind, alcoholics or drug addicts or vagrants'. This rather vague condition has been clarified in the very important European case of *Winterwerp v Netherlands* (1979) in which the minimum standards for the detention of persons of 'unsound mind' have been defined as:

- The patient must be reliably shown by objective medical expertise to be of 'unsound mind';
- The disorder must be of such a nature as to justify detention; and
- The disorder must persist throughout the period during which the patient is detained.

Subsequent cases have also shown that patients should not be detained if nothing can be done for them medically – and, since our statutes must not conflict with the European Convention, it will be seen later that this provision may have to be interpreted fairly liberally.

Thus far, although we have seen that the treatment of mental ill-health demands something of a unique dual control by government and the medical profession, we have demonstrated no ethical conflict such as was suggested in our opening paragraph. The attitudes currently adopted can be accommodated under the umbrella of the Kantian ethos[2] which can be loosely seen as being founded on respect for the individuality of the person and on the importance of maintaining the dignity of that person. Nonetheless, it is impossible to deny that some forms of mental disorder have effects on others, which may range from simple disturbance to outright dangerousness. As a result, our approach to the management of mental disorder must include an element of communitarian ethic which may, at times, conflict with the interests of the individual. Thus, mental health law is almost unique – 'almost' because much the same principles apply to public health law – in that it has to bridge this apparent ethical divide, and it is fair to say that it has great difficulty in pleasing everyone in its attempt to do so. We will see, however, that the legal process of compulsory detention is

---

[1] There are, in fact, separate Mental Health Acts for England and Wales on the one hand (currently the 1983 Act) and for Scotland (currently the 1984 Act) but, for the sake of simplicity, we will be referring to the 1983 Act only unless there is a specific distinction to be made.

[2] Immanuel Kant, a German philosopher (1724–1804) whose influence on medical ethics has been profound.

closely linked to danger to the public. For the present, we can summarise the criteria which must be met before a person can be detained against his or her will as:

- There must be a mental disorder which warrants detention in hospital;
- An element of risk to the safety of the patient or of others must be present; and
- There is no alternative to detention in hospital as an effective means of avoiding that risk.

A patient may, of course, consent to treatment provided he or she has the capacity to do so but, in between, we have a relatively ill-defined group of persons who are admitted to hospital on an informal basis. An informal patient can be roughly classified as one who, while not actually consenting to admission, does not object to being detained. Such patients make up the majority of those in our mental hospitals.

Definition of mental disorder

The scope of the legal management of mental disorder depends to a very large extent on diagnosis and it has proved very difficult to arrive at definitions which satisfy both legal and medical requirements. Section 1(2) of the 1983 Act defines mental disorder as:

> Mental illness, arrested or incomplete development of mind, psychopathic disorder and any other disorder or disability of mind

and it is unsurprising that this is popularly known as 'the broad definition'! Nevertheless, it is all that is required to render a person liable to compulsory admission to hospital for assessment of his or her condition and its application is bound to be based on subjective impressions. An example of the difficulties that may arise is given, say, by the old person living in insanitary conditions who, as we will see, could be detained under the National Assistance Act 1948, s.47. Clearly, however, such a person could be said to be suffering from 'any other disorder of mind'; he or she could, therefore, be detained in hospital under the Mental Health Act for assessment and this may, in fact, be the easier option for the medical practitioner.

Admission for treatment is, however, another matter and, for this purpose, the patient must be shown to be suffering from either mental illness, psychopathic disorder, mental impairment (nowadays more appropriately described as learning disability) or severe mental impairment and, in addition, persons with mental impairment must demonstrate abnormally aggressive or seriously irresponsible conduct before they can be detained – this will exclude the great majority of, say, those whose mental impairment is associated with Down's syndrome.

There are several difficulties still to be overcome. In the first place, mental illness – which, as we have seen, is a form of mental disorder – is, legally, undefined[3] but is generally taken by psychiatrists to involve the recognised psychoses such as schizophrenia, bipolar affective disorder, anorexia nervosa and organic brain diseases, but it can be stretched to include, for example, phobias – and, again, the subjective nature of definition can lead both the doctor and the lawyer into turbulent waters.

---

[3] Save in the Mental Health (Northern Ireland) Order 1986, art 3(1).

We have already mentioned (see Chapter 5) the case of *Re MB* (1997). In this case a woman who had a phobic fear of needles, refused a caesarean section for delivery of her foetus which was in the breech position. The Court of Appeal, after lengthy analysis, concluded that she was suffering an impairment of her mental functioning which disabled her and the doctors were free to administer the anaesthetic if that were in her best interests. Similar rather tortuous reasoning in the court of first instance hearing the very complex case of *St George's Healthcare NHS Trust v S* (1998) was, however, rejected by the Court of Appeal, which held, in brief, that the Mental Health Act could not be deployed to achieve the detention of an individual against her will merely because her thinking process was unusual, bizarre or irrational. A perfectly rational woman, which the court found S to be, could remain outside the ambit of the Act, notwithstanding her unusual thought processes – which leaves the onus of drawing the line between mental disorder and eccentricity firmly on the shoulders of the doctor.

What is, perhaps, an even greater difficulty stems from the truism that compulsory admission for treatment can only be logical if a treatment is available – and the Act specifically insists on adherence to this rule in the event of a diagnosis of psychopathic disorder or mental impairment. We can thus see that, insofar as psychopathy is something of a doubtful clinical entity, it may well not be treatable and, in that it is the form of mental disorder which provides the greatest danger to the public, the condition raises some of the most difficult legal and ethical issues associated with mental health law. Psychopathy, therefore, merits special consideration.

The problem of the psychopath

Psychopathy is defined in the 1983 Act as 'a persistent disorder or disability of mind which results in abnormally aggressive or seriously irresponsible conduct on the part of the person concerned'. Thus, a diagnosis may be both difficult to make and imprecise when made – there can be no uniform distinction between an aggressive and an abnormally aggressive person. Moreover, it may be difficult to distinguish between psychopathy and schizophrenia, and it is this which underlies a proportion of the many medico-legal problems associated with the former condition. The fundamental question is that of treatability. The seriously affected schizophrenic clearly satisfies the conditions for compulsory admission for treatment. Many would hold, however, that the psychopath is untreatable; both as a matter of logic and of statute, therefore, he or she cannot be detained under the Mental Health Acts and we are left with a potentially dangerous person at large among the public who cannot be isolated until he or she has committed a criminal offence. The libertarian ethicist might well say that this is as it should be and that this is precisely the sort of person that Article 5 of the European Convention on Human Rights is designed to protect. The communitarian, however, would point to the fact that many psychopaths are dangerous, that dangerousness can be anticipated and that the community has a right to be shielded from such danger. Indeed, the problem of the person with 'dangerous severe personality disorder' has been vexing the government and the Executive of both England and Scotland for some time.

Securing admission to hospital does not dispose of all the problems. We must then ask about the retention of a person who is no longer treatable; a situation which is often precipitated by a change in diagnosis from schizophrenia on admission to psychotic disorder on reconsideration. In the English case of Mrs A (*R v Canons Park Mental Health Review Tribunal, ex parte A* (1994)), the Court of Appeal held that the words in the statute 'appropriate for a person to be liable to be detained' did not necessarily involve a response to treatment and that an untreatable person did not have to be discharged. However, shortly after this, a similar Scottish case (*Reid* (1999)) went to the House of Lords, which reached the opposite conclusion – that the 'treatability' condition applied to both compulsory admission to and compulsory retention in hospital. In other words, an untreatable psychopath could not be retained in hospital against his or her will. Admittedly, the House found that, since Reid's control of anger improved in a hospital environment, he was responding to treatment and could, therefore, be retained. Nevertheless, it was not long before a supposedly dangerous man – a Noel Ruddle – who was restricted to hospital by the criminal courts for having shot and killed a man, was found to be untreatable and was discharged.

This precipitated an unprecedented media campaign and an equally remarkable flurry of activity on the part of the Scottish Parliament, which culminated in the first Act of the reconstituted parliament – the Mental Health (Public Safety and Appeals) (Scotland) Act 1999. The most important aspect of this relates to an appeal for release by a restricted patient – that is, a person who has been detained in hospital by way of a restriction order made in the criminal courts. In short, the Sheriff (see Chapter 1) must refuse an appeal against continued detention if he is:

> satisfied that the patient is ... suffering from a mental disorder the effect of which is such that it is necessary, in order to protect the public from serious harm, that the patient continue to be detained in a hospital, whether for medical treatment or not,

and the Act goes on to make it clear that 'mental disorder' includes 'personality disorder'. There is, thus, a clear recognition that the public interest can, on rare occasions, override that of the individual and, lest it be thought that this is a purely Scottish concern, it is noteworthy that the Westminster Parliament and government have been moving in the same direction; we discuss the pending legislation briefly below.

It was inevitable that the Scottish Act – and, with it, the impending English legislation – would be challenged as conflicting with Article 5 of the European Convention of Human Rights as now included in the law of the United Kingdom. This came by way of a case called *A v The Scottish Ministers* (2001) but the appeal against the application of the Act failed, largely on the grounds that it was not an abuse of human rights to introduce new law when it was urgently needed in order to protect the public from serious harm. 'It is hard to imagine', said Lord Rodger, 'a more compelling public interest than the protection of the public from violent or lethal attacks by persons with a prior history of homicide related to an untreatable mental disorder'. Given the ever increasing respect for individual freedom, this was, in many ways, a surprising decision, but it serves to illustrate forcefully the conflict between the interests of the individual and those of the community that we have identified as an ingrained feature of mental health law. There is evidence that the swing to communitarian ethics, which was such a feature of government thinking at the turn of the century, is being watered down. Nevertheless, we would wager that the new legislation, which is awaited as we go to press, will be designed so as to ensure the legality of removing dangerous persons from the community – whether or not their 'dangerousness' is treatable.

Premature release into the community

The preference for treating those with mental disorder within a normal, rather than a hospital, environment was a main driving force behind the Mental Health (Patients in the Community) Act which was passed in 1995. In consequence, the pressure is on clinicians to adopt community care and to discharge patients from hospital where this is feasible. The question then arises as to the degree of responsibility of the clinician in the event that such a patient causes harm to a member of the public – and the answer to this is, currently, uncertain.

By and large, and as we have already discussed in Chapter 6, before an injury sustained in such circumstances can be attributed to a failure in a duty to care, the possibility must be foreseeable, there must be a close association between the carer and the injured party (the 'proximity' test) and it must be just and reasonable that the duty is imposed on the carer. The case of Mrs Palmer (*Palmer v Tees Health Authority* (1998)) gives us some insight into how the courts will consider the situation under discussion. Mrs Palmer's 4 year-old daughter was abducted, sexually abused and murdered by a man with a personality disorder who had been discharged from hospital, allegedly without adequate investigation of his likely dangerousness; she sued the Health Authority in negligence. In summary, the court held that, although the outcome was foreseeable, the case failed the proximity test because the victim did not come into a category of persons at distinctive risk from the actions of a third party – simply being a member of the public living in the same area, or even being a child living in the same area, was not enough. And as to fairness, how could the hospital be expected to warn the population at large? As was said in the Court of Appeal, you cannot warn someone of a risk if you do not know whom to warn.

Admittedly, *Palmer* does not tell us what would happen if there had been a closer relationship between the patient and his victim. We can get some further insight from the case of *Clunis v Camden and Islington HA* (1998). Clunis was diagnosed as having a schizo-affective disorder. On being discharged from hospital, he stabbed another man to death and was subsequently convicted of manslaughter. Clunis then took the innovative step of suing the hospital for allowing him out and, thus, causing him to be further detained as a result of the homicide. Once again, the complaint failed, largely on the grounds that it was neither fair nor reasonable to hold the authority responsible for the unfocussed actions of a man undergoing aftercare. *Clunis* left the question of whether a doctor owes a duty of care to a patient in certifying that he or she is fit to be detained under the Mental Health Act undecided. Even so, the existing authorities suggest that a doctor is very unlikely to be found responsible for the actions of his or her patient unless, possibly, the identity of the potential victim was clearly known to the responsible doctor.[4] The probability is that questions of negligence would then be decided on the principles derived from the *Bolam* case – which we have discussed in Chapter 6.

---

[4] Although, as we write this, the recent and only partially reported case brought by Ms Akenzua, whose close friend was murdered by a man known to be a dangerous criminal, leaves us rather less confident about this.

Changes for the future

As we write this, drafts of new Mental Health Bills have been issued by both the Westminster and the Holyrood Parliaments. It is, therefore, impossible to say with certainty what changes in the legislation lie ahead. We can, however, make some predictions.

In respect of the present topic of dangerousness, some of the Westminster indicators seem to have lapsed. At one time, the introduction of a Dangerous People with Severe Personality Disorder Bill, coupled with a white paper – *Reforming the Mental Health Act*, which spoke of dealing separately with those who need treatment primarily in their own interests and those who needed treatment because of the risk that they posed for others – suggested something of a Draconian change of direction. This may or may not have abated. Meantime, mental disorder is likely to be defined as: 'any disability or disorder of mind or brain which results in an impairment or disturbance of mental functioning'. This clearly includes personality disorder. Moreover, conditions justifying compulsory admission to hospital will include: 'in the case of a patient who is at substantial risk of causing serious harm to other persons, that it is necessary for the protection of those persons that medical treatment be provided to him'. Thus, the treatability test is abandoned – and there are to be no Mr Ruddle's South of the Border.

Against these rather specific concerns, the general tenor of the proposed legislation is now dominated by consideration for patients' rights. All treatments are to be managed by way of care plans controlled by clinical supervisors; long term treatment will be subject to approval by a Mental Health Tribunal whose decisions can be appealed to a Mental Health Appeal Tribunal; and to assist in the process, patients are to be represented by nominated persons backed by mental health advocates. All of this is to be covered by a statutory Code of Practice.

Despite this apparently patient-centred approach, there is little doubt that the way is open to include more public health in the management of mental health and this has caused some concern. But it is the practitioners who will administer the new Act and it is for them to ensure that this is not carried to extreme. We tend to the view that the new regime will be more caring and more patient oriented than was the last – although it cannot be over-emphasised that a degree of paternalism is inevitable in the treatment of the mentally ill. This is recognised in the fact that a doctor – albeit not the corporate Health Authority – who treats a patient within the confines of the Act, and who does so in good faith and with reasonable care, is immune from either civil or criminal proceedings unless leave to bring an action is sanctioned by the High Court. The patient is, however, at liberty to seek a judicial review – that is, a court's appraisal of the actions of a public body – of the reasonableness or legality of a hospital's actions. The mass murderer Ian Brady, for example, was able to have the propriety of his being force-fed considered by the Court – albeit unsuccessfully. This access to judicial review is used relatively often and remains the bulwark defence of the patient's human rights.

TREATMENT OF THE MENTALLY DISORDERED

The fact that a person is admitted for compulsory treatment does not give the doctor a free therapeutic hand. In the first place, the new regulations will insist on the preparation of a care plan for all 'registered' patients – and this applies both to formally and informally detained persons. Moreover, the care plan must be approved by the Mental Health Tribunal which it is expected will be established in both England and Wales and in Scotland and, before applying for such approval, the patient's clinical supervisor must consult his or her 'nominated person' and any carer. Subject to strict conditions, the clinical supervisor may amend the care plan. It should be noted, however, in passing, that a care plan can consist of no more than detention in a hospital environment – the psychopath can, therefore, be admitted for treatment despite the fact that his or her condition is fundamentally untreatable.

The more important limitation from the medico-ethical perspective, however, is that non-consensual treatment given under the Mental Health Acts is restricted to treatment for the mental condition – lawful provision of other treatment depends on whether or not the patient has the capacity to consent. The difficulties here are, first, that doctors naturally want to give the treatment that they consider necessary and, second, that judges are, in general, disinclined to override what are seen to be, at base, clinical decisions. As a result, there have been a number of court decisions which can be seen as being, at best, opportunistic. Many of these have been associated with forced feeding of persons suffering from anorexia nervosa which have been discussed in greater detail in Chapter 5. Classic examples include the court in *Re KB* (1994) deciding that refusal of treatment, including feeding, in anorexia nervosa is a manifestation of the underlying mental disorder and that the treatment of symptoms by way of forced feeding is of the same quality as treatment of the underlying condition and the Court of Appeal supporting this view in *B v Croydon Health Authority* (1995), where a psychopath's determination to harm herself was thought to be manifested in a refusal to eat. Such reasoning, which might be seen as bordering on sophistry, may well solve the immediate problem but it does little to support the concept of consistent legal principle. There is, indeed, evidence that such decisions will become unacceptable – the increasing use of mental health advocacy and the involvement of 'nominated persons' to oversee the interests of the incapax are likely to stem what some might see as incremental erosions of the mental patient's autonomy.

But what of treatment for conditions that have no possible connection with the person's mental state, such as abdominal surgery? Until recently, there has been no way by which someone could consent to treatment on behalf of an incapacitated adult as the courts of England and Wales no longer have what is known as the *parens patriae* jurisdiction – that is, the authority to look after the State's vulnerable adult citizens.[5] There have, however, been two recent major changes. In Scotland, the Adults with Incapacity (Scotland) Act 2000 now lays down a specific chain of authority – including the patient's medial practitioner, his or her appointed welfare attorney, a specially nominated medical arbitrator and the courts – whereby treatment of any sort may be provided. Second, the proposals for England and Wales detailed in the draft Bill of 2002 are that the incompetent patient's medical supervisor will be able to provide treatment so long as he has consulted the patient's nominated person; the latter will have the power of veto if it appears that the patient would have refused that particular treatment.

---

[5] The authority does, in fact, still subsist in Scotland.

Thus, although the position in Scotland appears to have been resolved by legislation, the absence of legislation in England and Wales means that, at the moment, a doctor can treat a patient who cannot consent only under cover of the doctrine of necessity. How, then, is necessity to be defined? The legal concept can be translated as meaning that the treatment is reasonable and that it is in the patient's best interests that it should be given – indeed it has been said that the doctor who did not treat when necessity demanded it could be held to have been negligent. In general, the patient's medical best interests will be judged on *Bolam* principles which we have described in Chapter 6 – that is, that a responsible body of medical opinion would have followed the same course. While this may be self-evident in most cases, there will clearly be cases where such a professional standard is put in doubt, either by virtue of the severity of the intervention or because of its secondary effects. In these circumstances, the doctor would be well advised to seek the advice of the courts, mainly on the grounds that, while the doctor may decide on the patient's best *medical* interests, it may take a judge to determine his or her best *overall* interests. We have noted above that the court cannot consent on behalf of the patient; what it can do is to declare that the proposed action will not be unlawful and, in the event, this comes to much the same thing. There are, in fact, occasional circumstances in which the courts *must* be involved; at present, in England and Wales, these comprise sterilisation of the incapax and withdrawal of nutrition and hydration from persons in the permanent vegetative state.

In addition, we must note that there are some treatments for mental disorder which cannot be given other than with special safeguards. These will include, if the draft Bill becomes law, any surgical operation for destroying brain tissue or for destroying the function of brain tissue and electroconvulsive therapy – although the Minister can add to this list if necessary. The former – neurosurgery for mental disorder – will be, and is, covered by a very extensive list of requirements involving opinions from both medical and concerned lay persons if the patient is capable of consenting; a similar set of opinions backed by a declaration of lawfulness by the High Court, or the Court of Session in Scotland, will be needed in the event that he or she is not able to consent or refuse. Electroconvulsive therapy in the absence of an emergency will be lawful only if expressly authorised by the Mental Health Tribunal which will be set up under the new Act. The comparable Scottish position is likely to be governed by the authority of a medical practitioner who is specifically designated for the purpose by the Mental Health Commission.

The most important single thread running through all that we have said in this chapter is the over-riding importance to the way treatment is given to the patient's capacity to consent and it is to that aspect that we now turn.

CAPACITY

The concept of capacity is of importance beyond the sphere of mental health. It can be limited by status, this being particularly so in the case of the child. We have discussed this in detail in Chapters 4 and 5. Loss of capacity due to unconsciousness from whatever cause is probably the most important aspect from the point of view of the generalist physician or surgeon. Provision of treatment in such cases is subject to the legal doctrine of necessity, which we have dealt with above and under the heading of consent. We are left, then, with loss of capacity due to mental disorder and, although a young person may suffer from, say, a learning disability, we will address the problems from the point of view of the conscious and uncoerced adult.

Capacity in the adult

Capacity to consent to treatment is all-important to its validity. The basic rule is that an adult will be assumed to have that capacity and such a person has what is virtually an absolute right to consent to or to refuse treatment – and the decision as to the latter is binding on the doctor. The main exception is that no-one can give valid consent to an action which will cause him or her severe harm and which is contrary to his or her best interests. Thus, consent to being a live cardiac transplant donor would not make the operation lawful; similarly, consent to a lethal injection does not legalise euthanasia. Short of such extremes, however, consent, as we have already seen, precludes an action against the doctor for assault – as Lord Donaldson once famously put it, consent provides a flak-jacket, or bullet-proof waistcoat, for the healthcare professional.

Conversely, refusal of treatment is now also seen as the competent patient's absolute right and it is important to note that competence and rationality are not inter-changeable terms and can exist independently in the same person. Once again in Lord Donaldson's words, this right persists even if a refusal may risk permanent injury to health or to premature death – 'it matters not whether the reasons for the refusal were rational or irrational, unknown or even non-existent and this is notwithstanding the very strong public interest in preserving the life and health of all citizens'. This was demonstrated vividly in the relatively recent case involving *Ms B v An NHS Trust* (2002) which we have discussed in Chapter 5.

The presumption of mental capacity is, however, rebuttable. How, then, are we to make a decision when it is disputed? The *legal* ground-rules have been laid down in the case known as *Re C (mental patient: medical treatment)* which was heard in 1993. Here, a man confined to Broadmoor Special Hospital with a diagnosis of paranoid schizophrenia sought a declaration that he was capable of refusing amputation of his gangrenous leg and an injunction restraining the hospital from amputating his leg without express written consent. In the event, Mr Justice Thorpe considered that C's rejection of amputation seemed to result from sincere conviction; his grandiose delusions were manifest but there was no sign of inappropriate emotional expression. Of major importance, the judge accepted a three stage test of competence which involved:

- comprehending and retaining treatment information;
- believing it; and
- weighing it in the balance to arrive at a choice – i.e. there must be *actual* understanding.

The clinician will, no doubt, say that this analysis does little save confirm what is already good medical practice; certainly, it leaves the assessment of capacity firmly in the subjective hands of the individual doctor. Nevertheless, the test has taken on the mantle of rubric in the courts and it remains a useful guide to follow in any case that is likely to be questioned in court.

Needless to say, such questions are most likely to arise in the case of refusal of treatment where the autonomy of the patient clashes with the doctor's professional imperative to do what he or she thinks is best in clinical terms. What does seem to us to be important is that this type of confrontation should not deter the doctor from his or her correlative obligation to provide the patient with sufficient information on the basis of which to make a genuinely considered, or informed, refusal.

STERILISATION OF THE INCAPACITATED

Sterilisation is that form of therapeutic intervention which bids fair to place the greatest strain on the relation between ethics and non-consensual treatment of the patient who lacks capacity. It is, therefore, unsurprising that, as we have noted, it is a matter on which the courts insist that they are consulted before such a procedure is undertaken – unless, that is, sterilisation is no more than an unfortunate side effect of treatment for another condition. The case known as *Re GF* (1992) is sufficient authority to render a hysterectomy for carcinoma of the uterus, for example, inherently lawful.

Some would say that even this is not beyond doubt and, indeed, the whole arena is strewn with uncertainty, not the least of which involves the question of whether sterilisation, itself, can be regarded properly as medical treatment. Certainly, it is traditional to speak in terms of 'therapeutic' and 'non-therapeutic' sterilisation, but it takes only brief reflection to appreciate how artificial this distinction can be. A young woman with learning disability may be said to 'have a phobia to menstrual blood' - in which case a hysterectomy could be seen as an appropriate treatment. But, given the circumstances, it will often be difficult to distinguish this from an inability to manage one's personal hygiene; 'treatment' would, then, be essentially for social reasons and hysterectomy would be far harder to justify. On the other side of the coin, consider the same type of incapax who in danger of becoming pregnant and who we have discussed, briefly, in Chapter 1. Tubal occlusion might, then, be an available option but one which many would say was unjustified on purely social grounds. Again, however, others would say that, without the operation, her lifestyle would have to be seriously curtailed and that this might well be against both her social and medical 'best interests' – or, in the alternative, it could be asked: wherein lies the essential difference between preventive medicine and medical treatment ? True, we have the further options of depot contraception or the use of an intra-uterine device. But, then, we have to throw the inherent contraindications to both into the decision-making balance pans. The interested reader is referred to the cases of *Re S (Adult patient: Sterilisation)* (2000) and *Re Z (Medical treatment: Hysterectomy)* (1999) in which all these arguments were aired – and which, incidentally, provide a useful insight into the modern courts' attitudes to expert opinion. We doubt if we need to delve further in demonstrating the difficulties of making a clear distinction between medical and social indications for sterilisation save, perhaps, to emphasise the point by considering the case of the male. There can be no *medical* advantage whatsoever to the Down's syndrome male in being rendered sterile – if he was not so already; as a result, the courts will never authorise such an intervention – for which, see *Re A (Medical treatment: Male sterilisation)* (1999).

The whole of the above discussion rests, however, on a more fundamental question - is there a right to procreate ? This debate originates in the judge's reference to 'the basic human right of a woman to reproduce' in the 1976 case of *Re D* which is probably the index case in the field. Since then, such a right has been widely assumed but, at the same time, its *nature* has been seriously questioned. The proposition appears flawed as it stands – many would hold that there can be no right when there is no corresponding obligation to satisfy that right. Perhaps more importantly, one has to dig deeper and establish the true meaning of 'reproduction' – is it simply a physiological event or should it be interpreted holistically so as to include not only the production but also the rearing of children ? A well-known quotation from the very important House of Lords case *Re B* (1987) goes to the heart of the question:

> To talk of the 'basic right to reproduce' of an individual who is not capable of knowing the causal connection between intercourse and childbirth ... [or who] is unable to form any maternal instincts or to care for a child, appears to me wholly to part company with reality.

Lord Hailsham's language may have been over-strong, but the point to be taken is that, once again, the issue is that of the extent of the *individual* incapax' incapacity – there can be no blanket approach and each case must be decided on its own merits.

What, then, is the true nature of this universal woman's right that the courts guard so jealously ? It is, surely, a right not to have her ability to reproduce – and her choice to use that ability – removed in an arbitrary manner and, certainly, not for the intentional benefit of others. In other words, like all modern medical ethics, this right is grounded in the autonomy of the individual. Current evidence is that the courts rely on and apply this principle with increasing emphasis; authority to sterilise the woman with learning disability is likely to be granted in the future only with correspondingly increasing concern for her right to bodily integrity and her capacity to choose.

CONCLUSION

It is apparent that the management of the mentally disordered is based on a series of compromises. It is also inherently paternalistic, something which is inevitable and which was recognised in the original doctrine of *parens patriae* – that is that the monarch is the parent of his or her people and has parental responsibility for those who are incapacitated. The first compromise, then, lies in the attempt to constrain that paternalism so as to give maximum effect to the individual human rights of an incapax. Thus, in order to protect incompetents from the vicissitudes of life, the State must retain the right to confine them. At the same time, however, they must be guaranteed that their freedom will not, itself, be unreasonably curtailed.

This leads to the second necessary compromise, that is, the balancing of an individual right to freedom against the public need for protection from the person who is dangerously mentally disordered. There is no doubt that, relatively recently, the authorities became greatly influenced by considerations of public interest. The legislation that is currently being developed shows that, although there is a continuing concern, this extreme attitude is being modified; but the difficulties are expressed in the relatively acrimonious debate that surrounds the Bills going through Parliament in both England and Wales and in Scotland.

Finally, we note that the law must protect incompetents from assault but must, at the same time open the way for lawful, non-consensual assault in the form of medical treatment. We have seen that this is currently in an unsatisfactory state of resolution. Nevertheless, it has been addressed in Scotland by way of the Adults with Incapacity Act and much the same route is now planned for England and Wales. We will have to wait and see what solutions are reached in all these areas while, at the same time, sympathising with those who have to steer between the medico-legal equivalents of Scylla and Charybdis.

CASES REFERRED TO IN THE TEXT

A (Medical treatment: Male sterilisation), Re (1999) 53 BMLR 66.

A v Scottish Ministers 2001 SC 1.

B (A minor) (Wardship: sterilisation), Re [1987] 2 All ER 206.

B v Croydon Health Authority [1995] 1 All ER 683.

C (adult: refusal of treatment), Re [1994] 1 All ER 819.

Clunis v Camden and Islington Health Authority [1998] 3 All ER 180.

D (A minor) (Wardship: sterilisation), Re [1976] 1 All ER 326.

GF, Re [1992] 1 FLR 293.

Gillick v West Norfolk and Wisbech Area Health Authority [1985] 3 All ER 402.

KB (adult) (mental patient: medical treatment), Re (1994) 19 BMLR 144.

MB (an adult: Medical treatment), Re [1997] 2 FLR 426.

Ms B v An NHS Hospital Trust [2002] 2 All ER 449.

Palmer v Tees Health Authority (1998) 44 BMLR 88.

R v Canons Park Mental Health Review Tribunal, ex parte A [1994] 2 All ER 659.

R v Collins, ex parte Brady (2000) 58 BMLR 173.

Reid v Secretary of State for Scotland [1999] 1 All ER 481.

S (Adult patient: Sterilisation), Re [2000] 3 WLR 1288.

Winterwerp v Netherlands (1979) 2 EHRR 387.

Z (Medical treatment: Hysterectomy), Re (1999) 53 MLR 53.

FURTHER READING

Birmingham L. 'Detaining dangerous people with mental disorders', *British Medical Journal* 2002; 325: 2.

Department of Health. *Making Decisions*, 1999, Cm 4465.

Grubb A, Pearl D. 'Sterilisation and the courts', *Cambridge Law Review* 1987; 46: 439.

Jones MA, Keywood K. 'Assessing the patient's competence to consent to medical treatment', *Medical Law International* 1996; 2: 107.

Mason T, Jennings L. 'The Mental Health Act and professional hostage taking', *Medicine, Science and the Law* 1997; 37: 58.

Munro E, Rumgay J. 'Role of risk assessments in reducing homicides by people with metal illnesses', *British Journal of Psychiatry* 2000; 176: 116.

Tyrer P, Carey P, Ferguson B. 'Personality disorder in perspective', *British Journal of Psychiatry* 1991; 159: 463.

Stauch M. 'Rationality and the refusal of medical treatment: A critique of the recent approach of the English courts', *Journal of Medical Ethics* 1995; 21: 162.

van Staden CW, Kruger C. 'Incapacity to give informed consent owing to mental disorder', *Journal of Medical Ethics* 2003; 29: 41.

16

THE LAW AND THE ELDERLY

Projections for the future are always difficult but the Office for National Statistics states that the proportion of persons over the age of 65, which reached 16 per cent of the population in 1996, is expected to go on rising quite steadily so that the proportions of those aged more than 65 and those younger than 16 will be much the same in about 15 years' time. After this, there will be more old people than young. Very soon, it seems, there will be as great an overall need for 'elder' law as there is for child law.

When one adds to this that the elderly are, almost by definition, on the downslope of health and that, as a result, they become increasingly frail and vulnerable with time, one can appreciate even more clearly the need for their protection within a medico-legal context. And yet, what little legal involvement there is tends to aim at containing 'difficult people' rather than at recognising the autonomy of the aged and improving their self-esteem. The difficulty of so doing, of course, lies in the fact that all peoples' mental and physical capacities degenerate with age – and do so relatively steadily, albeit at different rates. At the same time, the capacity to generate income fails, savings get eaten away and poverty increases. The ageing person becomes progressively a greater emotional and financial drain on his or her family – and since women over 75 outnumber men by something like 2:1, we can effectively speak of 'her' for the remainder of this chapter.

Where, then, is this ageing woman to go? Ideally, she should live on her own, but the combined internal and external forces described above make this a strictly limited option. She can stay with her family. We will return to the problems that raises later on but, meantime, it need only be noted that children have no legal obligation to support their parents. Beyond that, the duty to care for the elderly who do not require hospitalisation is now vested firmly in the Local Authorities. It will be convenient to outline here the legal extent of that duty and its effectiveness.

ARRANGEMENTS FOR LIVING

The majority of the elderly would probably want to continue an independent existence for as long as possible. Independence need not, however, be absolute and a complex bundle of 'social security' allowances, intended to encourage a home environment for as long as possible, is available. These are subject to restrictions as to the degree of disability, age and other considerations, which it is impossible to describe in detail here. The most important, however, is the disability living allowance which is divided into care and mobility components. The allowance is payable if the person is so severely physically or mentally disabled as to require the constant attention of another person by day or prolonged or repeated attention – or watchful awakeness – at night. Disability living allowance is payable only if the disability arose before the age of 65; otherwise, it is replaced by attendance allowance which carries no age limit and is payable to the person who qualifies for it. In addition, invalid care allowance, which is intended to soften the disadvantages accruing to those caring for the elderly, is payable directly to a person who is regularly, and substantially, engaged in caring for a severely disabled person and who is not, otherwise, in 'gainful employment'. A notable feature of this allowance is that it is payable to spouses, partners and daughters.

These are generalised benefits. As regards the individual, the local authority has a primary duty to provide services in the home which will enable a person who needs them to carry on independently for as long as is practicable. This includes not only the provision of what is generally seen as 'home help' but also fitting appliances and carrying out adaptations to the house. Even so, the duty is only to 'make provision for' such services and the provision of improvement grants is discretionary. Moreover, such services are not necessarily free; local authorities will make a charge that is based on the individual's ability to pay. Indeed, it will be seen that, as the financial implications increase, so does the local authority become less anxious to 'foot the bill'. Thus, responsibility for the next step to dependence – a move to 'sheltered housing' where, in addition to the building being specially modified for occupation by the elderly, some sort of centralised assistance is provided to a group of persons in need – is shared to a varying proportion by the local authority, housing associations and the private sector, while the next-stage incremental move – to residential care homes – is now dominated by the last – although the difficulties of running such homes on an acceptable commercial basis has resulted in a serious shortage of available places.

As a consequence, the quality of residential care varies although minimum standards must be met in order to achieve registration under the Care Standards Act 2000 and 'care homes' as a whole are subject to supervision by the National Care Standards Commission.

Residential care homes are designed to accommodate that twilight population of old people who are unable to manage entirely for themselves but who are, at the same time, not sufficiently either mentally or physically disabled as to need accommodation in nursing homes. The anticipated needs of such persons vary enormously and meeting them is often an administrative and emotional minefield. Human nature being what it is, conditions can seldom be Utopian and there have been several sensational tales of elder abuse in homes run by both the public and the private sector. This may well be equally true of the nursing home whose occupants will certainly be more demanding of time and understanding. It is to be noted, however, that the Secretary of State now keeps a list of those regarded as unfit to care for the vulnerable elderly and persons on the list are, of course, excluded from working in registered care homes. Occasionally, what might in other circumstances be seen as abuse may be passive and virtually forced on administrators. For example, elderly persons may have to be confined to bed with siderails lest they fall and involve the home in a lawsuit in respect of personal injuries brought by relatives of the patient.

Responsibility for care homes is divided. In general, residential care homes are registered with the local authority while nursing homes are controlled though the health authority – although there are express regulations which dictate co-operation and load sharing where this will be economical. In either case, the administrator of the home is bound by statute to make regular reviews of conditions in the home and to make such necessary improvements as are possible. Moreover, the Care Standards Act of 2000 stipulates that all residential homes and nursing homes are registered and are subject to inspection – and this, of course, includes those homes that are provided by the private sector. Redress for wrongs alleged by residents or their representatives may be sought by claiming a breach of statutory duty – although much of the legislation allows for fairly wide discretion and success via this route might be difficult to achieve. Actions in negligence or trespass to the person (assault in Scotland) may be raised against the home itself or against individual workers. Occasionally, recourse may be had to the Local Government Ombudsman who may be able to recommend payment of compensation, which would not be available through the other avenues.

The residential home is designed for those who are found, after a careful assessment of their needs, to be unable to maintain themselves in their own homes but who do not need continuous nursing care. By definition, therefore, the residential home offers no nursing care – the statutory duty of the administrator is only to provide access to such medical and nursing attention as would be available were the patient being treated at home. Clearly, there may be grey areas between, on the one hand, assisted housing and residential care and, on the other, between residential and nursing care. Thus, a careful assessment of the infirm or aged person's needs is an essential part of the scheme and this involves a multidisciplinary approach which is attained through the co-ordination of the various agencies involved in the care of the elderly. A person's need for nursing care must, for example, be based on the opinion of a medical practitioner as well as that of the local authority.

But the difficulty of distinguishing the type of care needed can create considerable confusion and, indeed, even some hardship. Effectively, the division of responsibility leads to something of a struggle between the local and health authorities to avoid that responsibility – the coffers of neither are bulging with excess wealth and the financial demands upon both increase inexorably. Until comparatively recently, care of the aged could scarcely be regarded as a Governmental priority and care of the aged sick is seldom an attractive backdrop for ambitious consultants or hospital managers, who will complain that some 20 per cent of their beds are occupied by persons aged over 75. The elderly are, then, caught in the crossfire – and the problem is multicentred.

We have noted that the number of care homes is decreasing. As a result, it is increasingly difficult to discharge vulnerable patients from hospital and, at the same time, ensure that they have adequate facilities. The resulting 'bed blockage' is a real problem not only for those awaiting discharge but also for those awaiting admission. To counter this, the Government is in the process of providing intermediate care beds and intermediate places but the effect of these has yet to be assessed. On the other side of the coin, there is no reason why nursing care should not be provided by the local authority – and it often is. The difficulty was that nursing care then became subsumed within social care, the provision of which is subject to payment based on a means test.

This anomaly – which was a clear contradiction to the principle of 'cradle to the grave' protection by the National Health Service – was recently addressed in the test case of *R v North and East Devon Health Authority, ex parte Coughlan* (2000). Here, a severely disabled woman protested that the closure of the purpose built NHS home in which she lived, and her consequent enforced transfer to the care of the local authority, were unlawful actions. The Court of Appeal accepted this claim on the grounds that Ms Coughlan's needs were primarily health needs for which the health authority was responsible. The health authority was entitled to close some facilities, such as nursing care, which could then be taken over by the local authority but, in Ms Coughlan's case, her needs went beyond what could be expected of the nursing care provided by the local authority. This was limited to those services which came as part of the 'package' of residential care that we have described above – and the corollary was that, unfair or not, a charge could be made for such services. In other words, it was the quality, as defined by the 'residential home package', and the quantity – that is, how much nursing could reasonably be provided by the local authority – that would define the difference between what might be described as 'social care' and 'healthcare'. Unfortunately, but inevitably, the Court had to admit that the defining line could be blurred. But Ms Coughlan's case now makes it clear that continuing treatment must be funded free at the point of receipt if the patient's need is primarily for healthcare that is of sufficient quality and quantity as to justify it. The NHS must also be responsible for the 'difference' between the costs of social care and the more extensive healthcare.

This important decision is now in the process of being implemented via a directive issued by the Department of Health, and nursing care will be provided free of charge to all those in residential care homes as from 2003. Accommodation and social care are, however, still subject to a means test when not wholly provided by the NHS. It is generally estimated that some 40,000 homes are sold each year in order to pay for residential care but further recent regulations exclude the value of a person's home when assessing his or her capital assets for the first 12 weeks of such care. The Scottish parliament has gone a long way to rectifying the anomalies in the system by passing the Community Care and Health (Scotland) Act of 2002. Section 1 of the Act states that local authorities are not to charge for the social care provided by them if the social care is personal care, personal support or nursing care – whether or not this is provided by a registered nurse. It was inevitable that the financial implications of the Act should be hotly debated; there has, however, been insufficient time to indicate whether or not this was justified.

Money, money, money!

It will be seen that the social security net currently operated by the local authorities represents a brave effort to ensure that the elderly, and especially the elderly sick, are not simply left to live on the good will of their families or to die in isolation. But social security is not, of itself, a charity. We have seen that the majority of services, at least in England and Wales, are provided on the basis of capacity to pay for them.

Not only are the qualifying conditions generally rigorous but the 'means' on which the ability to pay are based are, to say the least, not generous to the individual in receipt of services. Thus, for example, the local authority will demand full payment for services if the recipient's capital assets exceed £18,500. Only when these have been reduced to £3,000 will it be accepted that she need no longer contribute to the benefits. While this may, at first sight, appear to be despotic, one must, in all fairness, mention the alternative view which points to the fact that the provision of free social services for the aged benefits not so much the old person but, rather, his or her heirs. Looked at in that way, this particular 'obligation' becomes far less compelling in nature.

Moreover, it has to be admitted that the local authority's purse, like that of the health authority (see Chapter 2), is not, and never can be, bottomless. As a result, many of the local authority's duties are defined as being *discretionary* and, in the nature of things, discretion and apparent injustices go hand in hand. The case of *R v Gloucestershire County Council, ex parte Barry* (1997) is one such instance and is important because it went all the way to the House of Lords where it was decided only by a majority of 3:2. The bare bones of the story are that the central allocation of funds to Gloucestershire County Council was reduced by £3 million. The Council, in its turn, withdrew various services from 1,500 disabled residents. Mr Barry, who represented the affected persons, had been assessed as 'needing' help with cleaning, laundry and shopping and he required the provision of community meals. He protested to the courts when his cleaning services were withdrawn and his laundry services reduced. In effect, the argument came down to the interpretation to be placed on the word 'need'. Mr Barry contended that, having been assessed as needing these services, his need remained the same unless his personal condition improved. His need was something that was unaffected by extraneous circumstances and the Council was, therefore, acting unlawfully in withdrawing the services on grounds which were not his concern. This has an undoubted ring of logic – as Lord Lloyd said in the House of Lords: 'Every child needs new pair of shoes from time to time. The need is not the less because his parents cannot afford them'.

The other side is, of course, that it is unrealistic to suppose that an authority can conjure up financial resources from an empty money box. There must be a balancing of the severity of the need against the availability of resources or, put another way, it is acceptable that the stringency of the tests for eligibility for services can be less or more severe according to whether the Council has more or less money to distribute – and that was their Lordships' majority view. Many might well feel that, while this is an acceptable argument when one is *allocating* resources, it loses much of its force when one is *altering* that allocation. Nevertheless, the message from Mr Barry's case reinforces that which we derived in Chapter 2 – the courts are very unlikely to argue with the responsible authority, be it a local or a health authority, when it comes to 'rationing' resources. But we suspect this is no more based on principle than on the uncomfortable fact that there is no reasonable alternative.[1]

---

[1] The law is not, now, quite as clear as it was insofar as a case concerning the special educational needs of a child has been decided on the basis that the authority cannot plead poverty in order to evade its duties. The solution to the problem lies in the rather legalistic distinction between the powers and the duties of a particular authority.

LIVING WITH THE FAMILY

As we have already noted, there is no obligation on children in the United Kingdom to take care of their elderly parents, yet a very large proportion undertake the task, many with great success. In others, however, the ideal becomes something of a mixed blessing. A female Chinese student once said to one of us: 'In my country you should never marry the eldest son for it is his duty to look after his parents – and his duty will quickly become my duty'. Much depends on the personalities involved, and it has to be remembered that one of a 'caring' couple will have no intuitive, genetic or child-hood relationship with the old person. Affluence also plays its part – the larger the house, the easier will be the discharge of any responsibility. At the same time, the pos-sibility of substantial inheritance may be the trigger for abuse of the elderly relative. This is hardly the place for a detailed discussion of family relationships; it need only be said that the conditions for elder abuse may well be established and the evidence is that it occurs with increasing frequency. Even so, it has to be repeated that this is not solely a matter of the home environment – some forms of elder abuse occur in much the same way in care homes.

Which reminds us that the assessment of the occurrence of this type of abuse lies in its definition. Physical abuse resulting in demonstrable injury is probably uncom-mon – certainly much less common than is seen in child abuse. Passive, emotional abuse in the form of isolation or failure to provide attention is far more likely and most people would include verbal abuse as part of the spectrum. Moreover, abuse may be unconscious – how many of us have never lowered our voices to avoid granny hearing while failing to appreciate the emotional turmoil that this induces in an old person?

It must also be asked what redress the old person has if she *is* abused? True, she may, as in any walk of life, bring an action for trespass to the person or assault. True, a criminal action for assault may be available, and, conceivably, she might be able to claim false imprisonment. But to succeed by any route would require evidence and, by and large, this would be available only in the event of serious physical ill-treatment which, we have noted, is, anyway, uncommon. Moreover, even if the old person is aware of her rights – which is, in itself, unlikely – the gateway to redress is effect-ively blocked by her aggressors who will, in practice, have complete control of her communications.

Given that the local authority has, currently, no mandate to enter premises with a view to protecting vulnerable adults, the general practitioner or, through him or her, the health visitor, remains the most likely detector of abuse of the elderly – and pleas for awareness of the condition are appearing in the medical press with the frequency they did in respect of child abuse 20 or so years ago. The doctor can, in serious cases, arrange for admission to hospital for assessment. He or she can also report the case to the social services or to the police, but the latter, in particular, must seldom be appro-priate. Advice from the charity Action on Elder Abuse is that the doctor does not have to prove that abuse has taken place – only that there is reasonable cause to suspect it. Here, however, we must reiterate an important caveat. We have seen in Chapter 3 that, at base, the doctor owes a duty of confidentiality to his patient and it would be wrong to *assume* that she has no objection to that duty being breached. Permission must be obtained if it is at all possible; very good reasons must be available to justify action on the grounds of necessity alone – it is all too easy to make matters worse. All in all, abuse of the elderly is poorly considered by the existing law and the Law Commission, which is established to review controversial areas of the law, has recommended extension of the local authority's powers with a view to improving the protection of the elderly comparable to the standards that are available in the USA. The government may be taking action in the not too distant future, although it is unfortunate that the Age Equality Commission Bill, introduced in 2001, lapsed because of the dissolution of Parliament.

'I WANT TO BE ALONE'

We have seen that both medical and social security opinion is to the effect that the elderly person should, so far as is possible, be encouraged to live an independent life. But, 'so far as is possible' clearly indicates a limit to the policy. In other words, there may well come a time when the elderly person is at such risk that independence should be discouraged in his or her own best interests. This conclusion, however, gives rise to considerable ethical uncertainty. First, it is implicit in the scenario that the person still *wants* to live his or her own life. Rejecting this preference, or altering their mind, must involve a degree of coercion and it is an important requirement of the Human Rights Act 1998 that a citizen is entitled to freedom of association subject only to national legislation that can be fully justified. Secondly, his or her best interests are being decided by an outside party – for, again, the individual sees his or her best interests as being to be left in peace. There is little doubt that the existing law accentuates these difficulties.

The National Assistance Act of 1948 states, at section 47, that persons

a. who are not mentally ill but who are suffering from grave chronic disease or, being aged, infirm or physically incapacitated, are living in insanitary conditions, and
b. who are unable to devote to themselves, and are not receiving from other persons, proper care and attention

may be removed to suitable premises – that is, a hospital or other place such as a residential home. Removal can be effected in the interests of the person concerned or, significantly, 'for preventing injury to the health of, or serious nuisance to, other persons'.

It will be seen that, other than that the person at risk has no recognised mental illness, the nature of the person's mental condition is not considered in section 47 which is, essentially, aimed at the recalcitrant old person who is an offence to his or her neighbours. While sympathy for the latter may be a natural reaction, many would doubt the ethics of using such draconian measures in the circumstances. True, the old person may be living in insanitary conditions, but it could be argued that the local authority already has the power to send in the cleaners and can use ancillary methods under the public health laws to improve conditions while, at the same time, preserving respect for the old person's autonomy. It is also to be noted that the section gives no directions as to treatment and, in any case, the order can remain in force for only 3 months – although it is, of course, permissible to find some other means of restricting the subject's independence meantime.[2] For these, and other, reasons, section 47 is used remarkably rarely but, objections notwithstanding, it, or something very like it, is still needed. The problem, as we all know, is that the world of the aged becomes progressively more difficult and unfair as time goes by. Even the most vocal advocate of libertarian values will be forced to admit that there will be times when something has to be done to balance our moral tolerance of individual cussedness against the interests of the community. Section 47, which was conceived as a protection for the elderly against oppressive officialdom, may yet be the best of a choice of evils.

What is the alternative? Effectively, it is to invoke the powers under the Mental Health Act of 1983, in particular section 135,[3] which allows a policeman to enter a house and, if necessary, to remove a person to a place of safety. To obtain a warrant for this to be done, an approved social worker must have reason to suspect that a person believed to be suffering from a mental disorder:

a. has been or is being ill-treated, neglected or kept otherwise than under proper control; or
b. being unable to care for him- or herself, is living alone.[4]

It is to be noted that the approved social worker need only *suspect* that the old person is *believed* to be suffering from a mental disorder and is at risk – indeed, not being medically qualified, he or she can do little more. As a result, such an order can last for only 72 hours but, during that time, procedures for compulsory admission for medical assessment under what is currently section 2 of the Mental Health Act can be put in motion. Detention must cease after 28 days unless the person is shown to be suffering from one of the statutory forms of mental disorder that will allow continued detention for treatment. Section 135 is not, therefore, achieving compulsory detention by way of the back door and it is, in fact, seldom used. Much more commonly, emergency admission to a mental hospital or admission for assessment will be sought from the beginning, the reason being that conditions for such admissions overlap very considerably with those underlying the use of section 47. The use of the Mental Health Act in any form, however, places the eccentric or the confused elderly person in the same category as the mentally abnormal and, although it is unjustifiable to do so, many would see this as a stigma. All in all, we take the view that the use of what is, at least to an extent, a ruse to achieve the same end is more morally questionable than is the use of section 47. Although they were uttered in a completely different set of circumstances, the words of the Court of Appeal in the case *Re MB* (1997) – which we have discussed at various points in this text – merit repetition in the present context:

> The Mental Health Act cannot be deployed to achieve the detention of an individual against her will merely because her thinking process is unusual, even apparently bizarre and irrational, and contrary to the views of the overwhelming majority of the community at large.

---

[2] Removal can be effected under emergency powers but the limit is, then, reduced to 3 weeks.
[3] Or under the Mental Health (Scotland) Act 1984, s.117.
[4] The conditions for the use of similar powers in Scotland are slightly more demanding in that a mental health officer must have previously been refused entry.

Problems abound in the management of the 'difficult' elderly and it must be admitted that good intentions rarely provide the perfect solution to them. The underlying driving force must, at the end of the day, be the avoidance of ill-will or bad faith, yet the law is surprisingly ill-equipped to cope with either.

MEDICAL TREATMENT AND THE ELDERLY

We have seen in Chapter 2 that, outside a 'free market', there has to be some sort of regulated distribution of health resources. We have also concluded that there is no universally satisfactory solution to the problem. As a result, Health Authorities and individual doctors tend to adopt arbitrary criteria and one common ploy for distinguishing between those who are to receive treatment and those who will not is 'rationing' on the basis of age.

'Age' in this context is not necessarily 'old age'. The courts have, for example, upheld the right of the health authority to deny *in vitro* fertilisation (see Chapter 8) to a childless woman on the grounds that she was aged 37. The Authority claimed that the results of IVF were so much less satisfactory when carried out in women coming to the end of their child-bearing years that it was medically unsound to offer the service. This, then, can be seen as a medical decision taken by a medical authority for medical reasons and, as such, may be acceptable on ethical grounds, although it is not uncontentious. There is no reason why similar logic should not be used in old age when the outcome of treatment is directly related to the patient's age, although it is, in many ways, surprising how seldom this applies. Given that the underlying condition is the same in each case, the *results* of an operation, say, on the stomach are remarkably similar in patients aged 45 and 75.

Providers of medical care are, however, on far less firm ethical ground when allocating resources using age as the *sole* determinant, irrespective of medical indications, and one would hope that this seldom occurs. Nonetheless, it does happen and it is a policy that is driven by little more than public intuition. Ask a member of the public whether a treatment of strictly limited availability should be given to a person aged 27 or one aged 67, and he or she will almost always opt for the former irrespective of the expected outcome. But the question goes deeper than intuition. Respected philosophers have suggested that, in a world of inevitable shortfalls in medical resources, society should plan to balance these against the length and quality of life and should accept that its duty to the elderly is discharged by its efforts to avoid *premature* death. In short, according to this argument, society is justified in refusing to spend a high proportion of its healthcare resources attempting to turn old age into permanent middle age. Justice is, however, one of the four major criteria that are held to define ethical medical practice and the profession must ask itself whether it is served by such an age-related choice.

In the first place, as outlined in Chapter 2, it is important to distinguish between the macro- and micro-allocation of resources. The former is, essentially, a matter of governmental strategy – at the level of Strategic Health Authorities or Boards at the lowest. This is in the order of things that can be altered only via the ballot box. Despite the evident logic of the argument set out above, it is doubtful if any government could, in fact, survive while supporting such a negative attitude to medical care of the elderly. Even so, it is not impossible to imagine it occurring covertly. This has led many to believe that we should consider the need for an Age Discrimination Act designed on much the same lines as the existing statutes dealing with discrimination on the grounds of race and sex, for there is also abundant evidence that discrimination on the grounds of age exists in fields other than healthcare, for example, in employment. For the present, however, we can only note, as above, that steps have been taken in this direction which suggest that the Government is now positively motivated towards care of the elderly but that no relevant legislation is currently in force.

We are, here, far more concerned with microallocation which, in general terms, is a matter of adjudicating a competition for resources at the individual level. In such circumstances, an adjudicator is as likely as not to fall back upon what has been called the 'fair innings' argument – in essence, that the old person has had his or her share of days in the sun and should, if necessary, give way to someone who has yet to be so fortunate.

This is a seductive argument in that it is so simple but it is not difficult to see that it cannot be applied without, at least, some limitation. It must, for example, be admitted that, if everyone is entitled to a minimum 'innings', that should rightly include some years' rest in the pavilion. It might – it *just* might – be conceded that a person aged more than 80 should surrender a scarce resource to a younger person. However, what we cannot claim is that a person aged 50 has had a 'fairer' innings than one aged 40. Moreover, it cannot be said that the enjoyment of life deteriorates in steady linear fashion after peaking, say, in young adulthood. The twilight years may, in fact, be the most valuable in a person's life. And this, again, draws attention to the importance of respect for *any* autonomous life. We have no more right to base our respect for a person on the grounds of his or her age than we have to do so by reason of his or her economic status. Ask two persons, one aged 30 and one aged 50 what value they put on their lives on a ten point scale and each will probably give the answer 10. The conclusion is forced, therefore, that medical resources must be distributed on the basis of what has become known as 'age neutrality'.

'Yes,' the reader may well say, 'but all this assumes good health and that the older person *wants* to survive. She may, in fact, regard her life as being so intolerable that she welcomes the fact that she is to be denied life-saving treatment – she may even have read Chapter 5 of this book and have signed an advance directive to that effect.' All of which is true, but age and health status are independent variables and, although age and deterioration in health very commonly run together, it is perfectly possible to base treatment decisions on the latter while ignoring the former. It has already been noted that the doctor is under no compulsion to provide treatment that he or she regards as medically futile and this, in the present context, is most vividly seen in the use of 'do not resuscitate' (DNR) orders. We have already discussed such orders in Chapter 12, to which the reader is referred. The DNR order may well be the final act in the doctor/patient relationship. Raising one has, therefore, a particular ethical poignancy.

DISPOSAL OF THE DEAD

One of the few certainties in our existence is that we will all die and our bodies have, then, to be disposed of. It follows that the law in this area will affect us all and, depressing as it may be, it is appropriate to end this book with a short look at the regulation of burial and cremation.

Death certification

A death must be registered, and the first step in this process is the provision of a certificate as to the cause of death by a registered medical practitioner. There are some practical difficulties in what might be regarded as no more than a routine matter. In England and Wales, the practitioner must be able to certify that he or she was in medical charge of the deceased during the terminal illness – and the one who *can* do so may be absent at the time. It is widely believed that doctors cannot sign the certificate if they did not see the deceased during the last 14 days of his or her life;[5] and, of course, the cause of death can only be given 'to the best of [the doctor's] knowledge and belief'. Add to these the fact that the death must be reasonably *expected*, and it will be seen that a certificate cannot be given in a large number of cases despite there being no suspicious circumstances associated with the death. Thus, in addition to those in which there *are* grounds for suspicion, many palpably natural deaths are reported to the Coroner in England, Wales and Northern Ireland – the aggregate being, generally, something in the region of 20 per cent of all deaths. This may have some unfortunate side-effects. In the first place, the ultimate disposal of the body is likely to be delayed; secondly, it will very probably result in post-mortem dissection of the body in the public mortuary which, as has already been discussed, many close kin may find distressing; and, thirdly, the tongues of those who associate the Coroner's or Procurator Fiscal's office with criminality may be set wagging. Nonetheless, it has been authoritatively stated that the main function of the Coroner is to maintain the accuracy of the mortality statistics and many, though not all, may feel that these are small prices to pay for a proven system that is, additionally, designed to improve the detection of secret homicide.

It is to be noted that, in the event of a death having been reported to the Coroner, the Coroner's certificate replaces any medical certificate as to the cause of death. Even so, it has to be wondered whether the current medico-legal system, which is based on practises that are centuries old, succeeds either in disclosing secret homicide or in maintaining the accuracy of the mortality statistics. Current practice as to death certification is, admittedly, something of a compromise, the balancing factor being that it is fairly easy to operate – any alternative suggestions inevitably tend to increase the bureaucratic load. As we go to press, yet another consultation document has been distributed and its proposals have provoked an unenthusiastic response from the medical profession – we will have to await events.

The system in Scotland is rather simpler – largely because any doctor who feels able to do so may complete the certificate as to the cause of death. Moreover, the function of the Coroner's counterpart, the Procurator Fiscal, is, effectively, to do little more than eliminate criminality and medical negligence – the Fiscal has no responsibility for the mortality statistics. As a result, while many natural – especially *sudden* natural – deaths may still be reported to the Fiscal, the great majority will be dealt

---

[5] Though this is only strictly so if the doctor *also* did not see the deceased after death.

with at the medical level by the Fiscal's medical adviser who is empowered to issue a certificate of cause of death in appropriate circumstances.

Assuming a medical certificate is available, the doctor must either send it to the Registrar and provide a 'Notice to Informant' that this has been done or, more probably in order to ease the process, he will hand both to the informant – normally a relative of the deceased – who will go direct to the Registrar. The Registrar will then issue a certificate for disposal after registration.

Burial

We have seen that there is no property in a dead body or in unmodified body parts. However, although no-one actually *owns* it, the deceased's executors have a right to possession and custody of the body for the purposes of its disposal – and, interestingly, the *responsibility* for disposal rests with the executors rather than with, say, a spouse. Perhaps because of this, funeral and burial expenses have a priority claim on the dead person's estate and directions in the deceased's will as to the mode of his or her disposal cannot have binding force.[6] The rights of the executors and of other interested parties are, however, limited in the interests of public health. In general, the Community Health Medical Officer wields considerable power as to the storage and transport of the body of a person who has died from, or while suffering from, a disease that is notifiable under the Public Health Acts.

Everyone has a common law right to be buried within his or her parish church-yard or in a burial ground, the great majority of which are now administered by the Local Authority acting in its capacity of a Burial Authority. Again, however, very surprisingly, there is no general rule that insists that a body can only be buried in an 'official' resting place. By-laws and the laws governing, say, town and country planning or public decency may limit the choice of a place for interment but, at least in theory, the choice is open to the executors. The Registrar must be informed by way of a regulation notice as to when and where a person was buried or cremated but this is normally the responsibility of the superintendent of the burial ground.

It is, perhaps, worth mentioning that the law relating to the *disinterment* of a body is very strict and is covered by both common and statute law. Thus, one cannot, for example, disinter and remove the body of a relative simply because one is moving to another part of the country. The Coroner in England and the Sheriff in Scotland can, of course, authorise an exhumation but this is almost invariably associated with the administration of justice at either the criminal or the civil level.

Cremation

This leads on to the subject of cremation, for cremation is the one sure way of destroying the physical evidence pointing to negligence or criminality as a cause of death. As a result, disposal of the dead by way of cremation is far more strictly

---

[6] Exceptions to this rule apply when directions have been made under the Human Tissue Act (disposal of parts of the body) or the Anatomy Act (bequeathing the body for anatomical dissection).

controlled than is disposal by burial, the first major difference being that the burning of human remains other than in a certified crematorium is forbidden.

The procedure for cremation is best understood by consideration of the forms which have to be completed in order to comply with the regulations. First, a relative must apply for cremation and, in doing so, must indicate the wishes of the executors, provide details of the death and affirm that there is no suspicion of foul play or need for further examination of the body. A statement by those in medical charge of the deceased must be included and the application has to be countersigned by a house-holder who knows the applicant. Form B must be completed by the medical attendant who has 18 questions to answer as to the manner of death. He must certify that there is no need for further inquiry and must, further, certify that he or she is not related to the deceased and has no pecuniary interest in the death. Major importance attaches to Form C which is a confirmatory certificate that has to be completed by a medical practitioner of at least 5 years standing who has no family or professional relationship with the doctor who completed Form B. He or she must state whether he or she has seen the body and whether a careful external examination has been conducted; failure to have done so will almost certainly lead to rejection of the application. The 'second doctor' must have questioned at least one of five categories of person who were asso-ciated with the management of the person's last illness and must also certify that he or she is satisfied as to the cause of death. Finally, the dossier is examined by the Medical Referee – a practitioner who is nominated by the Crematorium and appointed by the Secretary of State for the purpose. The Referee must confirm that the regulations have been followed, that the cause of death has been established and that no further exam-ination is required. He or she has very wide powers associated with this conclusion – including the carrying out of a post-mortem dissection and reporting the death to the Coroner or the Procurator Fiscal if that is considered to be appropriate.

Form C need not be completed following a death in hospital when a post-mortem examination has been carried out by a pathologist who would have been qualified to complete the form and the results of the autopsy are available to the doctor signing Form B. The certificate of the Coroner or Procurator Fiscal replaces Forms B and C if the death has been the subject of a medico-legal inquiry.

Thus, it will be seen that the cremation regulations, again, represent something of a compromise between an effort to prevent the concealment of crime while, at the same time, minimising inconvenience to the general public. The question then arises – do they succeed in their primary aim? Anyone looking at the various forms will appreciate that their usefulness depends in very great measure on the good faith and honesty of those who complete them – in particular, the doctors. The answer to the question is, then, 'yes, they probably do – except when the doctors, themselves, are involved'. Most readers of this book will be aware of the activities of the notorious Dr Shipman who was found guilty of the murder of at least 15 of his patients. The first part of the official report of the public inquiry into his practice, chaired by the judge Dame Janet Smith, has now been published, but much work remains to be done before the complete picture and final recommendations emerge. Nevertheless, it seems that the roots of his success in evading justice are embedded, at least in major part, in a failure to observe the spirit of the cremation regulations. But that still leaves us wondering what, if anything, can or should be done about it. Very large numbers of persons regard cremation as the most efficient and environmentally friendly method of disposal of the dead. At the same time, there are very few medically qualified serial murderers. Undoubtedly, the law on death certification and disposal of the bodies needs reconsideration and possible strengthening. But it would probably be a mistake radically to alter a system which has served the public reasonably well for many years by way of a knee-jerk response to a single maverick practitioner.

CASES REFERRED TO IN THE TEXT

MB (an adult: medical treatment), Re [1997] 2 FLR 426.

R (adult: medical treatment), Re [1996] 2 FLR 99.

R v East Sussex County Council, ex parte Tandy (1998) 42 BMLR 173.

R v Gloucestershire County Council, ex parte Barry [1997] 2 All ER 1.

R v North and East Devon Health Authority, ex parte Coughlan [2000] 3 All_ER 850.

R v Sheffield Health Authority, ex parte Seale (1994) 25 BMLR 1.

FURTHER READING

Buchanan DR, Mason JK. 'The Coroner's office revisited', *Medical Law Review* 1995; 3: 142.

Ebrahim S. 'Do not resuscitate decisions: Flogging dead horses or a dignified death?', *British Medical Journal* 2000; 320: 1155.

Evans JG, Tallis RC. 'A new beginning for care for elderly people?', *British Medical Journal* 2002; 322: 807.

Harris J. *The Value of Life*, 1985 London, Routledge.

Hobson SJ. 'The ethics of compulsory removal under Section 47 of the 1948 National Assistance Act', *Journal of Medical Ethics* 1998; 24: 38.

Hunt RW. 'A critique of using age to ration healthcare', *Journal of Medical Ethics* 1993; 19: 19.

Nair P, Mayberry JF. 'The compulsory removal of elderly people in England and Wales under Section 47 of the National Assistance Act and its 1951 Amendment: A survey of its implementation in England and Wales in 1988 and 1989', *Age and Ageing* 1995; 24: 180.

National Health Service. *The NHS plan: a plan for investment, a plan for reform*, Cm 4818-1, 2000.

Rivlin M. 'Should age based rationing of healthcare be illegal?', *British Medical Journal* 1999; 319: 1379.

Tonks A, Bennett G. 'Elder abuse', *British Medical Journal* 1999; 318: 278.

INDEX

Fashioning Alice

Bloomsbury Perspectives on Children's Literature

Bloomsbury Perspectives on Children's Literature seeks to expand the range and quality of research in children's literature through publishing innovative monographs by leading and rising scholars in the field. With an emphasis on cross and inter-disciplinary studies, this series takes literary approaches as a starting point, drawing on the particular capacity for children's literature to open out into other disciplines.

Series Editor:
Dr Lisa Sainsbury, Director of the National Centre for Research in Children's Literature, Roehampton University, UK.

Editorial Board:
Professor M. O. Grenby (Newcastle University, UK), Dr Marah Gubar (University of Pittsburgh, USA), Dr Vanessa Joosen (Tilburg University, The Netherlands).

Titles in the Series:
Adulthood in Children's Literature, Vanessa Joosen
The Courage to Imagine: The Child Hero in Children's Literature, Roni Natov
From Tongue to Text: A New Reading of Children's Poetry, Debbie Pullinger
Ethics in British Children's Literature: Unexamined Life, Lisa Sainsbury
Rereading Childhood Books: A Poetics, Alison Waller
Literature's Children: The Critical Child and the Art of Idealisation, Louise Joy

Forthcoming Titles:
Metaphysics of Children's Literature: Climbing Fuzzy Mountains, Lisa Sainsbury
The Styles of Children's Literature: A Century of Change, Peter Hunt
Irish Children's Literature and the Poetics of Memory, Rebecca Long
The Dark Matter of Children's "Fantastika" Literature, Chloé Germaine Buckley